# Health Transitions and the Double Disease Burden in Asia and the Pacific

T0264897

Chronic diseases – cardiovascular disease, cancer, chronic respiratory disease and diabetes – are not only the principal cause of world-wide mortality but also are now responsible for a striking increase in the percentage of sickness in developing countries still grappling with the acute problems of infectious diseases. This "double disease burden" poses demanding questions concerning the organisation of health care, allocation of scarce resources and strategies for disease prevention, control and treatment; and it threatens not only improvement in health status but economic development in the many poorer countries of the Asia Pacific region.

This book presents an historical account of the development of the double disease burden in Asia and the Pacific, a region which has experienced great economic, social, demographic and political change. With in-depth analysis of more than fifteen countries, this volume examines the impact of the double disease burden on health-care regimes, resource allocation, strategies for prevention and control on the wealthiest nations in the region, as well as the smallest Pacific islands. In doing so, the contributors to this book elaborate on the notion of the double disease burden as discussed by epidemiologists, and present real policy responses, whilst demonstrating how vital health is to economic development.

*Health Transitions and the Double Disease Burden in Asia and the Pacific* will be of great value both to scholars and policy makers in the fields of public health, the history of medicine, as well as to those with a wider interest in the Asia-Pacific region.

**Milton J. Lewis** was a Senior Research Fellow in the School of Public Health, 1989–2006 and is now at the Menzies Centre for Health Policy, University of Sydney, Australia.

**Kerrie L. MacPherson** is an Associate Professor of History, the Kadoorie Institute, University of Hong Kong.

# Routledge advances in Asia-Pacific studies

# Health Transitions and the Double Disease Burden in Asia and the Pacific

Histories of responses to non-communicable and communicable diseases

**Edited by Milton J. Lewis and Kerrie L. MacPherson**

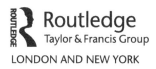

LONDON AND NEW YORK

First published 2013 by Routledge

2 Park Square, Milton Park, Abingdon, Oxon OX14 4RN
711 Third Avenue, New York, NY 10017, USA

*Routledge is an imprint of the Taylor & Francis Group, an informa business*

First issued in paperback 2017

*British Library Cataloguing in Publication Data*
A catalogue record for this book is available from the British Library

*Library of Congress Cataloging in Publication Data*
Health transitions and the double disease burden in Asia and the Pacific : histories of responses to non-communicable and communicable diseases / edited by Milton J. Lewis, Kerrie L. MacPherson.
　　p. cm. – (Routledge advances in Asia-Pacific studies ; 14)
　　Includes bibliographical references and index.
　　1. Epidemiology–Social aspects–Pacific Area. 2. Communicable diseases–Pacific Area. 3. Chronic diseases–Pacific Area. I. Lewis, Milton James. II. Macpherson, Kerrie L., 1950–
　　RA650.7.P16H43 2012
　　614.4'25–dc23　　　　　　　　　　　　　　　　　　　　2012011799

ISBN: 978-0-415-57543-0 (hbk)
ISBN: 978-1-138-10912-4 (pbk)

Typeset in Times New Roman
by Wearset Ltd, Boldon, Tyne and Wear

# Contents

# Illustrations

**Figures**

**Tables**

# Contributors

**Gabriel G. Carreon** has worked with the New South Wales Health Department and is a Fellow of the Royal Australian College of Medical Administrators.

**Wan-Yuen Choo** is a Senior Lecturer in the Department of Social and Preventive Medicine, Faculty of Medicine, University of Malaya, Malaysia.

**Paul T. Cohen** is Associate Professor and Honorary Senior Research Fellow in the Department of Anthropology, Macquarie University, Sydney, Australia.

**Michael J. Dibley** is an Associate Professor in International Public Health, School of Public Health, University of Sydney, Australia.

**Mahito Fukuda** is a Professor in the Graduate School of Languages and Cultures, Nagoya University, Japan.

**Jaime Galvez Tan** teaches at the University of the Philippines College of Medicine.

**Peter Heywood** is Honorary Professor of International Health at the University of Sydney, Australia.

**Tang Kim Hong** is the deputy head of the Epidemiology Department and the Division of Community Health, Pham Ngoc Thach University of Medicine, Ho Chi Minh City, Vietnam.

**Terence H. Hull** is J.C. Caldwell Professor of Population, Health and Development at the Australian National University, Canberra, Australia.

**Margaret Jones** is a Research Associate at the Wellcome Unit for the History of Medicine, University of Oxford, UK.

**Stephen R. Leeder** is a Professor of Public Health and Community Medicine at the University of Sydney and Director of the Menzies Centre for Health Policy (formerly the Australian Health Policy Institute).

**Milton J. Lewis** was a Senior Research Fellow in the School of Public Health, University of Sydney, 1989–2006, and is now at the Menzies Centre for Health Policy (formerly the Australian Health Policy Institute), University of Sydney, Australia.

**Meng-Kin Lim** is Associate Professor of Health Policy and Management, Yong Loo Lin School of Medicine and Director of Alumni Relations, National University of Singapore.

**Wah-Yun Low** is Professor of Psychology at the Medical Education and Research Development Unit, Faculty of Medicine, University of Malaya, Malaysia.

**Vicki Luker** is Executive Editor of the *Journal of Pacific History* and a Research Associate of the State, Society and Governance in Melanesia Project at the Australian National University, Canberra, Australia.

**Kerrie L. MacPherson** is an historian of public health and diseases of China and Hong Kong at the Kadoorie Institute, University of Hong Kong.

**Angelo Manalo** introduced the first Problem Based Learning curriculum in the Philippines at the Mindanao State University College of Medicine where he was Dean, 1992–1997 and 2000–2006.

**Giselle M. Manalo** is on the staff of the International Public Health program at the Sydney School of Public Health, University of Sydney, Australia.

**Sailesh Mohan** has trained in medicine, public health and cardiovascular epidemiology. He is currently a Senior Research Scientist and Associate Professor at the Public Health Foundation of India, New Delhi. He has been a recipient of the CIHR Canada HOPE Fellowship Award and completed his postdoctoral fellowship training in cardiovascular epidemiology at the Departments of Medicine and Community Health Sciences, University of Calgary, Canada. His primary research interest is in chronic non-communicable disease epidemiology, particularly risk factors and their modification using population based strategies with specific focus on tobacco and hypertension control.

**Chirk-Jenn Ng** is an Associate Professor in the Department of Primary Care Medicine, University of Malaya, Malaysia.

**Chiu-Wan Ng** is a Senior Lecturer in the Department of Social and Preventive Medicine, Faculty of Medicine, University of Malaya, Malaysia.

**Thapin Phatcharanurak** is Assistant Professor in the Department of Sociology and Anthropology, Chiang Mai University, Thailand.

**K. Srinath Reddy** is President of the Public Health Foundation of India and was recently appointed foundation Bernard Lown Professor of Cardiovascular Health, Harvard School of Public Health. He is also an Adjunct Professor at the Rollins School of Public Health, Emory University, USA.

**Alberto Romualdez** is currently Dean, the Graduate School of Health Sciences at the Pamantasan ng Lungsod ng Maynila, Philippines.

**Amala de Silva** is a Professor in the Department of Economics at the University of Colombo, Sri Lanka.

**Richard Taylor** is Professor of Public and International Health at the University of New South Wales, Australia.

**Wen-Ting Tong** is a Research Officer at the Medical Education and Research Development Unit, Faculty of Medicine, University of Malaya, Malaysia.

**Nguyen Hoang Hanh Doan Trang** is Lecturer in Clinical Epidemiology, Pham Ngoc Thach University of Medicine, Ho Chi Minh City, Vietnam.

**Tran Tuan** is the Director of the Research and Training Centre for Community Development in Hanoi, Vietnam.

**Angelito Umali** is a program coordinator for the United Nations Population Fund in the Philippines.

**In-sok Yeo** is Associate Professor of History of Medicine at Yonsei University in Seoul, South Korea.

# 1 Health transitions and the double disease burden in Asian and Pacific countries

## Some introductory observations

*Milton J. Lewis and Kerrie L. MacPherson*

## Aims

The aim of our book is to offer historically oriented accounts and analyses of contemporary health transitions (including the double disease burden) taking place in countries of the Asia-Pacific region; economically, politically and demographically a very significant region of the world.

Chronic noncommunicable diseases (NCDs)[1] – in particular cardiovascular disease, cancer, chronic respiratory disease and diabetes – have recently caused a striking increase in illness and death in developing countries still grappling with a significant threat from communicable diseases (CDs). NCDs cause 60 per cent of deaths worldwide while 80 per cent of these deaths take place in low income and middle income countries. Moreover, they impact disproportionately on those people who are in the productive, younger adult and middle aged years. Because of heart disease, strokes and diabetes (to a great extent preventable diseases), in the next decade China and India will lose in national income an estimated US$558 and US$237 billion respectively. By 2020, NCDs are expected to cause 70 per cent of deaths in developing nations and to be responsible for 80 per cent of the global disease burden (Boutayeb 2006: 192; Narayan *et al.* 2010: 1,196).

The double disease burden (DDB) – the onset of significant mortality from NCDs while mortality from CDs remains high – has marked the health transition in the developing world. Developed countries had the historical 'luxury' of dealing with chronic diseases after much of the burden of communicable diseases had disappeared. Even so, some new CDs such as HIV/AIDS have in recent years produced notable morbidity and mortality. Moreover, some CDs may lead to NCDs; for example, the papilloma virus and the onset of cervical cancer.

The DDB in Asia and the Pacific and the problems that it poses for the organisation of health care, resource allocation, strategies for prevention, control and treatment, and the need for integrated responses to communicable and chronic noncommunicable diseases, will threaten not only the advancement of health status but the economic development of poorer countries in the region. We hope that analysis of the historical experiences of these countries will put 'flesh on the bones' of the DDB as discussed by epidemiologists; and provide further insights helpful to understanding of the DDB and to the formulation of more effective policy.

## Historical transitions relevant to health status

Three models have been proposed as important in understanding changes in health status in developed countries in the last century and a half or so. These are:

- the epidemiologic transition proposed in the early 1970s by demographer, Abdel Omran (1971); it involved a change in the pattern of diseases from the predominance of CDs to that of NCDs; soon after, medical sociologist, Monroe Lerner (1973) and, later, other scholars proposed that the epidemiologic transition was part of a health transition involving an advance in health status to historically unprecedented heights;
- the demographic transition, or the change from a regime of high fertility and high mortality in pre-modern societies to one of low fertility and low mortality in modern societies; this was proposed as early as 1929 by Warren Thompson, but did not become prominent until the 1960s; and
- the nutrition transition, the most recently formulated model, involves, from the late nineteenth century, more abundant and nutritionally better food (especially meat) for the mass of people in Western countries, a healthy change that promoted resistance to significant CDs; but in the course of the twentieth century, and more so in the second half of that century, in developed countries, greater consumption of saturated fat, salt and refined sugar that promoted illness and deaths from NCDs; 'fast foods' and other highly processed products (along with lower levels of physical activity) have carried the process further. Widespread use of tobacco, particularly manufactured cigarettes which became increasingly popular after the First World War, also caused NCD morbidity and mortality to climb. These deleterious changes in diet and growing use of tobacco (together with the widespread change to sedentary forms of work) are now occurring in low and middle income countries with the same parlous health consequences. The speed of change is such that both over- and under-nutrition are to be found across many such countries and within households (Popkin 2002: 205, 211; Caraher and Coveney 2004: 592).

By the late 1990s, following World Health Organization practice, health researchers were commonly describing the health transition taking place globally as 'the complex changes in patterns of health, disease, and mortality' resulting from 'demographic and associated economic and societal changes in a world population that is getting older' (Vorster *et al.* 1999: 341). We would want to add cultural and political changes to their economic and societal changes.

## Economic development and health

Economic development has been seen as central to the health transition experienced by high income, Western countries.

The Asia-Pacific region contains the full range of countries categorised by the World Bank by level of per capita income as; high income, upper middle income, lower middle income and low income. Thus, as an example of the first, there is Australia,[2] like Western European and North American countries, one of the original, high income nations and now enjoying one of the highest life expectancies at birth (LEBs) in the world. There is Japan, the first non-Western nation to achieve high income status and, like Australia, having one of the highest LEBs in the world.

There are the nascent, economic superpowers, China and India, the former now classified as an upper middle income and the latter as a lower middle income country. But both display great inequality of income between affluent and growing, urban upper and middle classes and poor village people who still live a largely subsistence lifestyle.

China's incredible economic growth since 1980 has lifted over 500 million people out of poverty and it recently surpassed Japan as the second largest economy in the world. Yet, the polarisation of wealth in China is one of the most severe in the world: where 5 per cent of Americans own 60 per cent of national assets, 1 per cent of Chinese hold 41.4 per cent of assets.

In the region we also have Sri Lanka, a lower middle income country like India, yet one that in modern times has had much better health outcomes. In fact, it has been a pioneer of the transition to lower mortality and higher life expectancy among developing countries in Asia and the Pacific; and indeed the world (Riley 2001: 132; WHO 2005: 168–169; Rodrik 2009: 2; *Weekend Australian*, 5–6 June 2010; Zoellik 2011: 1; ChartsBin 2012: 1).

The idea that economic and social factors are very important in determining health status has a long history in public health. In the first half of the nineteenth century before the failure of the politically progressive 1848 Revolutions in Europe, socioeconomic explanations of disease causation were being discussed in both France and Prussia. In 1820 Louis Rene Villerme (1782–1863), a leading figure in the early French public health movement, inquired into mortality differences between poor and wealthy districts of Paris. He explained the differences in socioeconomic terms and proposed improvements in working conditions and education for the poor as ways to reduce the gap in health status. In the 1840s a young Rudolf Virchow (1821–1902) (later, a very distinguished pathologist) and politically radical, Prussian medical colleagues called for scientific investigation of the effects of social and economic factors on health. Friedrich Engels, Karl Marx's collaborator, used vital statistics compiled by early English medical officers of health to show urban death rates were inversely related to social class.

After mid-century, leading English public health figure, Edwin Chadwick's (1800–1890) 'sanitary idea' shifted the causal focus, in this pre-germ theory era, to noxious vapours (miasmas) from decaying matter in the physical environment; and the solution was removal of the matter (and so the miasmas) through underground sewers (and drains) sluiced by an abundant supply of piped water. This was an engineering solution, even if implemented at the societal level, and reduction of social and economic inequalities seemed irrelevant.

From about 1890 the sanitary idea gave way to the idea of 'specific cause', as microbiologists identified the biological pathogens involved in more and more CDs. The new view was that particular diseases were caused by particular infectious agents and interruption of the chain of biological causality was the royal road to lower mortality. The laboratory rather than the socioeconomic and sanitary environments would now be the key to public health progress and a higher LEB;[3] while epidemiology had become the study of the effect of pathogens on the health of populations.

The era of infectious diseases lasted from about 1890 to 1950 and the aim was to identify the necessary and, if possible, the sufficient cause of a disease (the Henle–Koch postulates); although in the interwar years, the epidemiological work on pellagra (a nutritional deficiency disease) of Joseph Goldberger and Edgar Sydenstricker again pointed to the importance of the social and economic disadvantage, in this case giving rise to the deficient diets that produced the disease.

In the era of risk factors, 1950–2010, the focus of epidemiology shifted from CDs to NCDs as what were at first called the 'diseases of affluence' – particularly cardiovascular disease and cancer – came to dominate the patterns of mortality and morbidity in economically developed countries. The idea of necessary and sufficient causes gave way to that of risk factors. Multiple interacting factors cause these diseases with each factor increasing the probability of disease in an individual.

The focus was for a long time on multiple, proximate, biological, risk factors in the individual. But, more recently, recognition of the effect of macro economic, social and cultural factors has grown, particularly because of the demonstration of a social gradient (in social class) in mortality rates and in health status (Lewis 2003a: 4–6; Lewis 2003b: 211–212; Fairchild *et al.* 2010: 57).

Epidemiologist, Michael Marmot has put forward a number of propositions that arise from his work and the work of others like Richard Wilkinson (1996; 2006) on the social gradient in health status:

- differences in individuals' health reflect inherent features of their societies;
- the way a society is organised is a major determinant of health;
- social, economic and political factors influence significantly health status and life expectancy;
- psychosocial factors like isolation, as well as social status and lifestyle, help explain ill health; and governments can reduce inequalities in health between higher and lower social classes by assessing all policies for their impact on health;
- thus, disease rates will change with their social, economic and cultural environments;

- the social gradient in health status does not result from selection; in the main, social status determines health, not vice versa (Marmot 2000: 379–382; Marmot 2006: 2–4).

Wilkinson claims that in most high income countries material conditions – average living standards – have ceased to be key determinants of health; that social hierarchy itself is the key to differences in health status. Even if such countries become very much richer, social inequality will still produce a social gradient in health status with those of higher social status enjoying better health than those lower down the ladder (Wilkinson 2006: 341–356; Clark 2010: 4).

Some epidemiologists like Ezra Susser are now looking beyond the focus on individual risk factors to 'eco epidemiology'. In this approach causality is seen to operate at multiple levels: at the macro level, according to the distribution of wealth and social status (the emphasis on macro social and economic factors proposed by Marmot and Wilkinson); at the individual level, through personal attitudes and behaviour; and at the micro level, through cellular and molecular events. For a fuller understanding (and more effective interventions) causal levels must be integrated.

In addition, attention must be paid to causality over time, both at the individual and societal levels. The individual is affected by past as well as present biological and social experiences. Disease onset may reflect adverse experiences earlier in the individual's life course, even as early as '*in utero*'. At the societal level, the effects of history also operate. Disease trends are influenced by social and economic change over time. So knowledge of the historical context advances understanding of changes in disease patterns. Further, we suggest, history helps us understand collective responses to disease, and especially cultural and policy change. Thus, we believe the historically oriented analyses of health transitions provided by our contributors will advance understanding of the changes in health status and in policy in the various countries included in our book.

Modern scientific knowledge, of which epidemiology sees itself a part, is both generalisable and universally applicable. Epidemiology is an abstracting, universalising and statistical discipline and seeks to establish determinants of disease across time and place. History is strongly concerned with the particularity of phenomena associated with a specific time and place. History prefers complexity to generality; epidemiology, generality to complexity.[4] We may, then, look to history, with its emphasis on complexity, diversity and specificity, to complement the generalising capacity of epidemiology, in the study of health and disease.

We have asked contributors to our book to take cognisance of the epidemiologists' generalising picture but also to see what insights might be derived from using history, as a more richly contextual discipline, to trace the health transition (and policy responses to it) in their Asian or Pacific country. We might expect national histories of the health transition to present more idiosyncratic pictures with country-specific, historical factors influencing the particular path taken in the transition.

We support epidemiologist, Stephen Kunitz's claim that 'local knowledge' of the development of diseases still has explanatory value. Until the microbiological revolution of the later nineteenth century, medicine adhered to a very old tradition of concern with the qualities of particular patients and the diseases of particular places. The rise of modern biomedical science seemed to make irrelevant such particularistic concerns and the focus was henceforth on context-free generalizations arising from the new universally applicable knowledge. But, as Kunitz notes, we may still gain much 'mileage' from viewing diseases in their local or national contexts, even when we recognise 'some processes are universal'. Indeed, while we may prefer generalizations that are 'parsimonious', such generalizations may also be 'impoverished' (Kunitz 1994: 4–6; Lewis *et al.* 1997: viii; March and Susser 2006: 1379–1383; Susser and Morabia 2006: 15–19; Susser *et al.* 2006a: 415, 420; Susser *et al.* 2006b: 25–27).

Historian, James C. Riley has pointed out that the road to unprecedentedly low levels of mortality taken by European countries (and overseas transplantations of Europe like the United States and Australia) has not been the only route (see also Introduction to Chapter 2 on Australia in this book). This Western route has depended on vast economic development over the last 200 years or so. High levels of national wealth, together with great advances in scientific understanding of human diseases arising from increasingly expensive university and research institutions, and considerable growth of state intervention in health and social matters, played a key role in the massive reduction of mortality from CDs and, more recently, reduction of deaths from NCDs. Economic development provided the resources used by high income countries to achieve unprecedentedly high levels of LEB.[5] It provided individuals with a higher material standard of living (especially better nutrition); while it gave governments the revenue to fund large-scale, health-enhancing, physical infrastructure and to institute nationwide social welfare systems as well as nationwide health-care and educational services staffed by expensively trained and well paid professionals.

However, the route taken by some low income countries was different. Too poor to build costly physical, health and educational infrastructure typical of Western industrialized nations, they pursued social growth that induced cultural change; for example, villagers were instructed in how to dig simple pit latrines and taught personal hygiene practices in local elementary schools that not only spread basic literacy but a receptivity to scientifically based information about health. Schools produced cultural change that promoted health;[6] they engendered a more modern frame of mind. Of course, there was an economic cost but it was comparatively small because basic health and education services, being labour intensive, were relatively inexpensive in such low wage countries.

On this much simpler basis, in 1890–1930, a low income colony like Ceylon (now Sri Lanka) could begin, under a comparatively benign imperial regime, to raise LEB.

Social investments such as elementary education lowered mortality from widespread CDs,[7] especially gastrointestinal infections, tuberculosis and malaria. As noted already, this social approach did not require the large funding needed to create the underground water and sewerage systems of later nineteenth century European, North American and Australian cities. Moreover, the low income countries that pioneered the non-Western health transition might mix imported and domestic programmes and prefer one foreign tactic to another. Thus, from the 1870s, as it began to climb the life expectancy ladder, Japan employed vaccination to reduce mortality from smallpox, then a major cause of death, but did not substantially modernise sanitary systems until decades later (Sen 1999: 47–48; Riley 2001: 51–54; Riley 2008: 2–18).

The Indian State of Kerala (with a current population of over 30 million) also relied on social rather than economic development as the driver of health improvement:

- female as well as male literacy; greater female workforce participation;
- later marriage and lower fertility arising from family planning;
- basic health clinics (providing primary treatments, maternal and infant care and immunisation) located so they were easily accessible and modest in cost;
- food shops charging fair prices.

Kerala built on local historical advantages like the habit of boiling drinking water and the availability of basic schooling at village level. Another and major advantage was that the status of women was higher than in other parts of India because of the continuing strength of matrilineal practices. Traditionally, perhaps 50 per cent of the population followed matrilineal kinship rules. In South Asia, Kerala and Sri Lanka have stood out as places where women have enjoyed greater autonomy.

By the beginning of the 1990s,[8] where in India as a whole 64 per cent of males and 39 per cent of females aged seven years or older were literate, in Kerala, the figures were 94 per cent and 87 per cent. The much higher literacy rate and longer schooling of women led to health-promoting practices like births supervised by doctors, high immunisation levels and greater use of health centres. Such social growth conferred on the state the highest life expectancy (and the lowest fertility) in India (Caldwell 1991: 16; Caldwell and Caldwell 1994: 349; Sen 1999: 46; Riley 2001: 133; Manju 2007: 510).

Unable to afford expensive medical and surgical facilities (for the great bulk of the population at least) to deal with the disabling effects of NCDs, developing countries must rely heavily on prevention and health promotion to reduce the burden of remaining communicable diseases plus that of the quickly growing levels of NCDs. Even if Riley overstates the applicability of the historical lessons from Ceylon/Sri Lanka and Kerala to other developing countries – some critics have plausibly argued that they are exceptions rather than widely applicable models; and it is a fact that education and health services were far more developed in Ceylon than in any other British colony (Caldwell 2009: 421–423; Manderson 2007: 477) – his highlighting of the role of social investment (producing cultural change) reminds us that wealth and advanced technologies have not been the only significant ways to promote health status. In any case, he points to the great importance of popular involvement in health promotion as well as government commitment to such interventions: people with limited schooling were successfully taught about CDs and how to control them (Riley 2008: 169–170). It may augur well for teaching people with limited education in contemporary developing countries how to deal with issues around diet and life-style change that are vital to the control of NCDs today.

Policymakers in countries of the region have publicly indicated that they are well aware of the double burden. The Chinese Vice-Minister of Health, Wang Longde, has noted: 'Chronic disease death rates in our middle-aged population are higher than in some high income countries' (WHO 2005: xii). Twenty per cent of urban children seven to 17 years of age are overweight or obese. The total economic cost to China of heart disease, stroke and diabetes in 2005–2015 is expected to be US$550 billion. The global cost of treatment and prevention of diabetes alone is estimated to be US$490 billion by 2030. Another cost is lost productivity: in the United States, for example, the total cost of diabetes is put at US$174 billion of which 30 per cent, or US$58 billion, is due to lost productivity (Colagiuri 2010: 306).

In India where 2.5 million children succumb to infectious diseases annually, the population also has the highest rate of diabetes in the world. The Indian Minister of Health and Family Welfare, Dr Anbumani Ramadoss, has observed: 'In India ... public health advocacy to date has been mainly devoted to infectious diseases. However, we now have major public health issues due to chronic diseases that need to be addressed with equal energy and focus' (WHO 2005: x).

## The prevailing, risk-factor picture of determinants of NCDs

Contemporary health analysts commonly identify the underlying determinants of chronic diseases (the causes of the causes) as globalisation, urbanisation, ageing of the population and government policies on food, agriculture, trade, media advertising, transport and urban design and the built environment. Poverty may also play a role, especially through the poor health status of infants that impacts adversely on their adult health status.

As noted earlier, the more proximate causes of the main chronic diseases (heart disease, stroke, cancer, chronic respiratory diseases and diabetes) that can be modified are the following risk factors – unhealthy diet and excessive intake of sources of energy, physical inactivity and smoking. These translate into the intermediate risk factors – raised blood pressure, raised blood glucose, abnormal blood lipids and overweight and obesity (WHO 2005: 48–51).

For epidemiologists the relationship between the common, modifiable risk factors and the main chronic diseases holds across countries and the globe. However, as we have suggested above, understanding of health changes (including the DDB) in developing countries in Asia and the Pacific will also benefit from historical analysis at the level of the particular nation state. In this age of globalisation, although we must be concerned with the linkages between globalisation (some see as the ultimate 'upstream factor') and health, 'mid-range' analyses (at the national and subnational levels) remain significant, given the need to obtain empirical evidence of the effects of globalisation on community and individual health (Harris and Seid 2004: 42). In addition, it is clear that health policy itself is still very largely developed and implemented at the national and subnational levels.

Like Lincoln Chen and colleagues, we think that investigation of the modern health transition must move beyond established, risk factor epidemiology and demography and 'explore sociocultural, economic, political, historical, and public health dimensions of health change' (Chen *et al.* 1994: ix). There is in the real world no single health transition. Even though there are important common features, country-specific health transitions may be identified because the health and mortality changes take place in nation states with different cultural, social, economic and political conditions and with different histories of institutional and policy development (Lewis and Rapaport 1995: 211–212; Capstick *et al.* 2009: 1341).

## Notes

1 Psychiatric disorders and the dementias have not been included because, historically, sufferers were usually lodged in special psychiatric or aged care institutions separate from the mainstream health-care system; and, in any case, they are significant enough to require a volume of their own. They represent, in effect, a third disease burden faced by contemporary developing countries as they experience the health transition. Cardiovascular disease is a very old human affliction. Recently, evidence of atherosclerosis was found in Egyptian mummies dating back 3,500 years. Twenty-two mummies were examined, and hearts, arteries or both were identified in 16; of these nine showed evidence of calcium accumulation.The mummies were of members of the upper class whose diet included the flesh of cattle, ducks and geese. Moreover, since salt was routinely used as a preservative of meat and fish, some may have suffered from high blood pressure (*Australian*, 19 November 2009).
2 Almost all immigrants to Australia when the health transition commenced were from England, Wales, Scotland or Ireland which had already begun (or were beginning) their transitions. However, as outlined in the chapter on Australia, economic and social conditions for lower class people were better in Australia than in the immigrants' places of origin. Well into the twentieth century Australians enjoyed a higher life expectancy at birth than their English and Celtic 'cousins' (Riley 2008: 175–176).
3 Life expectancy is a hypothetical measure. It serves to indicate prevailing health and mortality conditions. LEB is the average number of years of life a newborn may expect to enjoy if the prevailing mortality trends continue (Last 1988: 45).
4 According to complexity theory, to gain useful knowledge when studying a complex phenomenon like human health, the inquirer must focus on the appropriate level of analysis. Thus, while the molecular level may be important for understanding some health issues, the public's health may still be improved without addressing health at the level of molecular events. Contemporary epidemiology commonly addresses health problems at the level of the individual. But, again, according to complexity theory, populations are more than collections of individuals; and the context in which the population is located may be fundamentally important. Because complexity research is characterised by feedback loops and non-linearity, the new epidemiological methods required 'will look less like a randomized controlled trial ... and more like complex

observational research such as evolutionary biology or cosmology' (Pearce and Merletti 2006: 517–518).

5  The first Western country to enter upon the modern health transition was Sweden. Interestingly, it employed, towards the end of the eighteenth century, social organisation and
effective leadership by the central government at least as much as a comparatively high
level of national income to initiate the transition. Thus, Sweden's per capita income
(1820) was $1,198 (in 1990 US dollars); that of England, another pioneer of the health
transition, was much higher; $1,706. What initially brought down mortality in Sweden
was a national programme of vaccination that controlled smallpox; then a major cause
of death. Compulsory from 1815, vaccination markedly reduced all-cause mortality
(Lewis 2003a: 3–4; Caldwell *et al.* 2006: 158; Riley 2008: 23–24, 175).Taking a very
much longer view of the history of life expectancy, some scholars have questioned the
weight commonly given to economic development as a driver. They have argued for a
larger role for genetic factors and natural selection. At the beginning of the stone-age
Agricultural Revolution, around 10,000 years ago, because of greater infection rates
due to the permanence and larger size of human settlements together with poorer nutrition due to lower meat intake, Neolithic farmers were both shorter and less long-lived
than had been Mesolithic hunter gatherers. LEB in the Mesolithic era was about 30
years but in the Neolithic period more like 20 years (see Caldwell *et al.* (2006: 51–63)
for a questioning of the widely accepted idea that mortality significantly increased in
the Neolithic era). Greater population density, domestication of animals, the intensification of the work effort required by agriculture and, probably, a poorer diet increased
both exposure and vulnerability to infectious and parasitic diseases, so increasing the
extrinsic mortality risk. In turn this offered an evolutionary advantage to individuals
who were genetically predisposed to greater somatic investment, repairs and maintenance (to stronger immune systems, DNA repairs, accurate gene regulation, antioxidants
and suppression of tumours). In the course of the Agricultural Revolution – the 10,000
years between it and the Industrial Revolution is long enough for significant evolutionary change – the gene distribution associated with intrinsic mortality risk (biochemical
and physiological decay during a lifetime) changed. Over time there was a greater representation in the population of individuals predisposed to somatic investment, repairs
and maintenance and as a result LEB in the longer run grew beyond its level in hunter–
gatherer society. This increased the probability of survival and advanced life expectancy. But there were regional fluctuations around the trend, arising from differences in
local environmental and climatic conditions. So LEB in Egypt was only 24 years in the
two centuries from AD 33 but was as high as 42 years in England at the end of the sixteenth century. Sedentary, agricultural society sustained population densities ten to 100
times those of hunter gatherer society. Pathogens of domesticated animals evolved into
human pathogens: smallpox from cowpox in cattle; influenza from pigs and ducks;
whooping cough from pigs and dogs; and human TB from bovine TB. Proximity to
human waste accumulations increased exposure to faecal–oral infections, especially
dangerous for infants. In the Roman imperial era, these 'new' pathogens were shared
between Eurasia and North Africa. But the Indigenes of Australia, the Pacific Islands
and the Americas were isolated from this long term exposure to these deadly microbes.
They had no opportunity to build up resistance and were very susceptible when from
the sixteenth century they began to have contact with Europeans. Central to the rising
wealth of Western European countries from the sixteenth century was urbanisation. The
urban part of the population grew from 3 per cent in 1520 to almost 18 per cent in 1750.
Initially, urbanisation drove down the LEB from about 40 years in the late 1500s to 33
in the late 1600s. But the greater extrinsic mortality risk in cities also encouraged the
growth in the population of those genetically predisposed to higher somatic investment.
This contributed to a fluctuating but slowly rising trend in the LEB in England after the
1720s. By 1830, it had again risen to about 40 years. The genetic selection and the
resulting, more robust 'biological infrastructure' then reinforced the longer term,

positive effect on the LEB of the huge economic development resulting from the industrialisation in the nineteenth century, even if the initial impact of unregulated industrialisation had been unfavourable to LEB. By the late nineteenth century, the historically unprecedented economic development of England had significantly raised the average standard of living (manifested especially in better nutrition for working class people) and funded major improvements in public sanitation and the purity of water supplies in urban areas, both of which reduced the extrinsic mortality risk from communicable diseases. In England from the 1880s there was an upward, long-term trend in the LEB. By 1901–1910, for males, it was 48.5 years and for females, 52.4 years (Lancaster 1990: 44; Lewis 2003a: 15–16; Galor and Moav 2005: 1–8). It should be noted that the above account, drawn largely from Galor and Moav (2005), relies in part on the idea that genetic selection has continued to play a very important role into recent times. This is at odds with the established view that sociocultural change replaced significant biological evolution about 40,000 to 50,000 years ago, before humans migrated out of Africa to other parts of the world (except for the spread of the lactose-tolerance mutation that allowed Europeans to consume dairy products without harm and the genetic defence against falciparum malaria among African peoples). Two anthropologists, well informed about genetics, have recently argued (against the established view and in support of the Galor and Moav position) that in fact human evolution has speeded up in the last 10,000 years since the birth of agriculture and cities and has responded to the changing sociocultural environment; biological as well as sociocultural change has been occurring in the modern era (Cochran and Harpending 2010: 1–23).

6  Richard Eckersley persuasively points out that contemporary epidemiology and population health in fact ignores culture as a system of meanings by which people interpret their world and so as a fundamental determinant of health. Culture is mainly regarded as 'a dimension of socio-economic status' (Eckersley 2011: 4–5).

7  Like Riley, economist, Amartya Sen is interested in historical examples of low income countries that used social growth, not economic development, to advance the quality of life including reduction of mortality. Such countries showed that basic education and health care were not luxuries only wealthier countries could enjoy. Thus, speedy reduction of mortality, at least from communicable diseases, could be achieved by these social 'support-led' processes as well as economic development. Sen has pointed out that Japan, the first non-Western country to undergo a modern health transition, enjoyed a higher rate of literacy than Europe when it began the process of modernisation after the Meiji restoration in the mid-nineteenth century. Industrialisation had not yet happened but this legacy of 'human resource development' much assisted subsequent economic development as well as increasing quality of life. Sen notes that the social, support-led development of publicly provided, basic education and health services directly raised the quality of life in some other low income countries, notably Sri Lanka. Declining mortality rates then promoted reductions in birth rates and reinforced the downward effect of female literacy on fertility (Sen 1999: 40–49, 90–92).

8  Recently, criticism of the 'Kerala model' (which showed that even with a comparatively low per capita income, an LEB of a developed-country level could be achieved) has been growing. Incompetence, corruption and lack of political will on the part of both Communist and Congress party governments have been blamed for the crumbling of the model. But there are other, structural problems arising from the very success of the model. Thus, an ageing population is putting heavy pressure on the health-care system, especially because of the costs of treating NCDs in hospitals, while primary care centres are now much less well-funded and are in any case ill-equipped to deal with the more complex needs of NCD patients just when NCDs have become leading causes of illness and death. Moreover, without industrial development there are too few employment opportunities for the well-educated population. Many Keralites must go overseas, particularly to the oil-producing countries of the Middle East, for employment

(as well as to other parts of India). The economy of the State is now very dependent on the financial remittances of these migrant workers (Meyer and Brysac 2009: 1–9).

## References

Boutayeb, A. (2006) 'The Double Disease Burden of Communicable and Non-Communicable Diseases in Developing Countries', *Transactions of the Royal Society of Tropical Medicine and Hygiene*, 100(3): 191–199.

Caldwell, B. (2009) 'Review of James C. Riley, *Low Income, Social Growth, and Good Health: A History of Twelve Countries*, Berkeley: University of California Press, 2008', *Bulletin of the History of Medicine*, 83(2): 421–423.

Caldwell, J.C. (1991) 'Routes to Low Mortality in Poor Countries', in J.C. Caldwell and G. Santow, eds, *Selected Readings in the Cultural, Social and Behavioural Determinants of Health*, Canberra: Health Transition Centre, National Centre for Epidemiology and Population Health, Australian National University, 1–46.

Caldwell, J.C. and Caldwell, P. (1994) 'Patriarchy, Gender, and Family Discrimination, and the Role of Women', in J.C. Chen, A. Kleinman and N.C. Ware, eds, *Health and Social Change in International Perspective*, Boston, MA: Harvard University Press, 339–371.

Caldwell, J.C., Caldwell, B.K., Caldwell, P., McDonald, P.F. and Schindlmayr, T. (2006) *Demographic Transition Theory*, Dordrecht: Springer.

Capstick, S., Norris, P., Sopoaga, F. and Tobata, W. (2009) 'Relationships between Health and Culture in Polynesia: A Review', *Social Science and Medicine*, 68(7): 1341–1348.

Caraher, M. and Coveney, J. (2004) 'Public Health Nutrition and Food Policy', *Public Health Nutrition*, 7(5): 591–598.

ChartsBin (2012) 'Country Income Groups (World Bank Classification)'. Online, available at: http://chartsbin.com/view/2438 (accessed 30 January 2012).

Chen, L.C., Kleinman, A. and Ware, N.C. (1994) 'Overview', in L.C. Chen, A. Kleinman and N.C. Ware, eds, *Health and Social Change in International Perspective*, Boston, MA: Harvard University Press, vii–xv.

Clark, P. (2010) 'Interview with Richard Wilkinson', *Public Health Today*, September: 4–5.

Cochran, G. and Harpending, H. (2010) *The 10,000 Year Explosion: How Civilization Accelerated Human Evolution*, New York: Basic Books.

Colagiuri, R. (2010) 'Diabetes: A Pandemic, a Development Issue or Both?' *Expert Review of Cardiovascular Therapy*, 8(3): 305–309.

Eckersley, R. (2011) 'The Science and Politics of Population Health: Giving Health a Greater Role in Public Policy'. Online, available at: www.webmedcentral.com (accessed 8 September 2011).

Fairchild, A.L., Rosner, D., Colgrove, J., Bayer, R. and Fried, L.P. (2010) 'The Exodus of Public Health: What History can Tell Us about the Future', *American Journal of Public Health*, 100(1): 54–63.

Galor, O. and Moav, O. (2005) 'Natural Selection and the Evolution of Life Expectancy'. Online, available at: http://sticerd.lse.ac.uk/seminarpapers/dg09102006.pdf (accessed 24 February 2010).

Harris, R.L. and Seid, M.J. (2004) 'Globalization and Health in the New Millenium', *Perspectives on Global Development and Technology*, 3(1–2): 1–46.

Kunitz, S.J. (1994) *Disease and Social Diversity. The European Impact on the Health of Non-Europeans*, New York: Oxford University Press.

Lancaster, H.O. (1990) *Expectations of Life: A Study in the Demography, Statistics, and History of World Mortality*, New York: Springer-Verlag.

Last, J.M. (1988) *A Dictionary of Epidemiology*, New York: Oxford University Press.

Lerner, M. (1973) 'Modernization and Health: A Model of the Health Transition'. Paper presented at annual meeting of American Public Health Association, San Francisco, November.

Lewis, M.J. (2003a) *The People's Health*, Volume 1, *Public Health in Australia, 1788–1950*, Westport, CT: Praeger Press.

Lewis, M.J. (2003b) *The People's Health*, Volume 2, *Public Health in Australia, 1950 to the Present*, Westport, CT: Praeger Press.

Lewis, M., Bamber, S. and Waugh, M. (1997) 'Preface', in M. Lewis, S. Bamber and M. Waugh, eds, *Sex, Disease, and Society: A Comparative History of Sexually Transmitted Diseases and HIV/AIDs in Asia and the Pacific*, Westport, CT: Greenwood Press, vii–ix.

Lewis, N.D. and Rapaport, M. (1995) 'In a Sea of Change: Health Transitions in the Pacific', *Health and Place*, 1(4): 211–226.

Manderson, L. (2007) 'Review of Margaret Jones, *Health Policy in Britain's Model Colony: Ceylon (1900–1948)*, Hyderabad: Orient Longman, 2004', *Bulletin of the History of Medicine*, 81(2): 477–478.

Manju, N. (2007) 'Health Status of Women in Kerala: Beyond Indicators', in C.C. Kartha, ed., *Kerala: Fifty Years and Beyond*, Thiruvanathapuram: Gautha Books, 505–521.

March, D. and Susser, E. (2006) 'The Eco- in Eco-Epidemiology', *International Journal of Epidemiology*, 35(6): 1379–1383.

Marmot, M. (2000) 'Social Determinants of Health: From Observation to Policy', *Medical Journal of Australia*, 172(8): 379–382.

Marmot, M. (2006) 'Introduction', in M. Marmot and R.G. Wilkinson, eds, *Social Determinants of Health*, Oxford: Oxford University Press, 1–5.

Meyer, K.E. and Brysac, S. (2009) 'India: The Kerala Model'. Online, available at: http://pulitzercenter.typepad.com/untold_stories/india-the-kerala-model/ (accessed 5 July 2010).

Narayan, K.M.V., Ali, M.K. and Koplan, J.P. (2010) 'Global Noncommunicable Diseases: Where Worlds Meet', *New England Journal of Medicine*, 363(13): 1,196–1,198.

Omran, A.R. (1971) 'The Epidemiologic Transition: A Theory of the Epidemiology of Population Change', *Milbank Memorial Fund Quarterly*, 49(4/1): 509–538.

Pearce, N. and Merletti, F. (2006) 'Complexity, Simplicity, and Epidemiology', *International Journal of Epidemiology*, 35(3): 515–519.

Popkin, B.M. (2002) 'Part ii. What is Unique about the Experience in Lower- and Middle-Income Less-Industrialised Countries Compared with the Very-High-Income Countries? The Shift in Stages of the Nutrition Transition in the Developing World Differs from Past Experiences!', *Public Health Nutrition*, 5(1A): 205–214.

Riley, J.C. (2001) *Rising Life Expectancy: A Global History*, Cambridge: Cambridge University Press.

Riley, J.C. (2008) *Low Income, Social Growth, and Good Health: A History of Twelve Countries*, Berkeley, CA: University of California Press.

Rodrik, D. (2009) *One Economics Many Recipes: Globalization, Institutions and Economic Growth*, Princeton, NJ: Princeton University Press.

Sen, A. (1999) *Development as Freedom*, Oxford: Oxford University Press.

Susser, E. and Morabia, A. (2006) 'The Arc of Epidemiology', in E. Susser, S. Schwartz,

A. Morabia and E.J. Bromet, eds, *Psychiatric Epidemiology: Searching for the Causes of Mental Disorders*, Oxford: Oxford University Press, 15–24.

Susser, E., Schwartz, E. and Morabia, A. (2006a) 'Eco-Epidemiology', in E. Susser, S. Schwartz, A. Morabia and E.J. Bromet, eds, *Psychiatric Epidemiology: Searching for the Causes of Mental Disorders*, Oxford: Oxford University Press, 415–421.

Susser, E., Schwartz, S., Morabia, A. and Bromet, E.J. (2006b) 'Searching for the Causes of Mental Disorders', in E. Susser, S. Schwartz, A. Morabia and E.J. Bromet, eds, *Psychiatric Epidemiology: Searching for the Causes of Mental Disorders*, Oxford: Oxford University Press, 25–30. Also, *Weekend Australian*, 5–6 June 2010.

Thompson, W.S. (1929) 'Population', *American Journal of Sociology*, 34(6): 959–975.

Vorster, H.H., Bourne, L.T., Venter, C.S. and Oosthuizen, W. (1999) 'Contribution of Nutrition to the Health Transition in Developing Countries: A Framework for Reseach and Intervention', *Nutrition Reviews*, 57(11): 341–349.

WHO (2005) *Preventing Chronic Diseases: A Vital Investment*, Geneva: WHO Press.

Wilkinson, R. (1996) *Unhealthy Societies: The Afflictions of Inequality*, London: Routledge.

Wilkinson, R.G. (2006) 'Ourselves and Others: For Better or Worse: Social Vulnerability and Inequality', in M. Marmot and R.G. Wilkinson, eds, *Social Determinants of Health*, Oxford: Oxford University Press, 341–356.

Zoellik, R.B. (2011) 'Opening Remarks at the Conference on China's Challenges for 2030'. Online, available at: http://worldbank.org/en/news/2011/09/03 (accessed 30 January 2012).

# 2 Two health transitions in Australia

## The Western and the Indigenous

*Milton J. Lewis and Stephen R. Leeder*

## Introduction

As noted in the introductory chapter, James C. Riley has identified two different historical forces driving the modern health transition. The first was economic growth, the driver for high income Western countries like Australia; the first countries historically to experience the health transition; and, the other was social growth, the driving force in certain low income countries that, more recently, pioneered the health transition in the non-Western world.

Riley identifies 12, non-Western, low income countries that in the six decades or so from 1890 entered on their own health transitions by reducing mortality from gastrointestinal infections, tuberculosis (TB) and malaria using a variety of factors that facilitated social growth: primary education; inexpensive, basic public health measures; wider access to basic health care; better popular knowledge of common health risks; and direct participation by people in public health improvements. This outstanding achievement took place largely in the era before high-technology products like antibiotics and DDT (dichloro-diphenyl-trichloroethane) were available to them.

Four of the 12 countries are located in the Asia-Pacific region – Japan, South Korea, China and Sri Lanka.[1]

While social rather than economic growth was the driver common to the four, the path to lower mortality was influenced notably by the economic, political, social and cultural conditions peculiar to each country. The comparative study of national histories shows the journey to higher life expectancy for a particular country was determined by the range of means available when the transition began, what could be afforded and what interventions from among the many possible were pursued. Thus, Japan initially chose not to follow the powerful example of England and invest a great deal in sanitary systems; rather, it used vaccination to reduce mortality from smallpox, then a major cause of death. In Sri Lanka and China, governments promoted the education of their peoples in simple ways of disease prevention and provided basic (sometimes very basic) health care; although government in the first case was benign, British colonial and, after independence, democratic progressive, while in the second it was authoritarian socialist.

Japan initiated its health transition about 1890, the first non-Western nation to do so. Compulsory school attendance was introduced in 1886, but Japan had a higher literacy rate than Europe even before modernisation began with the Meiji restoration in the mid-nineteenth century. After the Second World War, Japan's very strong growth in life expectancy was assisted by the extra public expenditure made possible because the United States took responsibility for its national defence and by a notably egalitarian income distribution. About 1978, Japan replaced Sweden as the country with the highest life expectancy in the world (Sen 1999: 41; Riley 2008: 2–18, 37–38, 53–64, 161–173; Ventres 2008: 1943).

In contrast to these Asian pioneers, Australia, like the other wealthy Western countries, used its high income to fund the means to initiate a health transition among its majority, European population. Moreover, communicable diseases (CDs) were largely brought under control before chronic non-communicable diseases (NCDs) became too burdensome.[2]

Yet, in our focus on the role of wealth we should not underestimate the importance of social developments like elementary schooling in bringing down mortality from CDs in Australia. Even in the large cities, it was not just a matter of costly water and sewerage systems or milk pasteurisation plants that reduced CD mortality from gastrointestinal infections and bovine TB; as for malaria, it was never a major threat. Individual behaviour change through hygiene education (in schools and informally through the printed word) and attitudinal change concerning the need to banish 'dirt' and germs played their part. In the late nineteenth century, a new generation of literate Australian mothers was ready to act on scientific information about infant care provided by health experts rather than on traditional advice from female kin or neighbours. This was cultural change fostered by social investment in basic schooling.

In the second half of the twentieth century, cultural changes in the population at large concerning diet, smoking and physical activity were significant counters to epidemics of heart disease and lung cancer.

However, in the much poorer health of Indigenous people, especially in rural and remote communities, Australia faces something not unlike the problem of the double disease burden (DDB) now being encountered by low income, Asian and Pacific countries.

After a discussion of the encouraging history of the health transition in European Australia – the great mortality decline and the attainment of one of the highest levels of life expectancy in the world – we will analyse the depressing history of the health transition in Indigenous Australia. But in more recent years there is reason for hope. While the gap in health status between Indigenes and other Australians remains substantial, it has narrowed. Further, new ideas are emerging from bitter, often ideologically driven debates about what will improve the quality of life and life chances of Indigenous people, especially in remote communities. These ideas have significant implications for how in the longer term the gap in health status might be permanently closed.

## Changes in European mortality from the beginning of settlement in 1788

Australia, only settled by Europeans in 1788, was not among the very first of Western countries to enter upon the health transition. In the period from the 1770s to the early 1800s, Denmark, France, Sweden and England were the first to start on that historically momentous journey. Australia, along with the Netherlands and New Zealand, began the journey in the 1860s.

From an early date Australia had a comparatively high life expectancy at birth (LEB). It averaged (in New South Wales (NSW), the original colony) 44 years for males and 47 years for females in 1856–1866; and 47 and 50 respectively in 1860–1875. Australia enjoyed a notable advantage over the 'mother country' (England and Wales) from the mid-nineteenth century to about 1950; for example, in 1901–1910, LEB was 55.2 years for males and 58.8 years for females whereas in England and Wales it was 48.5 and 52.4 years respectively (Lancaster 1990: 44; Taylor *et al.* 1998a: 29–30; Caldwell *et al.* 2006: 158; Riley 2008: 175–176).

By 2007, Australia was one of the healthiest countries in the world. Its LEB of 79 years for men and 83.7 for women was surpassed only by Iceland and Japan with 79.4 and 79.2 years respectively for men, and Japan and France with 86 and 84.4 respectively for women (Australian Institute of Health and Welfare 2010: 28).

Australian age-standardised mortality began to fall from about 1860, only 70 odd years after European settlement began; and there was a sustained fall from 1880, although the rate of decline slowed notably after 1930.

Sharp fluctuations are common in the nineteenth century but disappear after the noteworthy spike caused by the influenza epidemic of 1919 (part of the pandemic of 1918–1920). The fluctuations resulted from localised epidemics of infections. Indeed, from the 1830s, cyclical outbreaks of the common childhood infections took place as the population grew large and dense enough from free immigration and a high birth rate.

The first major outbreak of measles occurred in 1834–1835, with whooping cough and scarlet fever epidemics soon after. Influenza outbreaks, connected to pandemics, occurred in 1836–1838, 1847 and 1850, while enteric infections became endemic as the pace of urban development quickened from the 1850s.

Mortality from TB (a very significant cause of death) declined from the 1880s in tandem with the fall in all-cause mortality. National TB mortality rose from 120 per 100,000 population in 1850–1880 to 150 in 1881–1890, but fell to 100 in 1901–1910, and to 42 in 1931–1940. There was a sharp decline after the Second World War – from 28 deaths per 100,000 in 1948 to 0.33 at the end of the 1990s.

In 1875–1950 in England and Wales, more than 40 per cent of the reduction in overall mortality was due to the fall in deaths from communicable diseases (one-quarter to one-third of which was from the decline in mortality from TB); 13 to 16 per cent to the fall in deaths from bronchitis, pneumonia and influenza (infections often led to death from bronchitis or pneumonia in the pre-antibiotic era); and 7 to 11 per cent to reduction of deaths from diarrhoea and enteritis. A similar pattern of CD mortality developed in Australia.

The steady reduction in Australian deaths from CDs that began in the late nineteenth century continued in the twentieth. About 50 per cent of the decline in mortality from CDs in the twentieth century took place between the 1900s and the Second World War; that is, before the penicillin era. A steep fall occurred from the 1940s to 1960 with further falls in the 1960s and 1970s, at the height of the antibiotic era. A plateau at a very low level formed about 1980. A slight rise commenced in the late 1980s and this was very largely due to male deaths from HIV/AIDS.

Male and female mortality rates for communicable diseases fell from 159 and 117 per 100,000, respectively, in 1922 to 90 and 61 in 1939. They fell to a trivial five and three in 1980 (Proust 1991: 228; Taylor *et al.* 1998a: 28–34; Taylor *et al.* 1998b: 38–41; Najman 2000: 22–26, 35–37; Bi *et al.* 2002: 62; Lewis 2003a: 49, 225).

The decline in male all-cause mortality ceased in 1945–1970 and in females in 1960–1970. An epidemic of NCDs was responsible. An epidemic of cardio-vascular disease (CVD) began in the mid-1920s. Deaths increased quickly until the mid-1950s and then the mortality curve flattened (because a slow rise in male deaths was matched by a slow fall in female deaths). From the 1970s both sexes experienced a speedy decline in mortality.

CVD continued to be the major cause of death in Australia. From 22 per cent of male and 25 per cent of female deaths in the early 1920s, CVD accounted for slightly less than 60 per cent of all deaths in the mid-1960s, and about 40 per cent in the late 1990s. The age-standardised male death rate rose from 385 per 100,000 and the female rate from 344 in 1922 to 783 and 511 respectively in 1970. They had fallen to 292 and 190 in 1997.

Female mortality from all cancers combined did not change much in the course of the twentieth century. But this cloaks contrary movements in mortality from major cancers – cancer of the stomach and uterus (including the cervix) declined but that of the lung, colon, pancreas and ovary increased.

Total male cancer mortality grew slowly to about 1950 after which there was a marked increase to the mid-1980s. In the 1990s there was a trend downwards for males and females, with the trend beginning earlier for the former. Almost all the sustained increase in the male rate was due to rising mortality from lung cancer although falling rates for cancer of the stomach and mouth were balanced by increasing rates for cancer of the colon (and rectum), pancreas and prostate, and leukaemia.

The cancer death rate was

- 154 per 100,000 for males and 155 for females in 1921;
- 176 and 147 in 1950;
- 242 and 143 in 1985;
- 217 and 133 in 1997.

Where cancer was responsible for 10 per cent of aggregate mortality in 1921, it accounted for 25 per cent in 1988, and almost 28 per cent in 1997 (Taylor *et al.* 1998b: 41–43; Najman 2000: 26–37).

In 2007, the leading causes of death, accounting for approximately 50 per cent of all deaths, were

- Coronary heart diseases 17.2% of male deaths and 15.8% of female deaths;
- Lung cancer 6.7% and 4.3%;
- Cerebrovascular diseases 6.4% and 10.4%;
- Chronic obstructive pulmonary disease 4.2% and 3.3%;
- Prostate cancer 4.2% and Breast cancer 4.0%;
- Dementias 3.4% and 7.3%;
- Colorectal cancer 3.1% and 2.8%;
- Diabetes 2.7% and 2.8%;
- Unknown primary site cancers 2.6% and defined heart disease 3.1%.

(Australian Institute of Health and Welfare 2010: 50)

## The role of social investment and cultural change in the mortality decline in Australia

Over the last six to seven decades, scholars have developed a succession of influential models to explain the great improvement in population health in Western countries (including Australia) in the last 150 to 200 years; and they have tended to assume these have validity in the rest of the world.

Scholars in the 1940s and 1950s accounted for the West's sustained mortality decline from the later nineteenth century in terms of medical advances and public health improvements. By the 1960s, with affluence spreading in developed countries from sustained economic growth and rivalry intensifying between the basically market-oriented governments of the West and the state planning-oriented regimes of the Communist world, the demographic transition model gained prominence; although it had been discussed by Warren Thompson in the United States as early as 1929. In this model economic growth was the principal force behind the mortality decline and health improvement. The transition was marked by a fall in mortality accompanied by a fall in fertility. These produced a decline in population growth that allowed a proportion of aggregate output to be invested in economic growth rather than simply consumed.

In 1971, demographer, Abdel Omran put forward the concept of the epidemiological transition. It amplified the concept of the demographic transition that began in the West after about 1650 when a cyclic pattern of growth in world population was replaced by exponential growth. He identified different disease patterns matching the three 'ages' of the demographic transition:

- first, the 'age of pestilence and famine' with high and fluctuating mortality from infectious disease (normal and pandemic) that works against population growth; there is high fertility and an LEB that fluctuates between 20 and 40 years;

- second, the 'age of receding pandemics' with progressively falling mortality from infections, sustained population growth, declining fertility and an LEB of 30 to 50 years; this is the modern era of industrialisation and historically unprecedented economic growth;
- and third, the 'age of degenerative and man-made diseases' when the LEB rises above 50 years and fertility becomes critical to population growth.

Others, notably Monroe Lerner in 1973, Jack Caldwell in 1990 and Julio Frenk and colleagues in 1994, suggested the epidemiological transition was best seen as part of a larger health transition.

Physician, demographer and medical historian, Thomas McKeown's publications from the 1950s to the 1970s reinforced the view that economic growth had been the driver of the transition to low mortality in nineteenth century, Western countries; and by implication it would play this role in other parts of the world. Rising incomes in nineteenth century Europe, even among working class people, and cheaper food supplied by large-scale, New World producers like Australia and Argentina, made for better nutrition and hence greater resistance to many CDs.

However, in the late 1970s, McKeown's hypothesis was challenged by Australian demographer Jack Caldwell who drew on his work in developing countries. Caldwell stressed the role of social and cultural factors, particularly elementary education of women. He pointed to Sri Lanka and the Indian State of Kerala (with annual per capita incomes of only US$320 and US$160–270 respectively) where politically driven, social investment had been able to reduce mortality. The education of mothers that made them better able to manage life challenges had driven the mortality decline in these Asian pioneers of the health transition in the developing world (Omran 1971: 513–516; Caldwell 1991: 1–4; Frenk *et al.* 1994: 27–28; Riley 2001: chapter 7; Caldwell *et al.* 2006: 160; Szreter 2007: 416–419).

As mentioned earlier, the break-through to lower mortality in Australia was also in part achieved by social investment in elementary education and the cultural change that ensued. We will discuss this by looking at the decline in the infant mortality rate (IMR).

The IMR in Australia fell from considerably above 100 per 1,000 live births in the nineteenth century to under ten at the beginning of the 1990s. About 40 per cent of this decline occurred by 1910 and 70 per cent by the 1940s.

The decline in the IMR in the decade from 1899 – 116 to 72 per 1,000 – was remarkable, although comparable falls took place in England, other parts of Europe and New Zealand. A great deal of the decline was due to a fall in deaths from diarrhoeal disease and associated conditions. The decline cannot be explained by the effects of organised infant welfare work because almost all of this was carried out at a later time. Public health measures like cleaner milk and water supplies and safer sewage and garbage disposal contributed by reducing the risk of infection in the domestic environment. Reduction in the size of families also contributed, helping make income go further and allowing mothers more time for care of individual children. Broadly in step with developments in Northern Europe and the United States, the Australian crude birth rate declined from the 1860s – from a little over 43 births per 1,000 in 1862 to 35 in 1877. It fluctuated around that figure till 1890 but fell to just above 27 in 1900.

The 'sentimental' value of children increased, and working class children were now becoming scholars not labourers under the new regime of compulsory, elementary education. The education of women was a significant contributor to the decline in infection-related deaths of infants and children. Mothers of this era were literate: in NSW, for example, where in 1861, 25 per cent who married signed with a cross, in 1911, only 0.6 per cent did so. It was not just a matter of literacy and access to books and other print media but cultural change – the planting of a receptivity to expert information that encouraged mothers to accept the advice of doctors and nurses.

Social investment in education and cultural evolution had a significant role, then, in the earlier phases of the permanent downward trend in the IMR in Australia. Here as in other parts of the Western world, weanling diarrhoea, involving a deadly synergism between infection and nutrition, decimated infant populations. Because of unhygienic, domestic environments and, often, nutritionally poorer substitutes for breast milk, working class babies were more at risk than babies of higher social strata. But many literate mothers, across all social classes, heeded advice from nurses and doctors about the need to breast feed, and where that was not possible, to use hygienically prepared and properly modified cow's milk (Quiggan 1988: 1, 19; Lunn 1991:131; Lewis 2003a: 50, 62, 152; McCalman 2009: 31).

## Accounting for the mortality decline in European Australia

Australia followed the two-stage, Western health transition with mortality from CDs declining notably before NCDs became the problem. The decline in deaths from infections that began in the later nineteenth century continued in the twentieth. The decline is sharper from 1942 to 1960 and results from the progressive introduction of antibiotics, the national campaign against tuberculosis and immunisation coming on top of longer-established, environmental health measures and social and economic improvements. But about 50 per cent of the fall in mortality from infections took place between the 1900s and the Second World War before these new medical measures were implemented. This gain in health status is very likely due to social, economic and cultural determinants to do with quality and availability of food, especially for working class people, education (producing attitudinal and behavioural changes) and housing; to specific public health measures like a safer water supply and safer sewage and garbage disposal (aided by the unplanned decline in fly populations as the combustion engine replaced the very many horses used for transport in urban centres), better commercial food hygiene and health education provided in schools and increasingly by health departments; and to declining fertility as smaller families became the norm.

As noted earlier, until about 1950, Australia enjoyed a mortality advantage over England and Wales which arose from better nutrition and less intensive industrialisation. In the nineteenth century overseas visitors were impressed by Australian working people's large consumption of meat compared with that of their counterparts in Europe where meat was something of a luxury. The average Australian consumed over twice that consumed by his/her equivalent in England and the United States, and four times that eaten by the average German or French person. Meat was commonly consumed at each meal. In 1897 Philip Muskett, a prominent physician and early commentator on Australian eating habits, observed Australians consumed an impressive 125 kilograms of meat per capita per year; fish was little eaten and only a few varieties of vegetables were regularly consumed.

Moreover, food was generally cheaper than in Europe and wage rates were high. T.A. Coghlan, NSW Government Statistician, observed in 1902 that where it took a worker on average 127 days a year to earn the cost of food in Britain, 148 in Germany and 142 in France, it took only 111 days in Australia. There is limited evidence that children and youths weighed more and were taller than their British 'cousins'. A 1923 study revealed Adelaide infants at birth and for the first ten months of life were heavier than English ones. It seems clear the average Australian was better fed, and so more resistant to many infectious diseases, than his/her counterparts in Europe (Coghlan 1902: 367; Teow *et al.* 1988: 61–62; Cumpston 1989: 100–103; Taylor *et al.* 1998a: 34).

Thus, the ready availability of protein from meat and, later, dairy products provided a nutritional advantage for colonial and early twentieth century Australians when CDs were the major threats to life. But from about the mid-1920s an epidemic of CVD began and Australia entered on the second stage of its health transition where NCDs dominate mortality, and its nutrition profile was called into question.

Deaths from CVD increased quickly until the mid-1950s. As mentioned earlier, the mortality curve then flattened, with male deaths increasing slowly and female falling slowly, until 1970 when deaths of both declined rapidly. By 1990, age-standardised death rates were at least as low as those around the mid-1920s. The CVD mortality decline was experienced by all age groups at the same time so it was a period, not a cohort, effect.

Prevention and treatment brought down CVD mortality. Dietary changes (reductions in intake of animal fat and salt) and declining tobacco use together with better, drug control of hypertension and treatment of existing cardiovascular disease worked to produce the decline in mortality, one of the speediest in the developed world. Another likely positive influence was the growing preference for less meat-dominated cuisines resulting from large-scale immigration from Southern Europe (the healthier 'Mediterranean diet'), Asia and the Middle East. Between the late 1930s and the early 1980s, meat and butter consumption had fallen significantly with butter replaced by margarine. However, given the industrial hydrogenation of liquid, plant-based oils into solid trans fats that underpinned margarine manufacture for years, how much it contributed to the downturn is open to dispute. Annual per capita consumption of carcass meat fell from 102 to 71 kilograms, butter from 15 to 4, while margarine rose from 2 (of which 0.4 was table) to 9 (table, 6.8) kilograms (Shergold 1987: 224–225; Walker and Roberts 1988: 161; Taylor *et al.* 1998b: 41; Lewis 2003b: 52).

A recent study has explained the spectacular fall in CHD mortality of 82 per cent for males and 84 per cent for females from a peak in 1968 to 2000 in terms of the combined effect of reductions in three population risk factors. Put more precisely, it may be said 74 per cent of the male decline and 81 per cent of the female result from reductions in these risk factors – diastolic blood pressure (BP), cholesterol and tobacco smoking. In males, reductions in BP accounted for 36 per cent of the decline, cholesterol 22 per cent and smoking 16 per cent; in females, 56 per cent, 20 per cent and 5 per cent respectively. For both sexes, reduction in serum cholesterol had the most impact in 1968–1979, while reduction in BP predominated in the next two decades to 2000. For males, the effects of reduction in smoking were more apparent in the 1980s.

Because the most notable reduction in cholesterol took place before lipid-lowering drugs were widely used, most of the reduction would appear to have been due to dietary change. Various policy initiatives in the 1980s helped reduce smoking prevalence – banning of tobacco advertising in the print media, on billboards and at sporting events, prohibition of smoking in workplaces, health promotion campaigns in the media, pricing and taxation, and stronger health warnings on cigarette packs. Medical practitioners' preventive work with individuals also contributed to reduction in CHD mortality. Some of the fall in BP resulted from reduction of salt intake. These gains are fragile. Obesity has risen as consumption of high fat, high salt, fast food and high sugar, soft drinks has increased in the last two decades.

As noted above, up to 1950 male mortality from all cancers combined grew slowly but then underwent a sustained linear increase until the mid-1980s when it levelled out. Lung cancer deaths are almost wholly responsible for this long-term increase in male mortality. The lung cancer death rate in males began to fall in the late 1980s. Both the rise and decline in lung cancer mortality are attributable to changes in smoking prevalence. The decline in lung cancer deaths may plausibly be put down to the combined effect of various tobacco control initiatives in the development of which Australia was a global leader.

As early as 1962 the Australian Medical Association, three Medical Colleges and the Victorian Anti-Cancer Council urged the Federal government to restrict advertising and promote education. Seven years later the National Health and Medical Research Council called for control of advertising, warnings on packets and an anti-smoking campaign. In the late 1970s, anti-smoking activists took more extreme, publicity-generating action such as defacing poster advertisements. In the 1980s, the Victorian government set up a Health Promotion Foundation funded by a tobacco tax. Other jurisdictions followed. These foundations replaced tobacco companies as sponsors of sporting and cultural activities.

In 1965–1991, cigarette consumption per adult declined by over 33 per cent, but during 1964–1976 it hardly changed. Then, from 1977, with a national ban on radio and television advertising in place, consumption declined just over 2 per cent per year. Smoking prevalence continued to decline: in 1995–2004, for males, from 29 per cent to 24 per cent, and for females, 23 per cent to 21 per cent. Tobacco control experts are now debating how to reduce it to 9 per cent by 2020 (Taylor *et al.* 1998b: 42; Taylor *et al.* 2006: 760–766; Chapman 1993: 429; Lewis 2003b: 55, 63–69; Lewis 2008: 232–233; Thomas 2009: 3, 8).

There is evidence (much better for more recent decades) of increasing prevalence of overweight and obesity in the twentieth century. Surveys of NSW school children (5–12 years) showed little change in mean body mass index (BMI) between 1901 and 1937. But where both girls' and boys' BMIs were 23.4 in 1937, by 1970 they were 24.4 and 24.3 respectively. National surveys of 1980 and 1983 revealed an increase even in that short time in overweight (BMI, 25–30) and obese (BMI, over 30) men from 41.4 per cent to 42.7 per cent and women from 31.5 per cent to 35.1 per cent. While the health consequences of being overweight are not so clear, being obese is universally accepted as a health hazard.

By 2008, an estimated 17.5 per cent of Australians were obese. By 2025, it is estimated 18.3 per cent will be obese. Obesity causes just under 24 per cent of type 2 diabetes, just over 21 per cent of CVD, 21 per cent of colorectal, breast, uterine and kidney cancer and 25 per cent of osteoarthritis (Walker and Roberts 1988: 163; Access Economics 2008: iii).

Between the 1900s and the end of the 1990s, mortality from diabetes (type 1 and 2) increased for males from 14.4 to 16.1 deaths per 100,000 population but decreased for females from 19.6 to 10.6. Mortality of under-19 year olds fell notably as treatment for type 1 diabetes improved with the introduction of insulin therapy in the 1920s, extensive patient education programmes in the fields of nutrition and self-management and preemptive treatment of diabetic coma; and after the 1980s, with the introduction of HbA1testing, home blood glucose monitoring, superior quality insulins and better blood pressure therapy. The trend in mortality of those 40 years and older (which tends to reflect the growing prevalence of type 2 diabetes) resembled that of the overall population. From 1980 to 2000, the prevalence of diabetes more than doubled, yet the mortality rate was comparatively stable because of better treatment methods and advances in medical technology. In the first decade of this century, the burden of disease attributable to type 2 diabetes continued to grow, and it is expected to be the leading cause of the disease burden by 2023.

Diabetes is rife among Australia's Indigenous population. It stands as a terrifying example of the effects of a nutrition transition occurring in the context of a society under heavy stress. Prevalence rates of type 2 diabetes are among the worst in the world. In the early 1990s, diabetes mortality was as high as 146 per 100,000 for males and 153 for females. For the period, 2003–2007, Indigenes were seven times more likely than other Australians to have diabetes stated on their death certificate (Bi *et al.* 2005: 272–276; Australian Institute of Health and Welfare 2010: x, 239).While genetic disposition may account for some of the problem, poor nutrition, obesity, excessive use of alcohol and other environmental factors dominate.

The modern nutrition transition in Australia may be seen as the result of both demand and supply factors. On the demand side, the greater number of women, especially married women, in the paid workforce – and hence increased pressures on their time and energy – has reduced the consumption of home-cooked meals in favour of processed 'convenience' foods, take-away foods and meals eaten in fast-food outlets, cafes and other venues outside the home.

On the supply side, the food service industry has expanded at a rapid rate. Where in 1956, 6 per cent of the household food budget was expended on food eaten away from home, it was 22 per cent in 1984 and over 30 per cent in 2000.

'Image' fast food chains have been basic to this change. Perhaps the best known (and among the earliest) are Pizza Hut, Kentucky Fried Chicken (KFC), and McDonald's. McDonald's opened its first establishment, selling hamburgers, in 1971. By 1987, it had 204 outlets. By 2008, it had 780 outlets (in 2007, A\$1.074 billion in sales), while Yum Restaurants had 560 KFC outlets and 270 Pizza Hut outlets. Three other significant companies are Competitive Foods with 340 Hungry Jacks and 49 KFC outlets (A\$804 million in sales), Quick Service with 400 Red Rooster and other cooked chicken outlets, and Domino's, the largest pizza retailer, with 434 outlets (A\$170 million in sales) (Webb and Manderson 1990: 156; Heywood and Lund-Adams 1991: 265–267; *The Australian*, 16 February 2009).

Foods high in fat and sugar are also marketed in other venues. The average supermarket offers over 1,800 snack food lines. A study recently done in Victoria found junk food in 93 per cent of school children's lunch boxes.

In mid-2009 the Health and Ageing Committee of the Federal Parliament's House of Representatives released its report on obesity, *Weighing It Up*. Noting over half of all adults were now overweight or obese, it pointed out the problem cost A\$8 billion in 2008 including the cost to the health-care system of increasing rates of diabetes, CVD and complications from surgical and other interventions.

Recommendations included:

- urban design initiatives such as walking trails to encourage more physical activity;
- teaching children about the value of healthy eating and exercise;
- the food industry and government work together on guidelines to reduce sugar, salt and fats in processed foods and develop uniform nutritional advice on food labels;
- public health campaigns to reduce obesity; and
- tax incentives to make fresh healthy food and access to physical activity more affordable.

In June 2009 speaking from an industry perspective, the Executive Director of the Advertising Federation of Australia, Mark Champion, endorsed the Committee's rejection of official bans on television advertising of fast foods on the grounds that they would not reduce consumption and might retard progress with introduction of healthier foods at fast food outlets. He welcomed the Committee's preference for industry self-regulation and cooperation between industry and government to reduce the advertising of unhealthy foods and drinks aimed at children. The food industry was as committed to reformulation of such products as the advertising industry was to communicating their benefits and those of fresh fruit and vegetables.

Seven fast food chains announced voluntary abandonment of fast food advertising to children, but several others including Domino's did not join the pact.

Public health and other critics were unhappy with reliance on industry self-regulation. Boyd Swinburn, Professor of Population Health, Deakin University said there were too many loopholes in the rules to protect children and they were really intended to pre-empt any stronger federal government action such as banning the screening of commercials altogether before 9 p.m. Jane Roberts from the Australian Council on Children and the Media pointed out the voluntary rules only applied to children's media so that advertising could be directed to families but still influence children. The voluntary guidelines included a ban on use of popular personalities in marketing to children under 14 years and on advertising in schools unless approved by school administrations. But they did not ban marketing of toys with junk food (condemned by many parents), although the food, not the toy, was to be the focus of the marketing.

As early as February 2010 the burger chain, Hungry Jacks admitted it had breached the voluntary industry code on advertising by screening advertisements for high fat food for children. In any case, good evidence has existed for some time that voluntary guidelines do not work. However, a coherent regulatory programme might be expected to reduce the growth of child and adolescent obesity quite quickly – perhaps within a year. Such a programme would need to include:

- banning all marketing of food targetting children;
- introduction of stringent food and physical activity requirements in schools;
- removal of junk foods and drinks from all state-funded premises;
- 'traffic light' food labelling, based on nutritional profiling, on all foods, drinks and meals irrespective of place of sale;
- use of fiscal measures to alter the prices of foods and drinks high in fat and sugar to the advantage of fruit and vegetables; and
- urban environmental requirements that favour pedestrians and cyclists.

Over the last decade-and-a-half there has been an abundance of reports on obesity; six in the last 15 years. But little Federal action – power over advertising and labelling lies with the Federal government – has resulted. The Howard Coalition government, 1996–2007, saw obesity as the individual's responsibility and, not surprisingly, the food industry agreed with this approach. The Rudd Labor government established yet another inquiry in early 2008. As already noted, the authors of its report, *Weighing It Up*, released in mid-2009, preferred industry self-regulation to government bans on advertising aimed at children (*Weighing It Up – Report on Obesity in Australia* 2009: no pagination; *The Australian*, 22 June 2009, 26 June 2009, 15 February 2010; Stanton 2009: 280–281).

## The course of Aboriginal mortality and the emergence of a double disease burden

Australian Aborigines are one of 5,000 Indigenous groups spread across 70 countries. The global total of Indigenes is at least 300 million and there is a heavy concentration in Asian countries. They generally suffer much poorer living standards and have less schooling, higher risk of disease and earlier deaths than the majority population. In addition to carrying these burdens, they commonly experience racial prejudice.

Indigenous Australians (Aborigines, 90 per cent and Torres Strait Islanders, 10 per cent) make up only 2.5 per cent of the national population (just over half a million people). About 32 per cent of Indigenous Australians live in large cities, 21 per cent in inner regional areas, 22 per cent in outer regional areas, 10 per cent in remote locations and 16 per cent in very remote locations. It is a young population with as few as 3 per cent aged 65 years or older, compared with 13 per cent of other Australians. Although lifestyles range from remote, tradition-oriented to urban, modern, and a number of Indigenes have entered well-paid professions like Law or Medicine, become academics or joined the higher ranks of the Public Service,[3] their general level of disadvantage is great. Their average household income is A$460 per week against A$740 for other Australians (2006); their unemployment rate is four times and imprisonment rate 16 times greater; and the difference in health status from other Australians is substantial (McNeish and Eversole 2005: 1–2; Eversole 2005: 29–31; Eversole *et al.* 2005: 262; Australian Human Rights Commission 2008: 2, 9; National Health and Hospitals Reform Commission 2008: 198–199, 207; Thomas 2009: 3).

While estimates differ, the total Aboriginal population in 1788 was probably about 315,000. Numbers fell rapidly after colonisation. The nadir was reached in the 1930s. The next decade saw the birth rate climb to a considerable 40 per 1,000 population. By the 1960s, the birth rate was still 35 per 1,000 and the mortality rate had declined from a long-standing high of 35 to 16 per 1,000 population. In the early 1970s, the total Aboriginal population was 116,000. By 2009, the Indigenous population was estimated to be 550,000, and it was much younger than the non-Indigenous with a median age of 20 years compared to 37 years.

A number of destructive factors resulting from European colonisation – new deadly diseases, frontier violence, loss of lands, and social and cultural collapse – produced this decline. Epidemics of diseases like smallpox were probably not as significant killers as endemic diseases interacting with social and ecological dislocation. There was also poor nutrition due to loss of land to settlers that restricted access to native plants and animals, and widespread adoption of a nutritionally poorer, European bushmen's diet of flour, sugar and tea (without milk) as well as fresh beef or mutton. Although the pre-contact diet was well balanced, periods of food scarcity were permanent aspects of traditional Aboriginal life.

Post-contact there was heavy use of alcohol and tobacco. Chest and bowel infections were common while there were high levels of female sterility and proneness to abortion from the widespread prevalence of introduced gonorrhoea and syphilis (Dane 1980: 95, 103; Moodie 1981: 157–158; Lewis 2003a: 20–25; Australian Institute of Health and Welfare 2010: 231–232).

By the First World War, NSW, Victoria and Tasmania were mainly concerned with people of part-Aboriginal descent where Queensland, Western Australia (WA), South Australia (SA) and the Northern Territory (NT) still had comparatively large populations of people of full descent. Five decades later, taking just WA and NT, we find Indigenous mortality rates were very high. In 1961–1964, the crude death rate in WA was 20 per 1,000 population and in NT, 18, when it was nine for other Australians. Infant mortality rates were respectively 75, over 140 and 22 per 1,000 live births. Gastroenteritis, dysentery, influenza and pneumonia were the prime causes of infant deaths.

In the same era in NSW, two of the four main causes of Aboriginal deaths were infection related – pneumonia (147 per 100,000 population but other Australians only 27) and gastroenteritis (86 per 100,000 as against only four for other Australians). CHD, CVD and cancer were also high on the list but at this point the mortality was much lower for Indigenes than other Australians: respectively, 133 to 256 per 100,000, 66 to 114 and 59 to 130 (Lewis 2003b: 244).

Other Australians were already experiencing epidemics of these NCDs as the second stage of the health transition typical of modern Western countries proceeded. However, as shown below, by the end of the twentieth century, the differences in the NCD mortality burden had reversed, and Aborigines were experiencing higher NCD death rates than other Australians.

Abuse of alcohol was, and remains, an important cause of premature mortality and excess morbidity. While many Aborigines are abstainers – 10 to 35 per cent of males and 39 to 80 per cent of females – a larger proportion of Indigenous than non-Indigenous drinkers consume excessive amounts. Alcohol directly causes about 10 per cent of Aboriginal mortality. It also contributes to the high levels of violence, accidents, crime and imprisonment,[4] and child abuse and neglect. The Productivity Commission found that between 1999 and 2008 reported cases of neglect increased from 16 to 35 per 1,000 children in Indigenous communities and from five to six in other Australian communities (Lewis 2003b: 232, 240–250; *Australian*, 3 July 2009). Prevalence of alcohol consumption and other behavioural health risk factors are generally higher for Aborigines,[5] although binge drinking is also a fast-growing habit among young, non-Indigenous adults.

Table 2.1 shows the higher prevalence across a range of significant risk factors including alcohol consumption experienced by Indigenous as against other Australians.

*Table 2.1* Age-standardised prevalence of NCD risk factors for people 18 years and older, Indigenous and other Australians, 2001

| Risk factor | Indigenous Australian (%) | Other Australian (%) |
|---|---|---|
| Current daily smoker | 49 | 22 |
| Alcohol consumption: | | |
| High risk | 7 | 4 |
| Exercise level: | | |
| Sedentary | 43 | 30 |
| Obese | | |
| (Body Mass Index of 30 or more) | 31 | 16 |
| Inadequate fruit intake* | 59 | 47 |
| Inadequate vegetable intake*# | 63 | 70 |

Source: adapted from Australian Institute of Health and Welfare 2006: 57.

Notes
* Data from non-remote areas only.
# Daily intake of three servings of vegetables or less.

Progress in health has been made. But the lower health status of Aborigines is clear in the widely cited gap of 17 years between Indigenous LEB[6] and that of other Australians. However, the gap, while still unacceptably high, is not in fact as great as this. Because of data limitations concerning Indigenous population estimates and death registrations, different methods may be used to establish Indigenous LEB.[7] Under the method preferred by the Australian Bureau of Statistics, the gap was 11 years – just under 12 years for males and 10 for females – although the male gap ranged from a low of nine years in NSW to a high of 17 years in NT, and the female, eight years in NSW to 13 years in NT.

Indigenous infant mortality rates have much improved: in WA, from 26 per 1,000 live births in 1991 down to 12 in 2005, in NT, from 25 to 16 and in SA, from 20 to 10. But they remain high compared with those of other Australian infants (2005): in WA, four, in NT, 11, and in SA, five.

The CD burden has been considerably reduced. Thus, mortality from pneumococcal pneumonia has fallen mainly because of vaccination programmes, as has the incidence of invasive *Haemophilus influenzae* type B in children and *Hepatitis B*. Hospitalisation rates for children with diarrhoeal disease have been reduced. New cases of TB fell from about 80 a year in the mid-1980s to fewer than 50 in 2001. There were 33 new cases in 2006.

However, Indigenes still suffer more CD mortality and deaths from injuries than other Australians. They suffer five times the CD mortality of other Australians; and three times the mortality from injuries. But it does not stop there. Although other Australians carry a significant burden of NCDs, Indigenes are now subject to an even greater burden; around 70 per cent of Indigenous mortality.

In more recent years, Aboriginal people have been experiencing something like a DDB, more usually identified as a key health problem in developing countries – high levels of poverty-related CDs together with high levels of NCDs.

That Aboriginal people suffer comparatively more from major chronic diseases than other Australians may be seen from the following: the standard mortality ratio (the number of Aboriginal deaths compared with the number of deaths to be expected if they had the same rate as other Australians) for circulatory system diseases is 3 for males and 2.5 for females; for cancers, 1.5 for both; for respiratory system diseases, 4 and 3.5; and for endocrine, nutritional and metabolic diseases (including diabetes), 7.5 and 10.5 (Thomson 2003: 489–491; Damman 2005: 70–71; Australian Bureau of Statistics 2005: 4–5; Australian Bureau of Statistics 2006: 1–5; Australian Institute of Health and Welfare 2006: 56; Australian Bureau of Statistics 2008: 5; National Health and Hospitals Reform Commission 2008: 197; Australian Indigenous HealthInfonet 2009: 1–4).

The larger NCD burden borne by Aborigines may also be seen in the greater number of years of life lost than other Australians.

Health status is determined by the interaction of social, cultural, economic, environmental and personal (genetic and behavioural) factors plus the quality and availability of health services. It is now widely accepted in public health circles that social and economic determinants – upstream factors – play a considerable part in establishing health status. They are interconnected and include income, education, employment, social support, living[8] and working conditions, and gender. Cultural factors including beliefs, customs and attitudes also influence health through personal and group behaviour and are especially important for Aborigines whose traditional culture was so vastly different from Western culture and so damaged by the encounter with European settlers.

But, in the last 40 years, since governments have expressed a commitment to addressing Indigenes' health problems, solutions have been difficult to find since they involve competing material and ideological interests, and demand priority setting between the health sector and other sectors, between prevention and treatment services, and between the short term and longer term.

Some researchers propose as much as 30 to 50 per cent of the gap in health status between Indigenes and other Australians is accounted for by social and economic factors. The balance is determined by access to health services, the health behaviour of the individual (cultural) and environmental factors (Thomson 2003: 492–494; National Health and Hospitals Reform Commission 2008: 205).

## Health policy for Indigenous Australians

In early 2008 the new Rudd Federal Labor government set up the National Health and Hospitals Reform Commission (NHHRC) to advise on reform of the Australian health system. One of the four themes it identified as defining the direction of reform was responding to health inequities. As to be expected, the group seen as suffering the most injustice was Indigenes (National Health and Hospitals Reform Commission 2008: 1).

*Table 2.2* Average years of life lost from chronic diseases, Aborigines and other Australians, 2001–2003

| Cause | Aboriginal males | Other males | Aboriginal females | Other females |
|---|---|---|---|---|
| CHD | 21.2 years | 12.1 years | 18.6 years | 8.6 years |
| Cerebrovascular disease | 15.0 | 10.0 | 13.7 | 8.8 |
| Lung cancer | 19.0 | 14.2 | 24.0 | 16.9 |
| Colorectal cancer | 16.3 | 14.7 | 20.6 | 15.2 |
| Diabetes | 22.9 | 19.7 | 14.2 | 11.2 |
| Chronic obstructive pulmonary disease | 15.0 | 10.0 | 18.9 | 12.0 |
| Kidney disease | 26.7 | 9.8 | 25.3 | 9.2 |

Source: Australian Institute of Health and Welfare 2006: 61.

The NHHRC proposed a variety of initiatives concerning Indigenes:

- the Commonwealth Health Department encourage intersectoral collaboration to reduce the impact of the social and economic determinants on Aboriginal health;
- additional funding for health services; increasing from $150 million in the first year to $500 million in the fifth year, and sustained at the latter level until the gap in health status was closed;
- provide comprehensive primary care services, greater investment in Aboriginal community health services that will allow development of enhanced organisational capacity;
- establish a National Aboriginal and Torres Strait Islander Health Authority to purchase high-quality and timely services for these peoples, channelling existing funding from mainstream sources such as Medicare and Closing the Gap investment, and the Office of Aboriginal and Torres Strait Islander Health; the Authority would be located in the health portfolio;
- education of health professionals to include specific modules on Aboriginal and Islander health to encourage more Indigenes to enter the health professions and to assist non-indigenous professionals to understand better special needs of indigenous patients;
- additional investment to build an Aboriginal health workforce;
- subsidise the cost of fresh food, especially fruit and vegetables, and nutrition education and promote healthy diets in remote communities (National Health and Hospitals Reform Commission 2008: 215–218; National Health and Hospitals Reform Commission 2009: 86–89).

The NHHRC recognised not only health-sector but wider, social and economic determinants of health status had to be addressed if the gap in LEB between Indigenes and other Australians was to be bridged. But it did not elaborate in nearly the same detail about how to address social and economic determinants – more difficult for governments to influence – as it did about determinants within the reach of health-sector action (National Health and Hospitals Reform Commission 2009: 95–96).

Attempts had already been made in the 1990s to identify the causes of the poorer health status of Aborigines compared with those of the Indigenes of the United States, Canada and New Zealand. American epidemiologist, Stephen Kunitz argued when central governments (not States or Territories) have responsibility for indigenous affairs, as has been the case in the United States, Canada and New Zealand, the health status of Indigenes has been higher.

Kunitz and Australian anthropologist Maggie Brady pinpointed three reasons for greater success in the United States than Australia. First, Federal administration there meant State equivocation about responsibility did not stand in the way of action; American like Australian States were historically very susceptible to pressures from non-Indigenes wanting access to the natural resources possessed by Indigenes. Second, the separation, from the 1950s, of health services from the United States Bureau of Indian Affairs provided protection for the services from continuing policy battles over natural resources. Third, the health services over time were able to marry primary, secondary and some tertiary care, as well as alcohol and other drug services, to public health services, so improving the quality of care provided. Finally, despite many breaches, Federal treaties with Indian tribes ultimately underpinned their claims to central government services. No treaties existed in Australia, and even after the Commonwealth assumed national responsibility, the States and Territories remained much involved (Kunitz 1994: 24–29; Kunitz and Brady 1995: 549–557; Lewis 2003b: 255; *Weekend Australian*, 28–29 November 2009; *Australian*, 30 November 2009).

Brady herself argues elsewhere that health interventions have been much influenced by two, significant historical themes of broader, Aboriginal affairs policy: cultural difference and equality. Since the 1840s, the basic aim of Aboriginal affairs policy has changed, first, from protection to assimilation into the general population and, more recently, to self-determination and self-management. We can see that in alcohol policy as in other health policy, these themes of difference and equality have been influential. The first official approach to Aboriginal alcohol use (which continued from the colonial era till the 1960s) was prohibition. Not only did this promote a harmful style of binge drinking but the right to drink became for Indigenes a powerful symbol of equality with other Australians.

Reacting against assimilation, Aboriginal activists in the 1960s called for recognition of the idea of cultural difference from other Australians, and as self-determination came to the fore in policy, community-controlled alcohol and other health programmes, separate from mainstream programmes, were publicly funded in the 1970s. With the idea and practice of cultural difference so politically potent, government health authorities in the 1980s and 1990s were reluctant to urge Aboriginal services to apply new, effective, mainstream treatments of alcohol misuse (based on the new model of harm minimisation) such as early, brief interventions through primary health care. Aboriginal treatment providers remained committed to the much more demanding treatment goal of total abstinence (arising from the older disease model of alcoholism). While excessive alcohol consumption, particularly by men, has remained a major problem deeply disruptive of social life, local initiatives by women's groups and land councils as well as health and legal services have enjoyed some success in reducing harm: for example, restrictions on the local supply of alcohol and community education about alcohol and other drugs.

Another significant influence has been the direction Aboriginal affairs took over more than a decade of the conservative Howard Federal Coalition government (to the end of 2007) when national representative bodies were disbanded and execution of policy handed back to mainstream Departments. This involved a watering down of the recognition of cultural difference and greater emphasis on the idea of equality and integration with mainstream Australian life (Brady 2007: 759–762).

The issue of the best balance in policy and practice between cultural difference and equality–integration remains largely unresolved. But over the last ten years, a new approach to improvement of the health and other aspects of the quality of life of Indigenes has been articulated by a small group of Aboriginal opinion-makers. They see good health status in the long term resulting from economic advancement based on participation in the mainstream economy and underwritten by a sound education that combines knowledge and skills needed for the modern world with coherent knowledge of traditional culture.

The more prominent exponents of this new approach – lawyer, Noel Pearson, anthropologist and academic, Marcia Langton, and former President of the Australian Labor Party, Warren Mundine – have argued that the pursuit of a rights-based approach to Aboriginal affairs that has been orthodoxy for liberals and progressives on both sides of politics over the last three to four decades has failed. Their position is supported by some older leaders like former chairman of the Northern Land Council, Galarrwuy Yunupingu, who in late 2009 talked of the need for Aboriginal people to escape from the prison of welfare dependency by creating jobs through self help (*Weekend Australian*, 7–8 November 2009).

According to Noel Pearson and fellow critics, the established, rights-based approach has led to a morally corrosive dependence on public welfare payments and to poor literacy and numeracy skills. These combined with excessive use of alcohol and other intoxicants, and high levels of domestic and communal violence, have trapped many Indigenes, especially in remote communities, in poor health, low LEB and intergenerational poverty. These critics say social dysfunction and undue isolation from mainstream life have to end. The substance abuse and violence must be eradicated as a necessary first step to the social order that will allow the teaching of the modern skills needed for employment in the real economy (*Sydney Morning Herald*, 19 August 2000; *Weekend Australian*, 6–7 December 2008, 13–14 December 2008, 3–4 October 2009, 7–8 November 2009; *Sun-Herald*, 10 May 2009).

At the same time, public health professionals have shown the health interventions that reduce mortality of other Australians from significant NCDs will also work with Indigenous people. Cultural difference does not stand in the way. One important example is from tobacco control. Thomas (2009) has shown that the seemingly intractable level of Indigenous smoking prevalence, responsible for 20 per cent of indigenous deaths and 17 per cent of the health status gap between Indigenes and other Australians, can be reduced by increasing funding for the tobacco control measures known to have worked with other Australians.

Noel Pearson sees quality education as the key to overcoming disadvantage in employment, housing, health and, ultimately, life expectancy. We noted earlier the capacity of education and literacy (leading to cultural change) to raise life expectancy in the face of low incomes in the countries that pioneered the modern health transition in Asia.

Pearson envisages quality education providing literacy in English and numeracy but also knowledge of Aboriginal languages and other aspects of traditional culture. Children would then be able to 'orbit' between the mainstream and indigenous worlds. He sees three possible futures for Aborigines as a minority, indigenous people in a developed country with an advanced welfare system

- continuing dependence on passive welfare that will simply perpetuate social and cultural 'pauperisation';
- maintaining cultural and linguistic diversity; but in the face of the over-whelming presence of the dominant society and economy, it is unrealistic to expect any revival of the traditional economy to be sustainable;
- the only viable future; combining real economic activities whether subsist-ence or modern with biculturalism and bilingualism; education being the key.

However, in remote Aboriginal communities, at present, many are not receiving even minimal education. Chronic truancy and parental 'anti-school' attitudes are deeply entrenched. In Wadeye, a large NT regional community of 2,500 people, more than half the population is under 18 years of age and 80 per cent of young adults are unemployed. But as few as 14 per cent of children of school age attend school four days out of five. Many experts believe an individual must attend at least 90 per cent of the time for a successful educational outcome to be achieved. The problem of truancy has multiple causes: an established culture of non-attendance, overcrowded homes occupied by troubled families, an environment full of alcohol and drugs, very mobile lifestyles and long-term lack of hope about improvement in social and economic conditions (*Weekend Australian*, 13–14 March 2010, 20–21 March 2010, 27–28 March 2010, 15–16 May 2010).

Marcia Langton shares Pearson's concern to see implementation of reform measures like quarantining of welfare payments to ensure children are properly nourished. She has been particularly outspoken about sexual abuse of, and viol-ence against, women and children.

She strongly endorses the arguments of anthropologist, Peter Sutton against rights-based policy. She believes his analysis has the virtue that it supports neither the Left's romanticisation of Aborigines as 'noble savages' nor the Right's advocacy of rapid integration into the modern economy whatever the cost (Langton 2009: iii–vi; *Weekend Australian*, 3–4 October 2009; *Sun-Herald*, 10 May 2009; *Weekend Australian Review*, 11–12 July 2009).

Sutton argues that he and other liberals and progressives who sought to pre-serve traditional culture by insulating Indigenes from the forces of modernisa-tion have been too slow to recognise the high cost to Aboriginal people's health and quality of life. Modernisation is not simply a swamping of Aboriginal culture by the majority culture. It is a complex, two-way process. Moreover, the cultural changes required to support advances in well-being are not well under-stood by anthropologists, the anointed experts in cultural change, and certainly not by politicians.

Sutton notes liberal-progressive Australians accept the need for modernisa-tion to overcome mass poverty and low health status in Asia and Africa. Yet, they oppose it in Aboriginal communities because it seems to imply modern values are superior to traditional ones (Sutton 2009: 1–13, 68–69; *Australian Literary Review*, 3 June 2009; *Weekend Australian Review*, 11–12 July 2009).

For him the liberal-progressive explanation of the poor health status of Indigenes – an explanation in terms of a history of domination and discrimination – is a partial one; and the solution of separatism is no solution when the problem lies in culturally embedded health behaviours that promote poor hygiene and poor diet; both of which contribute importantly to high rates of illness and death.

He recognises Stephen Kunitz's attempt to explain the lower health status of modern Aborigines compared with that of Indigenes in the United States, Canada and New Zealand as more compelling. He accepts Kunitz's argument Aborigines have suffered from the lack of the treaties which delivered better health services to Indigenes in these three countries. But, he cautions, this ignores the impact of more basic cultural, social and economic differences between Aborigines and these other Indigenes. Kunitz has in effect compared these four Indigenous groups on the basis of their common experience as victims of colonisation. He should also be comparing former nomadic hunter gatherers within all these nation-states; next, comparing hunter gatherers with pastoralists; and, then, with sedentary horticultural and agricultural peoples. This might well reveal cultural and social features of particular types of tribal societies that conferred advantages when encountering hegemonic, European settler societies (Sutton 2009: 117–143).

The issue of the extent and type of cultural change (as opposed to health-sector change) thought necessary to sustain a high level of Indigenous health and well-being remains unresolved. On this as other issues, Noel Pearson has taken a radical stand, saying if Indigenous people are to prosper (and significantly improve their health and well-being in the long term), individualism and self-interest, the Western values promoting economic development, must be encouraged but not at the expense of tribal or collective identity.[9]

Pearson claims social and economic structuralism, under which structural factors are held responsible for inequities and so it is futile to look to individual behaviour change to remove disadvantage, still dominates thinking about how to advance Indigenous quality of life. He argues individual behaviour change (individual agency), especially when expressed as engagement in real jobs in the real economy, must be encouraged if Indigenous people are to break out of the trap of welfare dependency.

He is certainly correct in recognising there is a fundamental and, in many ways, still unresolved issue for the social sciences in the question of the primacy of social structure or individual agency in determining human behaviour. The issue is obviously important for policy development as well as theory; and it is complicated by the fact that the two, most relevant social sciences have differed in their answers to this question.

Mainstream economics has generally emphasised individual agency while mainstream sociology has emphasised structure. Neoclassical economics focuses on utility-maximising, individual agents who interact in markets; it is largely unconcerned with social structure; and there is little room for government intervention so that in policy there is a clear preference for markets over state planning. There is an opposition, then, between individual agency and social structure as the driver of human affairs.

Some social theorists have sought to reconcile these last two. Sociologist, Anthony Giddens, for example, treats them as distinct but interdependent. In his 'duality of structure', agency reproduces but can also transform structures, although agents can function only within a structured environment. This is all very well at the level of theory but how it plays out empirically in the real world and, in particular, where the emphasis in policy should lie is not so clear (Jackson 1999: 545–553; *Australian*, 15 February 2010, 23 June 2010; *Weekend Australian*, 26–27 June 2010).

However, as discussed in the introductory chapter, the work of Michael Marmot, Richard Wilkinson and some other epidemiologists has pointed to the great significance of social relations in determining health status once national wealth has grown to a certain level. After countries enter a 'post-scarcity era', as all developed nations have, the degree of social inequality becomes critical in determining health status. Marmot has noted that observations of differences in disease rates within and between countries, rapid time changes in disease rates and social inequalities, and changing disease rates in migrant populations indicate the social environment is very important (Marmot 2006: 5).

## What may we conclude from Australia's historical experience of two kinds of health transition?

The drama of the health transition in Australia has been enacted on two stages with very different scripts. The encouraging script tells of a long-term transition by the European, majority society from a health profile compromised by infectious diseases and an LEB of about 48 years (1870) to one limited by non-communicable disorders but with an LEB of more than 80 years; one of the highest LEBs in the world. It is a script shared with other, high income Western nations. The other is a script that until the last few decades has been relentlessly depressing. It is about the destruction of small-scale tribal groups of nomadic, hunter gatherers with deaths due to zoonotic infections ('accidentally' transmitted), some chronic infections and infestations (that co-evolved with humans from the time of our primate forerunners), and violence and accidents, and their replacement by a fractured, poverty-stricken society of sedentary fringe-dwellers, beset by imported, deadly infections and massive, social, cultural and ecological dislocation (Lewis 2003a: 15–16; Riley 2008: 176). This disabled society, caught between tradition and modernity, endured high mortality from CDs. Its members did not share until very recently in the unprecedented growth in LEB enjoyed by the non-Indigenous majority.

In the last two decades or so Indigenous CD mortality has fallen but NCDs have become a heavy burden, now heavier for Indigenous people than other Australians. Indeed, Indigenous Australians are facing something like a double disease burden, better known as a feature of contemporary health transitions in developing countries in Asia and the Pacific.

A gap in health status between Indigenes and other Australians still exists. Currently the LEB of Indigenous people is just under 70 years for males and almost 73 years for females; respectively, 12 and ten years lower than for other Australians.

Nevertheless, there has been progress. Indigenous LEB has improved. Even in the worst-performing jurisdiction, NT, LEB increased from 52 years for males and 54 for females in the late 1960s to 62 and 69 years in 2005–2007. The Indigenous infant mortality rate (IMR) between 1991 and 2005 in WA, SA and NT fell from 26 per 1,000 live births to 12 in the first, 20 to ten in the second and 25 to 16 in the third. These are significant declines and are equivalent to reductions in the IMR of 41 per cent, 58 per cent and 46 per cent respectively.

In mid-February 2010, in his second annual report on 'Close the Gap' policy (the policy, costing \$5.5 billion over ten years, was announced after the national government's 2008 apology to Indigenous people for the past, forced removal of children from families), the then Prime Minister, Kevin Rudd, observed that generations of disadvantage cannot be overcome quickly. We very much agree. It has taken us two centuries to get into the mess with Indigenous people. It is likely to take some years more to find our way out. The extent of long-term, social, cultural and economic change required, and how best to reconcile tradition-oriented, communitarian values and behaviour with the individualistic norms and behaviour underlying activities in the mainstream economy, is not self-evident (Australian Bureau of Statistics 2006: 4; Australian Bureau of Statistics 2008: 4–5, 8; *Australian*, 12 February 2010). But we hope Noel Pearson's faith in a realistic marriage of education in modern skills of literacy and numeracy and in tradition-oriented culture is fulfilled.

Australia's non-Indigenous health transition stands in marked contrast to that of Indigenes. It has raised the LEB of non-Indigenous Australians to historically unprecedented heights and to almost the highest level in the world, although increasing rates of obesity and overweight threaten the further growth of LEB. There is no doubt high and expanding national income underpinned the enterprise. However, social investment in mass education played a not insignificant role in bringing down mortality from CDs in the later nineteenth and early twentieth century. Social growth in turn produced cultural change expressed as health-advancing attitudes and behaviour.

In recent decades other nations have looked to Australia's effective health preventive and promoting programmes (dependent for their success on the widespread existence of such health-focussed attitudes and behaviour) in tobacco control, immunisation and, to some extent, in nutrition for insights into what may be done about raising LEB. Viewed historically, health promotion programmes are in effect mechanisms to reinforce the health-focussed, cultural change initiated by elementary education and mass literacy in the late nineteenth and early twentieth century.

The programmes have encouraged the personal involvement of people in their own health improvement; a habit seen as increasingly important in control of NCDs. In the case of tobacco control, the state's mandatory powers of taxing and regulating individual behaviour and commercial activities have also been fruitfully employed. Health professionals are now calling for the application of such powers to reduce consumption of unhealthy foods and drinks in the hope of reducing overweight and obesity.

The histories of Australia's two health transitions – the Western and the Indigenous – support the growing global awareness that the better health of humans depends significantly upon a renewed attention to the ways in which we interact socially and culturally as well as economically; that is, to the social and cultural, as well as the economic, determinants of health status.[10]

We have discussed the emphasis placed by Caldwell on cultural change, more specifically, the education of women, in raising health status in Sri Lanka and elsewhere where women enjoyed higher standing. We have noted that Riley attributes the beginning of improvement in health status in Ceylon/Sri Lanka in the earlier twentieth century (while it was still a low income country) to this sort of social (rather than economic) growth; and we have argued that even in Australia, where economic growth led the way to high health status for the non-Indigenous population, social growth played a not unimportant supporting role and that cultural change accompanied this social growth. Moreover, epidemiologist, Richard Wilkinson argues that in contemporary, high income countries economic conditions are no longer a key determinant of health status; rather, differences in social status (social hierarchy itself) now sustains the social gradient in health; and social inequality may be expected to continue to manifest as inequality in health status even as already high average incomes rise further.

Thus, we suggest that social and cultural determinants may play a very significant role in the low income phase (in countries where women's standing is such that they gain access to modern, basic schooling) and in the very high income phase (if Wilkinson is right) of the modern health transition. Further progress in health demands that we look with fresh eyes at the role of social and cultural, as well as economic, factors, in Australia (both among Indigenous and non-Indigenous people) and beyond.

## Notes

1 The other countries are Costa Rica, Cuba, Jamaica, Mexico, Oman, Panama, the former Soviet Union and Venezuela.

2 Even in the interwar years, as Australia began to experience growing mortality from NCDs, mortality from infectious diseases remained comparatively high: thus, in 1935 when LEB was 65 years, the proportion of total mortality that was due to infections was 25 per cent while that due to CVD was 28 per cent. If cancer deaths are added, the proportion of total mortality attributable to these two NCDs was 40 per cent. In his chapter in this volume, Richard Taylor argues that in fact non-Indigenous Australians experienced, between the 1920s and the late 1940s, a double burden of disease.

3 A number of Indigenous people have also enjoyed success in the graphic and performing arts and as elite sports people. Some are now becoming entrepreneurs. Karen Milward, the head of Victoria's new Aboriginal Chamber of Commerce, set up to advise Aboriginal people about business matters, sees good export prospects for the marketing of iconic art and food products. In Sydney in July 2010, the Australian

Indigenous Chamber of Commerce awarded the inaugural First Australians Business Awards for the best-performing Indigenous businesses. In the 2010 Federal election, Ken Wyatt (Liberal party) was returned for the Western Australian seat of Hasluck. He is the first Indigenous member of the House of Representatives, and only the third Indigenous member of the Federal Parliament. In his maiden speech he attributed his political success very much to his good education. There have been Indigenous members of State and Territory Parliaments. A high point was attained in 2008 when the total reached ten: six in the NT, two in WA, one in Tasmania and one in NSW (*Weekend Australian*, 30–31 January 2010; *Australian*, 29 July 2010, 30 September 2010).

4  In May 2010, the Chief Justice of the NT, Brian Martin, announced against a background of heated public debate about 'soft' and 'hard' sentencing of Indigenous offenders that he would retire early. He observed that too many offenders, as children, had themselves been victims of violence and abuse, and it might take 25 years or more to break this intergenerational cycle. Indigenous academic Professor Marcia Langton said this was too defeatist. Federal Minister for Indigenous Affairs in the Rudd Labor government, Jenny Macklin, said there were no quick and easy solutions, while former Federal Minister for Indigenous Affairs in the Howard Coalition government, Mal Brough, said it would not take 25 years to find an answer but he did understand Justice Martin's despair as so many government initiatives had failed. In October 2010, Sue Gordon, a retired children's court magistrate, said that responsibility for child protection should be taken away from the NT government after an inquiry into child protection reported there had been total systemic failure and the responsible Territory Minister admitted remote Indigenous communities were in 'total collapse'. Indigenous leaders demanded adults in these communities assume control of their lives and their children (*The Australian*, 28 May 2010, 20 October 2010).

5  Some experts have argued for a significant role for genetic as well as behavioural factors in the NCD burden borne by Aborigines. Geneticist James Neel put forward the 'thrifty' genotype hypothesis in the early 1960s. It was based on the idea that having to adapt to recurrent food scarcity, hunter gatherer peoples like the Aborigines developed a genetically based capacity to deposit fat quickly in periods of abundance and this assisted them to survive the 'hungry' times. However, the advantage predisposed them to diabetes in the modern era when an excess of highly refined, carbohydrate foods is commonly consumed. Other scientists have proposed that pre-agricultural peoples like the Aborigines never acquired a gene protective against diabetes that agricultural populations in Europe, Asia and sub-Saharan Africa gained in their adaptation to mainly cereal diets (Cochran and Harpending 2010: 79–81).

6  A recent study of longevity in hunter gatherers found that in five, traditional hunter gatherer societies the LEB ranged from 21 to 37 years. So pre-contact, Australian Indigenes very probably had a LEB somewhere in this range. Sweden, the first Western country to enter upon the modern health transition, had in 1751–1759, about the time it began the transition, a LEB of 34 years (see also Note 5 in Chapter 1). The study found, further, that post-reproductive longevity was a 'robust' aspect of hunter gatherer societies. In the five ones studied, 26 to 43 per cent of people lived to 45 years; and life expectancy at the age of 45 varied between 14 and 24 years (Gurven and Kaplan 2007: 326, 332, 348).

7  A 1967 national referendum gave the Federal government for the first time the legal capacity to legislate for Aborigines and to count them in national population censuses. Under the Australian Constitution of 1901 such capacity had been lacking. While population data could now be collected, there were problems concerning data on mortality and other health indicators. Not until the mid-1980s did the Commonwealth and most of the States and Territories agree to include provision for identification of Indigenous people in four fundamental, health-related, data collections – birth and death registration systems and maternal/perinatal and hospitalisation inpatient statistics.

However, only in 1996 did all States and Territories include a question on Indigenous status in birth and death registration systems. Even so, there was no provision made at the time for their identification in medical certificates of death and perinatal death in NSW, Tasmania and the ACT (Australian Capital Territory). Mortality statistics, of course, combine cause-of-death data from medical certificates of death (or data supplied by the coroner) with demographic and other data recorded on death notification forms. The standard method of compiling life tables and so deriving life expectancy at birth (LEB) requires both complete and accurate data about deaths and an estimate of the population exposed to those deaths at the mid-point of the period. But Indigenous population estimates and death registrations still have limitations so the Australian Bureau of Statistics (ABS) has investigated four demographic methods for deriving the LEB: three indirect and one direct. After analysis of the 2006 data, the ABS recommended against use of the indirect methods because of two main concerns. First, estimates of coverage of deaths for 2001–2006 were notably lower than coverage for 1996–2001; an implausible result when compared to the observed data. Second, life expectancy estimates have been found to be very sensitive to the quality of the population estimates at the respective end points so that errors in the age distribution and level of either population estimate may result in very different life expectancy outcomes. It proposed employment of the direct method, as is done for derivation of the life expectancy of the non-Indigenous population, but with adjustment for under-coverage using the Census Data Enhancement Indigenous Mortality Quality Study. The higher Indigenous LEB results using this preferred method are listed in the text (Brady 1991: 182; Thomson 2003: 2–3; Australian Bureau of Statistics 2006: 1–5).

8  Former Minister for Indigenous Policy in the NT Labor government, Alison Anderson, recently pointed out that in remote communities the most basic preventive health measures like personal cleanliness could not be pursued because families lacked the means to do so: housing was run-down and crowded, with non-functioning bathrooms; and community laundries, if available, were not properly maintained. More recently, Alison Anderson called for abandonment of 'separatist' policies that have created Indigenous-only jobs and schools. She said they have limited members of remote communities to publicly funded, 'dead-end jobs' and sustained 'second-rate' schools the literacy and numeracy standards of which were unacceptably low. In December 2009, the National Partnership Agreement on Remote Indigenous Housing, funded by the Federal Labor government, had to be renegotiated because progress by the States and the NT was too slow to meet existing targets. But by mid-2010, a national total of 316 new houses had been built and 828 houses refurbished. Queensland, SA and Tasmania had failed to meet their targets by a total of 32 new houses. The NT had constructed 67 new houses and renovated 344, exceeding its targets (*Weekend Australian*, 22–23 May 2010, 29–31 May 2010; *Australian*, 15 July 2010, 11 November 2010).

9  In late June 2010, Jenny Macklin, Labor Minister for Families, Housing, Community Services and Indigenous Affairs, made clear the Federal government (which retains some powers over the NT) would manage welfare incomes of Indigenous and other Australians in the NT if children were being deprived of food and other necessities because parents were spending excessively on alcohol and other non-necessities. Noel Pearson defended this major policy change against criticism by a coalition of welfare and social service organisations the spokesperson for which claimed it was not only an attack upon human dignity but, wrongly, saw welfare as the cause of this behaviour when structurally based poverty was the true cause. Pearson blamed the pervasiveness of structural thinking about economic and social reform in university and bureaucratic circles for a long-term failure to appreciate that individual behavioural change such as that induced by income management was as necessary as structural change. For him structural factors establish the conditions under which welfare

dependency flourishes but change in individual behaviour can work against this induced passivity. A report to the Queensland parliament tabled in December 2010 seemed to show that Pearson-style, 'tough-love', welfare reforms (including income management and bans on alcohol) improved the quality of life in a number of remote Indigenous communities. School attendance climbed as high as 90 per cent, assault rates fell by 50 per cent and more people were employed on housing development projects (127 across ten communities). In August 2011 NT Aboriginal leader, Galarrwuy Yunupingu, a former Australian of the Year, publicly aligned himself with Noel Pearson in rejecting welfare dependence: 'Please, no more, please no more welfare handouts. It's a killer to the Yolngu society'. He also demanded 'real education' for Aboriginal children, saying the NT government was being racist when it set a target school attendance rate of only 34 per cent for Indigenous children when the target for non-Indigenes was 98 per cent. In a report on spending on Indigenous people (in recent years $3.5 billion a year) presented to the Federal Department of Finance in February 2010, the author, former head of the Federal Department of Veterans' Affairs, Dr Neil Johnston, wrote: 'The history of commonwealth policy for indigenous Australians over the past 40 years is largely a story of good intentions, flawed policies, unrealistic assumptions, poor implementation, unintended consequences and dashed hopes.' He was particularly critical of the capacity of State and Territory governments to implement effectively and efficiently policies and programmes. The report was only released for public scrutiny after a protracted legal challenge under Freedom of Information laws by the Seven Television Network (*Australian*, 21 June 2010, 23 June 2010, 17 December 2010, 8 August 2011).

10  Just as Noel Pearson has called for economic modernisation of Aboriginal society combined with preservation of essential aspects of traditional culture, so Sitaleki Finau and colleagues have discussed models of possible health transitions in Pacific Island countries different from the Western model based on maximum economic growth. One of their models that has some affinity with Pearson's is their 'Bridge model'. It would involve selective adaptation of traditional economic and cultural features including commercialisation of subsistence fishing and agricultural activities and use of traditional medicine along with Western medicine (Finau *et al.* 2004: 123–125). In his recently published *Aboriginal Self-Determination: The Whiteman's Dream*, Gary Johns, a former Federal Labor Government Minister and now an Associate Professor of Public Policy at the Australian Catholic University, goes further than Pearson. He calls for an end to the grand experiment of separate development and argues for full integration of Indigenes into the Australian economy and mainstream way of life, with culture becoming primarily a private concern. He thinks future commentators will see the era of self-determination, lasting from about 1970 to about 2006, as a detour from the basic process of integration of Indigenous people into non-Indigenous, modern society; a process that started with the advent of European settlement. In Johns' view, separatism could not hold change forever at bay. It could only offer false hope, while, sadly, depriving Indigenous people of the very skills needed to succeed in the modern world (Johns 2011: 15–74, 249–302).

# References

Access Economics (2008) *The Growing Cost of Obesity in 2008: Three Years On*, iii. Online, available at: www.accesseconomics.com.au/publicationsreports (accessed 20 February 2010).

Australian Bureau of Statistics (2005) *The Health and Welfare of Australia's Aboriginal and Torres Strait Islander Peoples*, 1–11. Online, available at: www.abs.gov.au/austats/ABS@.nsf/Previousproducts/A3F338E5C16568A4CA (accessed 9 September 2008).

Australian Bureau of Statistics (2006) *Discussion Paper: Assessment of Methods for Developing Life Tables for Aboriginal and Torres Strait Islander Australians*, 1–7. Online, available at: www.abs.gov.au/ausstats/abs@.nsf/mf/3302.0.55.002 (accessed 12 October 2009).

Australian Bureau of Statistics (2008) *The Health and Welfare of Australia's Aboriginal and Torres Strait Islander Peoples*, 1–9. Online, available at: www.abs.gov.au/AUS-STATS/abs@.nsf/39433889d406eeb9ca2570610019 (accessed 20 October 2009).

Australian Human Rights Commission (2008) *Social Justice Report*, Appendix 2: A Statistical Overview of Aboriginal and Torres Strait Islander Peoples in Australia, 1–24. Online, available at: www.hreoc.gov.au/social_justice/sj_report/sjreport08/app. 2.html (accessed 7 May 2009).

Australian Indigenous HealthInfonet (2009) *Reviews: Summary of Tuberculosis among Indigenous People*, 1–2. Online, available at: http://archive.healthifonet.ecu.edu.au/html/html_Healthspecific (accessed 12 February 2010).

Australian Institute of Health and Welfare (2006) *Chronic Diseases and Associated Risk Factors in Australia*, 56–62. Online, available at: www.aihw.gov.au/publications/phe/cdarfa06/c (accessed 15 October 2009).

Australian Institute of Health and Welfare (2010) *Australia's Health 2010*, Canberra: Australian Institute of Health and Welfare.

Bi, P., Parton, K.A. and Donald, K. (2005) 'Secular Trends in Mortality Rates for Diabetes in Australia, 1907–1998', *Diabetes Research and Clinical Practice*, 70(3): 270–277.

Bi, P., Walker, S., Parton, K.A. and Whitby, M. (2002) 'Secular Change of Australian All-Cause Mortality, 1907–1998', *Australian Journal of Primary Health*, 8(3): 58–66.

Bi, P., Whitby, M., Walker, S. and Parton, K.A. (2003) 'Trends in Mortality Rates for Infectious and Parasitic Diseases in Australia: 1907–1997', *Internal Medicine Journal*, 33(4): 152–162.

Brady, M. (1991) 'Drug and Alcohol Use among Aboriginal People', in J. Reid and P. Trompf (eds) *The Health of Aboriginal Australia*, Sydney: Harcourt Brace Jovanovich, 173–217.

Brady, M. (2007) 'Equality and Difference: Persisting Historical Themes in Health and Alcohol Policies affecting Indigenous Australians', *Journal of Epidemiology and Community Health*, 61(9): 759–763.

Caldwell, J.C. (1991) 'Routes to Low Mortality in Poor Countries', in J.C. Caldwell and G. Santow (eds) *Selected Readings in the Cultural, Social and Behavioural Determinants of Health*, Canberra: Health Transition Centre, Australian National University, 1–37.

Caldwell, J.C., Caldwell, B.K., Caldwell, P., McDonald, P.F. and Schindlmayr, T. (2006) *Demographic Transition Theory*, Dordrecht: Springer.

Chapman, S. (1993) 'Unravelling Gossamer with Boxing Gloves: Problems in Explaining the Decline in Smoking', *BMJ*, 307(6901): 429–432.

Cochran, G. and Harpending, H. (2010) *10,000 Year Explosion: How Civilization Accelerated Human Evolution*, New York: Basic Books.

Coghlan, T.A. (1902) *A Statistical Account of the Seven Colonies of Australasia 1901–1902*, Sydney: Government Printer.

Cumpston, J.H.L. (1989) *Health and Disease in Australia: A History* (ed. M.J. Lewis), Canberra: AGPS Press.

Damman, S. (2005) 'Nutritional Vulnerability in Indigenous Children of the Americas: A Human Rights Issue', in R. Eversole, J-A. McNeish and A.D. Cimadore (eds) *Indigenous Peoples and Poverty: An International Perspective*, London: Zed Books, 69–73.

Dane, S. (1980) 'Diet, Disease and Demography: Hunter-Gatherers in Arnhem Land', unpublished Honours thesis, University of New England, Armidale, NSW.

Eversole, R. (2005) 'Overview: Patterns of Indigenous Disadvantage Worldwide', in R. Eversole, J.-A. McNeish and A.D. Cimadore (eds) *Indigenous Peoples and Poverty: An International Perspective*, London: Zed Books, 29–37.

Eversole, R., Ridgeway, L. and Mercer, D. (2005) 'Indigenous Anti-Poverty Strategies in an Australian Town', in R. Eversole, J.-A. McNeish and A.D. Cimadore (eds) *Indigenous Peoples and Poverty: An International Perspective*, London: Zed Books, 260–273.

Finau, S.A., Wainiqolo, I.L. and Cuboni, G.G. (2004) 'Health Transition and Globalization in the Pacific: Vestiges of Colonialism?' *Perspectives on Global Development and Technology*, 3(1–2): 109–129.

Frenk, J., Bobadilla, J.-L., Stern, C., Frejka, T. and Lozano, R. (1994) 'Elements for a Theory of the Health Transition', in L.C. Chen, A. Kleinman and N.C. Ware (eds) *Health and Social Change in International Perspective*, Boston, MA: Harvard University Press, 25–49.

Gurven, M. and Kaplan, H. (2007) 'Longevity among Hunter-Gatherers: A Cross-Cultural Examination', *Population and Development Review*, 33(2): 321–365.

Heywood, P. and Lund-Adams, M. (1991) 'The Australian Food and Nutrition System: A Basis for Policy Formulation and Analysis', *Australian Journal of Public Health*, 15(4): 258–270.

Jackson, W.A. (1999) 'Dualism, Duality and the Complexity of Economic Institutions', *International Journal of Social Economics*, 26(4): 545–558.

Johns, G. (2011) *Aboriginal Self-Determination: The Whiteman's Dream*, Ballan, Victoria: Connor Court Publishing.

Kunitz, S.J. (1994) *Disease and Diversity: The European Impact on the Health of Non-Europeans*, New York: Oxford University Press.

Kunitz, S.J. and Brady, M. (1995) 'Health Care Policy for Aboriginal Australians: The Relevance of the American Indian Experience', *Australian Journal of Public Health*, 19(6): 549–558.

Lancaster, H.O. (1990) *Expectations of Life: A Study in the Demography, Statistics, and History of World Mortality*, New York: Springer-Verlag.

Langton, M. (2009) 'Foreward', in P. Sutton (ed.) *The Politics of Suffering: Indigenous Australia and the End of the Liberal Consensus*, Carlton, Victoria: Melbourne University Press, iii–vi.

Lewis, M.J. (2003a) *The People's Health*, Volume 1, *Public Health in Australia, 1788–1950*, Westport, CT: Praeger Press.

Lewis, M.J. (2003b) *The People's Health*, Volume 2, *Public Health in Australia, 1950 to the Present*, Westport, CT: Praeger Press.

Lewis, M.J. (2008) 'Public Health in Australia from the Nineteenth to the Twenty-First Century', in M.J. Lewis and K.L. MacPherson (eds) *Public Health in Asia and the Pacific: Historical and Comparative Perspectives*, 222–249.

Lunn, P. (1991) 'Nutrition, Immunity and Infection', in R. Schofield, D. Reher and A. Bideau (eds) *The Decline of Mortality in Europe*, Oxford: Clarendon Press, 131–145.

McCalman, J. (2009) 'Silent Witnesses: Child Health and Well-being in England and Australia and the Health Transition', *Health Sociology Review*, 18(1): 25–35.

McNeish, J.-A. and Eversole, R. (2005) 'Introduction: Indigenous Peoples and Poverty', in R. Eversole, J.-A. McNeish and A.D. Cimadore (eds) *Indigenous Peoples and Poverty: An International Perspective*, London: Zed Books, 1–26.

Marmot, M. (2006) 'Introduction,' in M. Marmot and R.G. Wilkinson (eds) *Social Determinants of Health*, Oxford: Oxford University Press, 1–5.

Moodie, P.M. (1981) 'Australian Aborigines', in H.C. Trowell and D.P. Burkitt (eds) *Western Diseases: Their Emergence and Prevention*, London: Edward Arnold, 154–167.

Najman, J.M. (2000) 'The Demography of Death: Patterns of Australian Mortality', in A. Kellehear (ed.) *Death and Dying in Australia*, South Melbourne: Oxford University Press, 17–37.

National Health and Hospitals Reform Commission (2008) *A Healthier Future for All Australians: Interim Report*, Canberra: Australian Government Printer.

National Health and Hospitals Reform Commission (2009) *A Healthier Future for All Australians: Final Report*, Canberra: Australian Government Printer.

Omran, A.R. (1971) 'The Epidemiologic Transition: A Theory of the Epidemiology of Population Change', *Milbank Memorial Fund Quarterly*, 49(4/1): 509–538.

Proust, A.J. (1991) 'The Waxing and Waning of Tuberculosis in Australia 1788 to 1988', in A.J. Proust (ed.) *History of Tuberculosis in Australia, New Zealand and Papua New Guinea*, Canberra: Brolga Press, 227–230.

Quiggan, P. (1988) *No Rising Generation: Women and Fertility in Late Nineteenth Century Australia*, Canberra: Department of Demography, Research School of Social Sciences, Australian National University.

Riley, J.C. (2001) *Rising Life Expectancy: A Global History*, Cambridge: Cambridge University Press.

Riley, J.C. (2008) *Low Income, Social Growth, and Good Health: A History of Twelve Countries*, Berkeley, CA: University of California Press and Milbank Memorial Fund.

Sen, A. (1999) *Development as Freedom*, Oxford: Oxford University Press.

Shergold, P. (1987) 'Prices and Consumption', in W. Vamplew (ed.) *Australians. Historical Statistics*, Broadway, NSW: Fairfax, Syme and Weldon Associates, 210–226.

Stanton, R. (2009) 'Who Will Take Responsibility for Obesity in Australia?' *Public Health*, 123(3): 280–282.

Sutton, P. (2009) *The Politics of Suffering: Indigenous Australia and the End of the Liberal Consensus*, Carlton, Victoria: Melbourne University Press.

Szreter, S. (2007) *Health and Wealth: Studies in History and Policy*, Rochester, NY: University of Rochester Press.

Taylor, R., Dobson, A. and Mirzaei, M. (2006) 'Contribution of Changes in Risk Factors to the Decline of Coronary Heart Disease Mortality in Australia over Three Decades', *European Journal of Cardiovascular Prevention and Rehabilitation*, 13(5): 760–768.

Taylor, R., Lewis, M. and Powles, J. (1998a) 'The Australian Mortality Decline: All-Cause Mortality 1788–1990', *Australian and New Zealand Journal of Public Health*, 22(1): 27–36.

Taylor, R., Lewis, M. and Powles, J. (1998b) 'The Australian Mortality Decline: Cause-Specific Mortality 1907–1990', *Australian and New Zealand Journal of Public Health*, 22(1): 37–44.

Teow, B.H., Wahlquist, M.L. and Flint, D.M. (1988) 'Food Patterns of Australians at the Turn of the Century', in A.S. Truswell and M.L. Wahlquist (eds) *Food Habits in Australia: Proceedings of the First Deakin/Sydney Universities Symposium on Australian Nutrition*, North Balwyn, Victoria: Gordon, 60–76.

Thomas, D.P. (2009) 'Smoking Prevalence Trends in Indigenous Australians, 1994–2004: A Typical Rather Than an Exceptional Epidemic', *International Journal for Equity in Health*, 8(37): 1–7.

Thomson, N. (2003) 'Responding to Our "Spectacular Failure"', in N. Thomson (ed.) *The Health of Indigenous Australians*, South Melbourne: Oxford University Press, 488–505.

Ventres, W.B. (2008) 'Review of James C. Riley, *Low Income, Social Growth, and Good Health. A History of Twelve Countries*, Berkeley: University of California Press', *JAMA*, 300(16): 1,943–1,944.

Walker, R. and Roberts, D. (1988) *From Scarcity to Surfeit: A History of Food and Nutrition in New South Wales*, Kensington, NSW: New South Wales University Press.

Webb, K. and Manderson, L. (1990) 'Food Habits and their Influence on Health', in J. Reid and P. Trompf (eds) *The Health of Immigrants in Australia: A Social Perspective*, Sydney: Harcourt, Brace, Jovanovich, 154–205.

*Weighing It Up – Report on Obesity in Australia*, House of Representatives Liaison and Projects Office, 2 June 2009. Online, available at: www.aph.gov.au/house/committee/haa/obesity/index.htm (accessed 30 January 2010).

# 3 Health transitions

## Hong Kong and China and the double disease burden

*Kerrie L. MacPherson*

## Introduction

Hong Kong, a British crown colony and free port since 1842, was returned to Chinese sovereignty in 1997. This marked the advent of the transitional period between the 'one country, two systems' political formula that guarantees the protection of Hong Kong's capitalist system and lifestyle for 50 years before China's 'socialist system and policies shall be practiced in Hong Kong' (Basic Law of the Hong Kong Special Administrative Region of the People's Republic of China, Article 5).

Hong Kong, with a population estimated to be (2011) 7.1 million people is a densely populated (6,540 persons per km$^2$) and highly urbanized territory measuring 1,104 km$^2$, will be integrated with a nation of 1.3 billion people, the largest nation in the world. Although Hong Kong and China share a human and ecological interdependence, they have diverged significantly since 1949 and the establishment of the People's Republic of China in their respective political, economic and social paths of development. Without comprehension of this political, social and economic reality, health status, health care structures and interventions, and their consequences cannot be properly understood. Health-related transitions (Frenk and Charon 1991), epidemiological (Omran 1971; Vallin and Meslé 2004)), demographic (Thompson 1929), nutritional and environmental, and the complex factors giving rise to them historically has generated considerable debate ranging from economic growth (Preston 1975), income disparities (Wilkinson 2005), urbanization (Harpham and Stephens 1991) and globalization (World Bank 1993; Woodward *et al.* 2001). Powerful as these imperatives are, governments confront serious administrative and ideological obstacles in tackling proximate and indirect causes of changes in population health. Inevitably these and other related issues shade into broad social questions that test the level of political competence necessary to deal with new obligations attendant to the economy of public health expenditure and their impact on the health of communities.

This chapter will examine the epidemiological, demographic, nutritional and environmental transitions in Hong Kong and China since the post Second World War period when high mortality from communicable diseases (CDs) was brought under control or eliminated and mortality and morbidity from chronic non-communicable diseases (NCDs) gained ascendancy. The approximate outline of these transitions can be identified in both China and Hong Kong in consonance with trends in both developed and developing countries, however, significant differences between Hong Kong and China as well as other countries in the world command further investigation. It is a story of uneven starting points as well as uneven political and societal adjustments to the challenges of advancing avowed public health agendas. Despite increasing resources, fiscal as well as medical and technological, responses to these transitions have highlighted the divergences in addressing the contingent consequences of these phenomena that have been linked to the rise of chronic diseases.

China has publicly admitted that it is faced with a double burden of disease, an acknowledgement that despite an epidemiological transition from CDs to NCDs, public health services and disease surveillance systems may be failing to adequately address either (Cook and Drummer, 2004). The environmental consequences to health, related to rapid and sustained economic growth fuelled by industrialization, are vital in understanding the protraction of the double disease burden when government engagement lags behind the recognition that environment and health are intimately interrelated (Wang *et al.* 2011).

Hong Kong has effectively controlled CDs and applied those historical lessons to the mitigation of NCDs. But it is faced with new or emerging infectious diseases such as SARS and H5N1 due to its position as an open global port city on the periphery of China. Historical differences in political, societal and health development aside, the regional environmental impact on public health and disease patterns continues to challenge Hong Kong's response to health questions that will in turn challenge its transition to integration with the mainland as a Chinese city.

## Pre-war and immediate post-war health in Hong Kong and China

The public's health as a political and societal responsibility was achieved in Hong Kong and China prior to the Second World War and rested on three legs: environmental hygiene and mechanisms to ensure its effectiveness; the transference of evolving modern (Western) public health care and delivery systems (as opposed to individual-based traditional and homeopathic medicine) dependent on epidemiological and biomedical tools to make significant downturns in and the control of infectious diseases as well as the identification of risk factors in the population; and sustained but modest economic growth. The confluence of these efforts was based on the establishment of civic institutions capable of advancing public health supported by increasing private and public initiatives and resources (MacPherson 1987). Epidemic or pandemic diseases with high mortality were an unrelenting feature of Hong Kong's and China's health profiles in the pre-war and immediate post-war period (MacPherson 1987; 2008).

As a benchmark it is worth reviewing briefly Hong Kong and China's health status and circumstances as of 1936, prior to the outbreak of the Greater East Asian War between Japan and China in 1937. Geographically, the colony consisted of: Hong Kong Island, ceded by China to Britain under the Treaty of Nanjing in 1842; Kowloon ceded in 1860; and the New Territories contiguous with Guangdong province leased in 1898 for 99 years – the trigger for opening negotiations for the return of Hong Kong in 1997. Hong Kong's population, to the best of pre-war statistics stood at 988,190 people, of whom 95 per cent were Chinese living primarily in the urban areas of Victoria City on Hong Kong Island and opposite the harbour in Kowloon. Approximately 100,000 people lived on boats and it was reckoned that 33 per cent of the population was born in Hong Kong. Population change was more dependent on in and out migration than on births and deaths and was directly affected by unstable political events in China as there was an average of more than 8,000 people arriving or departing daily (Medical and Sanitary Reports 1936: 4). Although registration of births and deaths was mandatory, enforcement was difficult and was only gradually implemented in the New Territories. Total registered births in the colony was 27,383 and the crude death rate was 27 per 1,000 population and the death rate for infants under one year of age stood at 372.42 a highly questionable figure since birth registration was easily evaded by the local population although the numbers of registered births doubled from 1932 to 1936. Children were sent back to China to live with relatives and the ill or dying often returned to their ancestral homes to expire.

There was also no systematic registration of sickness except for the returns relating to deaths and notifiable infectious diseases from the records of the government and other civil hospitals or clinics, and government-regulated Chinese charitable clinics and hospitals that offered traditional Chinese medicine (TCM) like the Tung Wah. From these sources it was estimated that respiratory diseases accounted for 39.7 per cent of all deaths, that is, broncho-pneumonia, pulmonary tuberculosis (TB), bronchitis and diarrhoea and infantile diarrhoea. Poverty and inadequate housing were noted in the medical report of that year as the causative factors. Cases of broncho-pneumonia may have been TB, as the death rate was 2.44 per 1,000 population and increasing rapidly creating a shortage of hospital beds for TB patients who accounted for over 30 per cent of all deaths and was Hong Kong's major health problem (Medical and Sanitary Reports 1936).

Advances to the sanitary infrastructure (including a potable water supply) were proceeding, though the bucket system for nightsoil removal still prevailed (and would still be used up until the early 1970s in some districts). The success of adequate drainage in the heavily populated areas of Victoria City (Hong Kong Island) and Kowloon across the harbour eradicated the incidence of malaria from the urban areas. Malaria was, however, rampant in the rural areas of the New Territories with a spleen rate of infection as high as 41 per cent of that population. Malaria was not a notifiable disease but the government Malaria Bureau was set up to control mosquito populations. Smallpox was a continual problem particularly spiking in the cold season and vaccination campaigns through the

Chinese public dispensaries and the St John's Ambulance services vaccinated over 274,784 people, mostly children, who were brought into the clinics after the lunar new year since spring was considered an auspicious date for vaccination. Plague had disappeared but an outbreak of Shiga dysentery occurred placing the milk supply under suspicion. To spread health information and to bring public health services out of the hospitals and to the public, the government created a scheme of district visits by public health nurses and travelling dispensaries visiting the villages three times a week in the rural areas.

The percentage of total deaths attributable to NCDs according to available statistics was low. Nephritis accounted for 3.69 per cent, heart disease for 3.02 per cent, followed by beriberi (a disease caused by nutritional deficiency), at 2.82 per cent. Funding for public health that included sanitary infrastructure, water supplies as well as medical services, accounted for 19.8 per cent of the total revenue of the colony. However, it should be noted that private sector and charitable medical provisions were not negligible, though not counted in the public record. From 1937 to 8 December 1941, when Japan invaded Hong Kong, the situation changed dramatically as a rapid influx of more than a half a million refugees from China strained the public health system. The Japanese ruthlessly forced one million people back to China, interned enemy nationals, appropriated civil and private hospitals, rationed medicines, systematically starved the remaining 600,000 people and neglected sanitary protocols all of which contributed to the outbreak of communicable and nutritional diseases (Selwyn-Clarke 1975: 101–103).

Immediately after the war, the government under emergency measures vigorously rehabilitated the colony; its infrastructure, water supplies and sanitation, food supplies, creating temporary or matshed housing and, particularly, its medical services. This was paramount since masses of refugees from China inundated the colony – over 1,760,000, many of whom were fleeing the civil war between the Nationalists and the Communists prior to the victory of the Communists and the establishment of the PRC on 1 October 1949 and the subsequent closing of the border. One unintended consequence was that many medical professionals, trained in foreign and nationalist government-funded medical schools in China, and now politically suspect for their 'imperialist' background, fled to Hong Kong where the government waived local medical registration requirements temporarily in order to meet the need for doctors.

China's health profile in 1936 bears some similarity to Hong Kong's in the cities and treaty ports like Shanghai opened to foreign trade and settlement since the introduction of western medicine and public health in the nineteenth century, but differed widely in the rural areas (where 90 per cent of the population lived) and the interior provinces. The establishment of the Republic in 1911 and the overthrow of the traditional dynastic system meant that modernization of the nation was key to creating a strong and independent nation and overturning the unequal treaties. Public health and medical modernization were viewed as essential to this state-building process of a nation of approximately 500 million people. With the nominal unification of the country by the Guomindang, the

National Health Administration was founded in 1936 to coordinate and rational-ize a patchwork of foreign, charitable and indigenous health care institutions, medical schools and medical standards, as well as expanding public health pro-vision and environmental hygiene throughout the nation (Yip 1995). Interna-tional cooperation in health was welcomed and China was an active member of the World Health Assembly of the League of Nations. State or socialized medi-cine was deemed necessary to redress a mortality rate thought to be four million people a year from infectious and parasitic diseases; an infant mortality rate in 1934 estimated to be nationally around 275 per 1,000 births; and a death rate of the overall population of 34 per 1,000 (Orleans 1972: 198). It is impossible with any precision at the national level to ascertain statistics of mortality and morbid-ity; however local, particularly urban statistics, showed that CDs, epidemic, pan-demic and endemic were rife (annual outbreaks of plague and cholera for example) and TB killed a reported 1.2 million people against an incidence of TB in excess of ten million people (Zhang and Elvin 1998: 523–533).

Increasing political threats from warlords in the north, communist agitation, Japanese invasion (a preliminary attack on Shanghai and invasion of Manchuria in 1931, the full-scale invasion in 1937), natural disasters such as the flooding in central China and the Yellow River (in 1931 and 1933) and famine, the attempt to grapple with competing claims of extraordinary circumstances and extraordinary epidemics with scarce resources challenged the government on all fronts (Wong and Wu 1936: 764–765). The Japanese occupied much of China from 1937–1945 with estimated casualties of up to 35 million people (*China Daily*, 15 August 2005). After the defeat of the Guomindang government and its withdrawal to Taiwan, and the establishment of the PRC, the diplomatically isolated communist regime was reliant on the former Soviet Union for expertise and aid to build the new China. This would help to guide the reorganization of the political economy and health care transformation until the Sino-Soviet split in 1959, and the Chinese path to socialism thereafter. Until the reforms in 1978–1979 and the 'opening up' of the economy, China diverged significantly from Hong Kong's path of develop-ment that arguably had an impact on health status.

## Hong Kong's epidemiological and demographic transition

In 1967–1968, for the first time since the founding of the colony, the leading cause of death was not from infectious, respiratory or intestinal diseases, but cancer, heart diseases and cerebrovascular lesions, diseases associated with an ageing population, despite the fact that 40 per cent of the population was under the age of 15 years and only 6 per cent over 60 years. The crude death rate dropped from 8.8 per 1,000 persons in 1949, to 5.1 per 1,000 in 1966–1967, and within the same time period the population more than doubled from 1,857,000 in 1949–1950 to 3,692,200 in 1966–1967. This was partly due to natural increase but more significantly from refugees fleeing the mainland. In the coming decades, fertility declined and longevity increased, a pattern associated with an epidemiological and demographic transition (MacPherson 2008: 20–24).

The principal reason for the epidemiological transition was the expansion of public health measures and infectious disease control. High priority was given to maternal and infant health services and the elimination of vaccine-preventable childhood diseases. Of signal importance, BCG vaccinations were given to all infants and small children to prevent TB in 1952 (the major cause of death in the pre-war period) a situation exacerbated after the war by the influx of refugees from China. Hong Kong was credited with pioneering supervised treatment (later known as directly observed treatment or DOT) to control TB. This was possible because of international cooperation in health and medical services and resources, and a public health policy remit 'to provide directly, or indirectly, low-cost or free medical and personal health services to that larger section of the community which is unable to seek medical attention from other sources' (Director of Medical and Health Services 1963–1964: 2). Modelled on the British National Health Service, this remit was deemed necessary since '50 per cent of the population was unable to afford unsubsidized outpatient treatment and 80 per cent unsubsidized hospital care' (Gauld and Gould 2002: 46). The government white paper, *The Development of Health Services in Hong Kong* (1964) laid out a ten-year plan for the expansion of hospitals and clinics including government subvented and charitable institutions. However, because 'the government did not have a differential charging policy, public health care services in effect became accessible to all Hong Kong residents regardless of income'. Subsequent economic growth, an increase in incomes and access to private sector health services proceeded, yet the subsidized health services 'policy has not been changed since 1974' (Liu and Yue 1998: 3).

Economic growth was predicated on the shift of Hong Kong's traditional role as a modest trading entrepôt with China before the war to a manufacturing and industrial base by geopolitical events: the end of the civil war between the Nationalists and the Communists and the establishment of the People's Republic of China in 1949, the Korean war and the trade embargo with China, the influx of refugees, including industrialists and their skilled workers from Shanghai and south China. However the masses of refugees, who were the bulk of the low-wage employees, created an unprecedented challenge to the existing health care system (such as the outbreaks of influenza in 1957 affecting 300,000 people, Cholera El Tor in 1961, and antibiotic-resistant TB), lack of housing provisions, education and welfare assistance. The situation became acute in the 1960s when social unrest (the riots of 1966–1967) in Hong Kong, encouraged by the radical policies of the Great Proletarian Cultural Revolution in China, elicited a social and economic policy shift of the colonial government. This may be summarized as a bifurcated public policy environment best exemplified by financial secretaries such as Sir John Cowperwaite (1961–1971) and his successors, who advocated for limited government, fiscal prudence, low tax regime and competitive free markets, and activist government by Governor Murray MacLehose (1971–1982) who recognized the need to invest in public-supported housing programmes (based on the British model) of New Towns development, transportation infrastructure, compulsory education, expansion to tertiary education (to invest in social mobility) and expanded welfare assistance to those in need, if social stability was to be maintained. The rule of law and the elimination of corruption in both the public and private sectors was targeted by the establishment of the Independent Commission Against Corruption (ICAC). Regardless of their philosophical differences, both policy frameworks adapted to local conditions had a direct impact on Hong Kong's health status.

According to World Bank analytical income categories (based on per capita income relative to GNP), Hong Kong grew from a lower middle income ranking in 1960 to a high income non-OECD world ranking by 1980. Thus, the demographic and epidemiological transition was coincident with economic growth and social and institutional policy changes, but arguably was preceded by medical and health care initiatives. Public medical and health care costs remained essentially the same as a percentage of total government expenditure (approximately 14.5 per cent) from the 1950s to the 1980s when a reevaluation of public health care structure and expenditures was impacted by the changing demographic and epidemiological profile. Hong Kong also transitioned from a manufacturing base to a high-end financial and services economy, no doubt helped by China's transition from a closed-door socialist command economy to a limited market economy with the reforms of 1978–1979, and the successful conclusion to the negotiations leading to the Sino-British Joint Declaration in 1984, the framework for the 'one country, two systems' policy delineating Hong Kong's reintegration with China.

## Hong Kong's NCD profile

Hong Kong's population of 7.1 million people has an estimated (2011) life expectancy at birth of 80 for men and 85.9 for women and ranks eighth in the world. The bulk of the population, 74.8 per cent, is between the ages of 15 and 64, while 13.5 per cent are over the age of 65 years and 11.6 per cent between the ages of zero and 14 years. The median age is 43.4, and 95 per cent of the population is Chinese. The birthrate is 7.49 per 1,000 of the population, below replacement rate, and the death rate is 7.07 per 1,000 population. Infant mortality is extremely low with 2.9 deaths per 1,000 live births. The decline in fertility is due to individual choice, not government policy as in China. Delayed marriage (average age of marriage for men in 2008 was 31.1 years and for women 28.8 years) and child-bearing, with 53 per cent of women in the workforce directly affect fertility rates (*The Standard*, 3 September 2010). Economic factors also play a role in fertility decline related to the rise in the standard of living and escalating costs, dense urbanization based on a limited land supply. Cramped living spaces play a role also since 90 per cent of the population live in flats less than $60\,m^2$.

The leading causes of age-standardized death are malignant neoplasms and diseases of the heart followed by pneumonia and cerebrovascular diseases. The four major preventable NCDs since 2006, account for 61 per cent of total registered deaths. It was estimated in 2006–2007, that 1,152,700 persons (16.7 per cent of the total population) suffered from chronic diseases; 48.9 per cent from hypertension, 20 per cent from type 2 diabetes and 11.7 per cent from heart diseases. Of that number, 58.8 per cent were 60 years or older. By 2031, government demographers expect that 25 per cent of the population will be 65 years or older. The demographic and epidemiological transition seems complete; however, the irreversible consequences of diminished ability that will affect an ageing population compromised by NCDs, will continue to call for medical ingenuity and a commitment to support quality of life outcomes.

### Cancer: the leading cause of death

There was no compulsory cancer notification system in Hong Kong until 1963 when the medical and health department began a voluntary reporting system. In 1964, cancer was the leading cause of death exceeding non-malignant diseases of the respiratory, circulatory and nervous systems as well as infectious and intestinal diseases. The increased incidence of cancer was attributed to a number of medical and non-medical factors: an ageing population, a decrease in the incidence of infectious, and non-malignant diseases due to major improvements in public health, improved diagnostic facilities and refined statistical surveillance, and the promotion of cancer awareness by health exhibitions held by the Kai-fongs (local mutual aid associations set up in 1949 to provide free or low-cost welfare, education and health services to refugees) and information disseminated by the Hong Kong Anti-cancer Society (Khoo 1965: 23). It was argued that early detection could cure one-third of patients diagnosed with cancer.

From 1983, when the Hong Kong Cancer Registry first computerized records, to 2007, the incidence of new cancers continued to rise by 2 per cent per annum and 60 per cent of all new cancers and 75 per cent of cancer deaths recorded were in people 60 years or older. In men the leading cancers are lung, colorectum, prostate, liver and nasopharynix, and in women, breast, colorectum, lung and liver cancers ('The Hong Kong Cancer Fund' 1993: 2,861–2,863).

The median age for diagnosis for all cancers today is 69 years for men (median age of mortality is 72 years) and 61 for women (median age of mortality at 74 years). However, age-standardized incidence consistently decreased for both genders with a downward trend in nasopharynx, oesophagus, stomach, lung and cervix and an increase in female breast, corpus ovary (33 per cent of cancers in women is gender-specific sites) and male colorectum and prostate cancers. These changes were partly attributed to socioeconomic and lifestyle factors and to technological changes in coding practices, the introduction and expansion of screening activities as well as general improvements in diagnostic procedures.

The leading cause of death in Hong Kong is lung cancer comprising 17.2 per cent of total cancer-related deaths. The incidence is highest among males aged over 50 years and the incidence ranks third for females. A downward trend has been observed primarily attributed to vigorous and continuous anti-smoking campaigns and legislation passed since the 1960s banning smoking on public transport and public institutions, increased taxation on tobacco products and semi-annual youth-targeted anti-smoking campaigns, more recently the 'I love a smoke-free Hong Kong' in 2005. Smoking-cessation services are provided by the Tobacco Control Office in the Department of Health and the Smoking Public Health Ordinance (Cap. 371) has fully come into effect in 2009 banning smoking in all public venues and public spaces. Daily smoking has dropped by 11.1 per cent in 2010, the lowest recorded in 30 years.

Nasopharyngeal and oesophageal carcinomas are of particular importance for Hong Kong and Asia generally. It was noted in the medical literature in China and in Hong Kong since the 1920s (Digby 1951: 254). In 1951, it ranked as the second most common cancer after cervical cancer and in 2007 ranks as the sixth cause of cancer mortality in males and females. Contributing factors for its occurrence in the Chinese population have ranged from opium smoking, charcoal burning in residences (no longer factors), drinking hot tea and soup, alcohol, salted fish, tobacco smoke and viruses (Digby 1951: 255–266). More recently, a 1992 study suggested that consumption of pickled vegetables with high concentrations of N-nitroso compounds was an attributable risk (Cheng *et al.* 1992: 1,317). The decrease in incidence therefore may be linked to changes in diet. In 2011, medical researchers at the University of Hong Kong and in Australia have found the Epstein Barr virus plays a role in nasopharyngeal carcinomas much like hepatitus B virus and liver cancer.

### Cancer and infectious diseases

The second leading cause of death in Hong Kong is cancer of the liver with 260,000 new cases reported annually (2007). The median age at diagnosis is 62 years for males and 72 years for females and mortality is 67 years and 75 years of age respectively.

Complicating the argument for an epidemiological transition was the relationship between CDs and NCDs that was not apparent from standard morbidity and mortality statistics or imprecise arguments that cancer was exclusively symptomatic as a disease of an ageing population. An aspect of the incidence of liver cancer was the fact that 47.7 per cent of the population had serologic markers of present or past infections for Hepatitis B virus (HBV) and that 80 per cent of hepato cellular carcinomas were attributable to HBV. Thus a major incidence of a CD (HBV) was responsible for a progression to a major incidence (and mortality) of an NCD (liver cancer) at around age 55–60 years plus and could only be prevented by vaccination of infants (with a persistent carrier state of 90 per cent). In 1983, the WHO consultative group on HBV made their recommendations for vaccinations and in Hong Kong resistance to universal vaccination of infants was predicated on financial grounds as well as safety concerns over a vaccine derived from human derived blood products that was triggered by the emergence of HIV/AIDS first notified in Hong Kong in 1984 (Yeoh 1986: 155–156). Dr E.K. Yeoh (later to become the first chief executive of the Hospital Authority in 1990 and Secretary of Health, Welfare and Food and at the forefront of the SARS epidemic in 1997) put it bluntly: 'By withholding vaccination from these infants and permitting them to be infected one is sentencing them to the cruel fate and anguish of waiting for a "liver death"' (Yeoh 1984: 19). When yeast-derived recombinant HBV vaccines became available, resistance evaporated and in 1986 infant vaccination at birth commenced and in the past two decades a decrease in incidence of HBV was recorded. Vaccination campaigns targeting the unexposed continue annually (Centre for Health Protection 2011).

The age-standardized incidence of cervical cancer in Hong Kong in 2010 is 9.7 per cent higher than the developed countries of the west and Australia particularly in older and poorer women and Hong Kong ranks second after the European Union in age-standardized mortality rates. The human papillonomavirus (HPV) is now considered 'as a necessary but not sole factor in cervical cancer' (Surveillance and Epidemiological Branch, Centre for Health Protection 2004: 9). In 2004, the government launched a surveillance and screening programme since 'most women who develop cervical cancer are not screened' (Surveillance and Epidemiological Branch, Centre for Health Protection 2004: ix). The death of popular singer and actress Anita Mui at age 40 in 2004 from cervical cancer and her public announcement of her condition in 2003 helped to bring the focus on timely screening for the general population. Prevention, as in HBV infections, is seen as the first line of defence in defeating the progression to cervical and liver cancers.

### *Heart disease, hypertension and cardiovascular disease*

Coronary heart disease (CHD) ranks as the second highest cause of death in Hong Kong after cancer since the 1960s, and accounts for 10 per cent of all deaths, though the death rate is lower than in most developed countries and in neighbouring Singapore. Risk factors, as expected, are high blood pressure, cholesterol, body mass index (BMI), smoking and diabetes. The mortality rate in the age group of 25–84 years decreased from 1989 to 2001. Dietary and fat consumption intake was found to be at recommended levels and the BMI of women decreased during this period, no doubt due to social pressures. Seventy-eight per cent of CHD mortality reduction from 1989 to 2001 was attributed to improved treatments, and 28 per cent was attributed to changes in population risk factors, for example decline in tobacco use after the 1970s (McGhee *et al.* 2009: 24–25). In 2009, an increase in CHD was noted in both male and female age-standardized death rates due to an ageing population, but also to stress. Stress, and the management of stress, has come under increased medical scrutiny due to several surveys that noted the high-pressured work environment as a contributing factor in developing CHD as well as a survey showing that 41.3 per cent of students admitted to having suicidal thoughts because of familial pressure to achieve scholastically to improve their families' socioeconomic position (Fu *et al.* 2004: 64; Fu and Hao 2003: 30).

The incidence of cerebrovascular disease (CVD) has remained steady as the fourth leading cause of death from 1981 to 2009 and comprised 8 per cent of all registered deaths in 2010. The age-standardized death rate due to CVD has dropped by more than half in the past two decades, but has increased in 2009 in persons aged over 60 years (Centre for Health Protection 2012). In 1998, the government launched the Elderly Health Service establishing 18 centres and 18 visiting health teams covering all districts to provide primary health care and healthy lifestyle promotions for the elderly. However, one troubling statistic is that 1.1 per cent of people aged 15 years and above had doctor-diagnosed CVD.

A 2003–2004 population health survey found that the prevalence of hypertension, an important risk factor for CVD and CHD, was 27.2 per cent of people aged 15 years and older, 5.2 per cent aged 15–24 years and 73.3 per cent aged 75 and above. The study revealed that 'less than two-thirds (62.9 per cent) of the people had their blood pressure checked by health professionals in the past five years' (Centre for Health Protection 2007). Of concern was the fact that the incidence of hypertension in people aged 25–34 years had doubled from 1999–2001. A survey of private doctors found that blood pressure tests were not routine (as many patients were asymptomatic) and the report urged private doctors to educate their patients on the risks of uncontrolled high blood pressure and how the condition could be managed not just by medication but by lifestyle changes in diet and exercise (Chan *et al.* 2006, 115–118). In 2008, to broad public support for proposals to improve primary care identified in the Healthcare Reform Consultation document, 'Your Health, Your Life', four task forces were established to address chronic diseases. In 2010, the *Hong Kong Reference Framework for Hypertension Care for Adults in Primary Care Settings* was published, the result of a collaborative effort of the Department of Health, the Food and Health bureau, the Hospital Authority, medical professionals and associations and university medical departments to revise standards of management and treatment reflecting changes in the population health profile.

### *Type 2 diabetes, metabolic syndrome and obesity*

Complex as environmental and genetic conditions are to the identification of determinants in a specific population for the development of metabolic syndrome and type 2 diabetes, age, family history and obesity were three identifiable factors in their development in Hong Kong (Chan *et al.* 2005: 51). Familial clustering and parental effect, particularly if the mother was diabetic (the impact of the intrauterine environment) was found to be significant and may account for an earlier age of onset (Lee *et al.* 2000: 1365–1368). It was noted that there was 'an alarmingly high prevalence of diabetic nephropathy' and that '30 per cent of patients admitted with stroke, heart failure, acute myocardial infarction or requiring renal dialysis have diabetes' (Chan *et al.* 2005: 51–52).

In Hong Kong, type 2 diabetes is the tenth cause of death accounting for 1.2 per cent of all deaths in 2009. An increase in age-standardized mortality rate was recorded from the early 1980s to 2000, and then it decreased slightly in 2001. A 2003–2004 population health survey found that 3.8 per cent of people aged 15 years and older reported that they had doctor-diagnosed diabetes (Centre for Health Protection 2007). Type 2 diabetes accounts for 97 per cent of all diabetes patients. The costs of care and treatment for diabetes patients consumed up to 3.9 per cent of the total health care budget in 2004 and 6.4 per cent of the Hospital Authority public sector expenditure on health (Chan *et al.* 2007: 455–468).

The second framework on diabetes arising from the Healthcare Reform Consultation document was published in 2010. Nevertheless, the private sector has made significant contributions to awareness, prevention and social support of diabetics. Diabetes Hong Kong, a charitable voluntary association was founded in 1996 to provide information, social and medical support for diabetics and their families, to encourage research and safeguard standards of care, and to liaise with national and international diabetes associations.

Metabolic syndrome (MES), that is, the assemblage of risk factors such as hypertension, high cholesterol, incipient diabetes, raised fasting blood plasma glucose, abdominal obesity leading to increased incidence of CVD and type 2 diabetes measured by the International Diabetes Federation (IDF) revised standards (2005) and the WHO revised BMI (body mass index) standards for Asian populations, has shown a threefold increase in Hong Kong Chinese from 1990 to 2000. In a 2001–2002 survey conducted by the United Christian Nethersole Service primary health care programme, the incidence of MES was 16 per cent in males and 13.4 per cent in females (Ko and Tang 2007: 1,115). An increased risk from MES was significant in males under 50 years of age and over 50 years in women, though a drop in rates of obesity (1.2 per cent) in women from 2004 to 2010 was encouraging. A comparison of studies done in the 1990s and 2002 of the working population showed a dramatic increase in central obesity in men from 12 to 27 per cent, whilst remaining fairly static for women (Ko 2010: 10). Obesity and related conditions were estimated to cost HK$3.36 billion annually in hospitalization costs or 8.2 to 9.8 per cent of the total public expenditure on health (Ko 2008: 74). The most worrisome statistic is the increase in obesity in children, from 16.7 per cent in 1996–1997 to 22.2 per cent in 2008–2009. An editorial in a local paper opined, '[T]he average flat has a tiny kitchen, which means many of us favour restaurants for meals. Tight public spaces and a low number of sporting and recreation facilities make exercising a challenging prospect'. The editorial also revealed that despite government focus on the 'fight against obesity', the 'Eat Smart' programme by government has only garnered 60 per cent of primary school participation and the youngest 'whom we are prone to spoiling, are most vulnerable' (*South China Morning Post*, 25 October 2010). Sedentary lifestyles, desk jobs requiring long working and study hours (to achieve academic excellence), lack of sleep, computers and television as major recreational activities, stress and lack of sleep, junk or processed food (Chinese, Japanese and Southeast Asian and western), all make contributions to an increase in BMI in both adults and children, an indicator of future risk for developing chronic diseases (Chan 2008: 87–90; Ko *et al.* 2007: 254–260; Centre for Health Protection 2005).

## Health care policy and funding

Health care financing has essentially remained unchanged since the 1950s, though health care policy has undergone a notable modification in recent decades reflecting changed priorities with the epidemiological and demographic changes and the rise of NCDs, the decrease in CDs, an ageing population and refined assessments of both policy and financing projections to meet future needs. As early as 1964, the director of medical and health services sparked a debate over acute, subsidiary and chronic or convalescent beds noting that a reorganization based on need and cost rationalization should be pursued (*Hong Kong Hansard*, 26 February 1964). There was recognition that despite epidemics of cholera or influenza that continued to plague the territory, an epidemiological shift was occurring.

Hong Kong has 41 public hospitals, 122 outpatient clinics and 13 private hospitals. Outpatient or primary care in the private sector in 2000–2001, accounts for 70 per cent of all these services with 15 per cent in the public sector at a subsidized rate, and the remaining 15 per cent of outpatient consultations provided by TCM practitioners. The 'two pillars' (public and private) of Hong Kong's overall health care financing was HK$39.1 billion in the tax-supported or public sector and 28.4 billion in the private sector. Specialist, tertiary and inpatient care is mostly delivered through the public sector. In 1990, the Hospital Authority (HA) was established to rationalize and coordinate hospital medical care, and 90 per cent of all hospital beds are managed by the HA. In 1997 (the year of the handover), the government commissioned a study from the School of Public Health, Harvard University, to make recommendations about reforming the system. One of the recommendations was compulsory health insurance which was roundly rejected by the majority of the public surveyed. The government in 2000, tried again with proposing a medical savings programme (with reference to Singapore and other Asian neighbours), but public consultation showed negative public support for the proposal (Bauhinia Foundation Research Centre Health Care Study Group 2007: 1–8).

Ultimately, to look forward to sustaining Hong Kong's health care system costs, a government-run medical insurance scheme has been floated in 2011, to public consultation and review. This modification to health care funding is in recognition of the demographic and epidemiological transition, without jeopardizing the low income subsidy that currently exists. What is important here is that any change to the existing system has to be vetted publicly taking into consideration the needs of the community (*South China Morning Post*, 9 July 2022).

## China's epidemiological and demographic transition

After the founding of the PRC in 1949, the reorganization of the political economy into a state-directed central planning regime included adopting the Soviet-style medical research and health care system to ration care and reduce inequalities. Health care was heavily subsidized by insurance schemes covering workers in state-owned enterprises and rural collectives, students, soldiers and government employees. Population mobility was strictly limited by workplace (*danwei*) and household (*hukou*) registration. Traditional Chinese medicine was integrated with 'western' or modern medicine. Foreign-funded or directed medical institutions were nationalized, and their personnel expelled and private practice was discouraged. A three-tiered hierarchical system was instituted where primary care was provided in the townships and rural communes and increasingly sophisticated services provided at higher administrative levels. Mass 'patriotic' health campaigns were launched to eradicate endemic, epidemic and parasitic diseases, and paramedical personnel (the barefoot doctors) were deployed to carry out vaccinations (including BCG shots for infants since an estimated 15 million people were TB patients and it was still the first cause of mortality in 1958), provide birth control, as well as environmental hygiene and pest control (Dimond 1971: 1555; Rifkin 1972: 143; Huang 1972: 240).

In 1949, life expectancy was reckoned to be around 35–50 years of age (depending on the source), approximately the same as Hong Kong's in the pre-war period. The first national census conducted in 1953, was flawed but it should be noted that demographic statistics were primarily used to implement the socialist and command economic reorganization or 'evenization' of society and a nation of 582.6 million people. However, the census did prompt a debate over China's fertility and the possible adverse effects on economic development. In 1957, the leadership promoted contraception and made sterilization legal, a policy that was downplayed in 1958, due to the labour demands of the 'Great Leap Forward' campaign of forced industrialization to surpass the west and collectivization of agriculture to serve that purpose (Orleans 1972: 198–200). The 'Great Leap Forward' proved to be catastrophic; coupled with natural disasters, an estimated 30 million or more people died from starvation in the 'three bitter years' (1958–1961) with a breakdown of public health measures. Yet, it was claimed in 1959, that because of the new health measures, infectious and parasitic diseases were 'brought under control' and preventive medicine was 'carried out with most satisfactory results' (Yeh and Chow 1972: 212). However, other data suggested that despite control schemes, TB mortality, the incidence of trachoma (ranked first in prevalence) and parasitic diseases, affected 280 million people or one of every two or three persons some with multiple infections in 1959. Schistosomiasis, endemic in a $7,770 \, km^2$ area south of the Huai river, affected ten million people. Evidence showed a link between infections and the later onset of colonic cancer (Huang 1972: 247, 257).

The shift in policies in 1962, to allow some privatization gave incentives to farmers to increase the food supply but ideological purity was back on the agenda when Mao Zedong faced challenges to his political authority and launched the 'Great Proletarian Cultural Revolution' in 1966, constituting the 'ten lost years' that directly affected medical and health care by closing medical schools, and reopening them in 1970, by abolishing examinations and diplomas, demoting medical professionals to non-medical personnel (committees of workers, peasants and soldiers) to run the hospitals and clinics, and supporting class warfare ('Red Guards' circulated the country by the millions funded by the State) all of which disrupted health care provisions including basic epidemiological statistics (Reynolds and Tierney 2004: 2141). In 1971, it was becoming apparent that China was beginning to suffer from a 'double disease burden'. The first American physician invited with several colleagues to visit China in 25 years noted that: 'Cancer is a major dread, and there is an increased incidence in the nasal passages, esophagus, and liver. Rheumatic fever is more common than in the United States; coronary heart disease and hypertension are quite common' (Dimond 1971: 1557).

In 1975, the 'four modernizations' (agriculture, industry, science and technology) were promulgated (Mao would die in 1976) to reverse the radical policies of the past decade. Medical examinations and remedial medical education were reconstituted and the reforms of 1978–1979 and China's 'opening up to the outside world' meant key policy changes to the socialist system, economic liberalization by the dismantling of the state-owned enterprises (a slow process but not to the central-level units), collective farms and their welfare provisions, fiscal decentralization and limited free market principles, allowance of private medical provision and fee-for-service and cost recovery in the public sector hospitals and clinics (with the exception of strategic and military medical services), all benchmarked against international standards (MacPherson 2008: 35–36). The reforms accelerated economic growth which averaged 9.5 per cent a year from 1978 to 2005 and China rose from a lower income ranking according to the World Bank analytical income categories to an upper middle income ranking of GNP per capita (World Bank 2011).

China's epidemiological and demographic transition appears to have begun in 1975 when life expectancy at birth was estimated to be nearly 70 years of age, due to the control of infectious diseases and conditions affecting maternal and prenatal health though there was wide variation between urbanized and rural regions. From 1990–2008, the rise in life expectancy slowed, due to changes in morbidity and mortality when CDs accounted for 27.8 per cent of all deaths in 1975 to 5.2 per cent in 2005 and NCDs (cerebrovascular, chronic obstructive pulmonary and cancers) rose to 74.1 per cent of all deaths from 41.7 per cent recorded in 1973. Rural western provinces, the most underdeveloped compared to the more urbanized coastal provinces have a higher incidence of CDs, and oesophageal and cervical cancers and injuries (Yang *et al.* 2008: 1,697). The demographic change was also related to fertility and national campaigns to promote birth control in 1972 (and delayed marriage), with minatory results. Strict birth control enforcement (including forced abortions) undergird the 'one-child policy' in the 1980s due to the rapid rise in births in the rural areas a by-product of economic liberalization (Scharping 2002: 29–80). The infant mortality rate decreased significantly from the 1970s; however, data show that in 1990, infant mortality for females was higher than males nationally; 33.71 per 1,000 live births compared to 29 per 1,000 for males. This sex ratio discrepancy was higher in rural areas than urban and 'likely accounted for' by 'unreliable data, female infanticide and abandonment, and unequal treatment of male and female infants' as well as sex-selected abortions (Xu *et al.* 1994: 242; Bannister 2004: 19–45).

## China's NCD profile

The 2011 (estimated) life expectancy at birth is 72.68 years for males and 76.94 years for females with 17.6 per cent of the population aged 1–14 years, 73.6 per cent aged 15–65 years and 8.9 per cent over 65 years. The median age is 35.5 years. The birthrate has dropped precipitously to 12.9 per 1,000 population as did the infant mortality rate of 16.06 per 1,000 live births. The death rate is 7.03 per 100,000 population and health care expenditure accounts for 4.6 per cent of GDP (2009) an annual change of 2.3 per cent (World Bank 2011). The population is rapidly ageing and the aged may reach 240 million or 17 per cent of the population by 2020.

NCDs account for 83 per cent of the 10.3 per cent of all recorded deaths from diseases annually and NCD mortality exceeds that of all G-20 countries. The main NCDs are CVDs, type 2 diabetes, chronic obstructive pulmonary diseases and lung cancer, all of which are expected to 'double or even triple over the next two decades, most of it during the next 10 years' in people over 40 years of age. As alarming as these statistics are, in 2011, 50 per cent of China's NCD burden already affected almost 50 per cent of the population under 65 years. In 2010, it was estimated that 580 million people 'had at least one modifiable NCD-related risk factor' and of that group, '70–85% were under the age of 65' (Wang *et al.* 2011: 1–3).

Rapid economic growth has meant an improvement to the general health of the population due to infectious diseases control and increased and improved nutrition; however, changes in diet such as increased salt and fat consumption with a corresponding decrease in the consumption of fruits and vegetables is having an impact on rates of hypertension and obesity. Rapid and sustained urbanization with an estimated 900 million people or 60 per cent of the total population living in cities by 2030, with corresponding lifestyle changes and exposure to environmental pollutants from the increase in motor vehicles, coal-burning power plants, manufacturing and industrial emissions (and an unreliable regulatory regime) are associated with more than 300,000 deaths and 20 million cases of respiratory illness from outdoor air pollution particularly detrimental to children's health and development (Millman *et al.* 2008: 620).

### Cancer

Prior to the founding of the PRC, the Chinese Medical Association urged the League of Nations in 1929, to create a special commission to investigate the prevalence and distribution of malignant neoplasms in China and its neighbours. In 1932, the Rockefeller-funded Peking Medical College opened its first tumour clinic and in 1935 conducted a survey of tumour incidence in hospital patients, the main source of epidemiological information before the founding of the PRC and the first national mortality survey in the 1970s. Cancer research was clearly emphasized in the 1956 national 12-year plan for scientific development and a national cancer conference was held in Tianjin in 1959, followed by conferences on specific cancers in 1960 (when Chinese scientists visited the USSR to learn from their cancer research programmes), and in 1964, a conference coinciding with the establishment of the Huanan cancer hospital in Guangzhou (King 1972: 264). Tumour registries were kept in cities like Shanghai and showed that in 1965, that cancer of the nasopharynx was 'the eighth most frequent malignancy in that region' (Yeh and Chow 1972: 226).

The incidence of cancer is complicated by the lack of national data but the results of three national morbidity surveys, in the 1970s, 1990 and 2006–2008 indicated that cancer ranked first in causes of mortality accounting for 27 per cent of all deaths in rural areas and 25 per cent in cities. The risk factors cited are the usual suspects – an ageing population, environmental degradation and a 'western lifestyle' (Zhao *et al.* 2010: 281). In 2009, the crude incidence of cancers in descending order of magnitude were of lung, stomach, liver, oesophagus, breast, colon, rectum, pancreas, bladder and leukaemia all showing a marked increase from decades earlier. A decrease was recorded in cervix uteri (the eighth most common cancer in women) in urban areas due to better access to medical facilities and ability to pay but not in rural regions or in central or western provinces where mortality was highest. The Ministry of Health and the All China's Women's Federation in conjunction with the WHO, launched a programme in 2009 to provide free cervical cancer screening for rural women aged 35–59 years. However, there is no access to HPV vaccine as yet which would be an important preventive measure (Li *et al.* 2011: 1152–1153). The first National Cancer Control Plan was inaugurated in 1986 and extended and refined in 2004 to improve quality of care and survival rates of cancer patients as well as to reduce the incidence and mortality of cancer. Several non-governmental organizations have been established recently, the China Anti-cancer Association and the Cancer Foundation of China, to promote cancer awareness and cancer prevention along the lines of similar organizations in Hong Kong and elsewhere (Ping *et al.* 2010: 283).

Lung cancer according to one study increased by 465 per cent over a 30-year period and was estimated by the WHO that one million people will be diagnosed with lung cancer annually by 2025, much of it attributed to smoking (Zhao *et al.* 2010: 281). Although China has signed the WHO Framework Convention on Tobacco Control, 28 per cent of the population smokes (301 million people) and control is hampered because the ministry that sells tobacco also oversees the implementation of the anti-tobacco treaty. The deputy director of the National Tobacco Control Office, Yang Gonghuan, stated: 'It's like a bunch of foxes in the chicken coop discussing how to protect the chickens'. The state-owned industry (China National Tobacco Corporation) generated 100 billion yuan in 1980 from taxes and profits rising to 513.1 billion yuan in 2009 though direct medical costs, and indirect costs – losses to years of life and productivity – mean that the 'net contribution of tobacco to China's economy is about minus 20 percent' (*Xinhua*, 2 June 2010). The rise in consumption of tobacco, illness and death attributable to that consumption, and revenues accruing to the state, coincided with changes in health care financing since the reforms of 1978–1979, when state subsidization of individual medical costs through state-owned enterprises and other state proxies was widely replaced by private insurance or out-of-pocket payments. The planned return to a national insurance scheme means that the costs will be generalized throughout the population.

*Liver cancer*

The relationship between liver cancer and environmental factors and infectious diseases is well documented. Cirrhosis was linked to polluted water sources, as well as parasitic infestations and nutritional deficiencies (Lin *et al.* 2000: 572; Yeh and Chow 1972: 226–227). But more substantial is the link between HBV infections and its prevalence with the later onset of liver cancer which kills 260 to 280,000 people more than TB mortality of 201,000 (WHO 2009). The PRC has the dubious distinction of having the 'greatest burden of chronic HBV infection in the world with a greater than 8% hepatitis B surface antigen (HBsAg) seroprevalence in a population of 1.3 billion people' more worrying is that '[V] ertical transmission at childbirth is the predominant route of chronic infection' (Chao *et al.* 2010: 1–2). The lack of knowledge about sterilization and the reusing of needles (including acupuncture needles) by undertrained 'barefoot doctors' may have contributed to the spread of HBV throughout the population. In 1992, a government programme was launched to provide HBV vaccinations to infants but the high costs discouraged compliance by the poor. In 2002, the vaccinations were given free to infants but this has not made significant inroads in reducing the rate of HBV infections and continues to expose a lack of knowledge about the infection amongst the general population and health care providers. Stigma associated with HBV infection has also played a role for persons who may have otherwise sought medical help since their HBV status was relayed to employers or schools by medical personnel. In 2007, the Ministry of Health and the Ministry of Human Resources and Social Security issued a directive that a person who was reported to have HBV infection or carrier status could not be denied employment or dismissal of employment because of HBV status (Chao *et al.* 2010: 9–10; Ping *et al.* 2010: 284).

*Cancer and the environment*

China has recognized the link between the increase in cancer incidence and the continued pollution of the environment, though there is still a division in practice between health concerns and environmental control faced with the rapid industrialization that has developed over the past 30 years. This is related to chemical and industrial pollution, lack of sewerage and enforcement of environmental regulations. The World Bank estimated that 750,000 people die prematurely annually from pollution of the land, water and air (Watts

2008: 1451–1452). *Aizheng cun* (cancer villages), that is, villages that have clusters of cancer deaths above the norm due to industrial pollution, began to emerge in the 1980s when industrialization was spurred by the economic reforms. These villages are mostly located in 11 middle and eastern provinces located on river systems. Although these villages have been reported in the press, there has been little formal government recognition of the long-term consequences of heavy metal exposure on the population. For example, in Hunan province the Liuyang river was used as a dump for toxic waste by a chemical company producing indium and people were exposed to heavy metal contamination leading to illness and death, and poisoning of the agricultural fields and irrigation water (*South China Morning Post*, 24 May 2011). Ironically, a solar manufacturing plant, part of the 'clean' energy solution, Jinko Solar Holding, was taken to task by local people in Haining, Zhejiang, for polluting their environment by their manufacturing processes (*Guardian*, 18 September 2011). Protests have escalated against polluting industries and the lack of government enforcement of environmental regulations affecting the air, water, land and food safety. Air pollution also affects Hong Kong because of the location of factories in the Pearl river delta (ironically, many owned by Hong Kong people) and the prevailing winds (MacPherson 2008: 42–45).

### *Heart disease, hypertension and cardiovascular disease*

'The profile of CVD among Chinese is much different from Caucasians … the incidence and mortality rates of cardiovascular disease were much higher than those of CHD in Chinese populations' (Ji *et al.* 2011: 1). The 'classical' risk factors are hypertension, smoking, overweight, hypercholesterolemia and age (the rate is higher in males than females and is related to the disparity in tobacco use). Heart disease was ranked first as the leading cause of death in 2009, killing 2.6 million people or '300 people on average every hour' with an annual cost of US$16 billion annually (Wang 2009). Mortality rates from stroke, for example, are four to six times higher than Japan, USA or France (Wang *et al.* 2011: 3). Hypertension, attributed to high salt intake and also simply a 'lack of awareness of the condition and one study indicates that doctors do not routinely give blood pressure checks' (Yang *et al.* 2008: 1,701). It is interesting to note, besides the fact that 24 per cent of people are unaware of the condition, that 'the percentages of those with hypertension that are aware, treated and controlled are unacceptably low'. Several factors are significant: many are unaware of the condition or the implications to their health from high blood pressure; many do not consider 'hypertension as a life-threatening disease but a life-long burden, so they would rather deal with it as late as possible'; 'many Chinese people believe that western medicines for hypertension are partially poisonous'; many feel once taking medication and symptoms recede that they are 'cured'; and, finally, medicines are costly and there is distrust of the medical profession because of government involvement in setting costs (Li and Wang 2010: 8241–8242).

## Type 2 diabetes, metabolic syndrome and obesity

Various surveys conducted in the 1980s, 1990 and 2000–2001 found a rising incidence of diabetes in the population. However, a large-scale study conducted from 2007–2008, showed a veritable epidemic of diabetes and pre-diabetes, a major risk factor for cardiovascular disease now China's highest cause of death. Diabetes affects 92.4 million adults (aged 20 years and older), 50.2 million are men and 42.2 million are women, and 60.7 per cent were undiagnosed with the disease. A further 148.2 million people were diagnosed with pre-diabetes (Yang *et al.* 2010: 1,090). The study confirmed that both socioeconomic status and metabolic risk factors, such as rising incomes, urban residence and lifestyle, lower educational level, diet, tobacco use, lack of physical activity, obesity (including central obesity), high blood pressure and insulin resistance, high cholesterol, family history of the disease, male gender and ageing were all associated with higher incidence of the disease. Other studies focusing on specific regions show similar results; a study conducted in southern China showed that MES was more prevalent in urbanized areas than rural, however, they found that females had at least one component of MES, recommending that only a 'population level strategy for prevention, detection and treatment of cardiovascular risk' would help to fight the epidemic (Lao *et al.* 2012). Other studies show that 'semi-urban' areas (this is difficult to factor since many cities include large suburban and rural hinterlands in their administrative statistical areas) are following the trend of the urban cores. Diabetes has also been shown to have a higher prevalence in people with liver disease, both serious but mostly preventive conditions (Hsieh and Hsieh 2011: 5,240–5,245).

Overweight and obesity, using Asian metrics, has increased by 39 per cent from 1992–2002, and in the largest cities 13 per cent of children aged 7–17 years were overweight. Caloric intake remained essentially the same from 1982–2002, and a study suggested that decreased physical activity, no doubt due to similar factors as in Hong Kong such as long study hours, computer use and television, lack of recreational facilities in the densely populated cities, helps to explain the rise in obesity in the young (Yang *et al.* 2008: 1701). What is clear, is that urban centres like Beijing or Shanghai, with growing affluence and food choices including western and Chinese fast food or heavily processed foods are facing the same challenges as Hong Kong (decades earlier) to cope with expanding waistlines (French and Crabbe 2010). Rural China, with a much larger population has lower rates of obesity partly because of limited 'access to and variety of foods'; a 'one country, but two eating systems' that has moderated the extent of the problem, though this may change dramatically in the coming years (*South China Morning Post*, 25 October 2010). According to a 2009 City Development Report, 50 per cent of the population will be living in cities and this will rise to 75 per cent by 2050, not counting peri-urban areas that will have a continuing impact on lifestyles, food choice and activity levels (*China Daily*, 12 May 2010). The problem is complex because of the legacy of the past, that is, starvation, malnutrition, micronutrient deficiencies and food hygiene and safety that were the goals of the national plan of action for nutrition in the 1990s. The challenges going forward include enhancing the previous action plan by addressing dietary patterns and lifestyle behaviour related to NCDs and issuing regulations to enhance quality control and consumer education through food labelling, not by reduction in food variety (Li 2010: 1–28).

## Health care policy and funding

The health care system and funding dramatically changed with the reforms of 1978–1979, from a state-controlled system of workplace, rural-collective based, welfare system (including old-age pensions, housing, workman's compensation, maternity and medical care) to a health insurance scheme jointly funded by employer and employee with socially pooled funds and personal medical accounts by the 1990s. The seventh five-year plan (1986–1991) devolved the state sector to provincial and local authorities to be funded through taxation, allowed for the legalization of private medical practice, the establishment of private hospitals and a reform of the state-controlled 'medicine production and circulation system'; a commitment to 'multiple forms' of health services. This policy was to help alleviate the fiscal burden on the state, to lower medical costs and inefficiencies, and allow for greater equity in the health system (Wong *et al.* 2006: 15–17). With the decollectivization of the countryside, revisions were made to the rural cooperative health care system, now supported or guided by the government, but devolved to the local level and individuals could opt to join on a fee-paying basis. Thus, 'China has a bifurcated health care system, namely, the urban and rural subsystems' (Wong *et al.* 2006: 11).

Counterintuitive as it is, China's rapid economic growth and rise in per capita income since the reforms of 1978–1979, has not translated well into better quality of health care, more equitable health care outcomes or increased public investment in the health care sector as might be expected, but seems to have followed socio-economic gradients, that also divide between rural versus urban residence and less developed and developed regions or provinces (Beijing, Shanghai and Guangzhou for example are large urban agglomerations that include rural population and rank as provinces administratively). Although overall life expectancy has increased dramatically since 1949, life expectancy continues to vary considerably between more affluent urban residents (Shanghai's life expectancy was 78 years) and poorer, more rural provinces (65 years) – a gap of 13 years. The same holds true for infant mortality rates, which show a fivefold disparity (Tang *et al.* 2008: 1494). Partly, this reflects the historical division and transitional process between the reforms of the rural and urban health care systems. Another aspect of economic reforms and development was the relaxation of the *hukou* system and the movement of large numbers of migrants to the urban areas to find jobs – over 220 million, or who have traded their land use rights for urban residence, thus losing their household welfare, educational, health care, housing and pension benefits and are often treated as 'second-class citizens' in the areas they migrate to. High costs of medical treatment deter them from seeking medical assistance (Watson 2009: 89).

The reforms as they developed have dramatically decreased the central government's spending on the health system relative to GNP and have escalated out-of-pocket payments, as hospitals and pharmacies, whether public or private, sought profits by raising fees to offset operational costs. It also affected other basic public health parameters such as environmental hygiene, clean water supplies, infectious disease control (an upsurge in STDs, antibiotic resistant TB, emerging and re-emerging diseases such as HIV, avian influenza, swine flu and SARS for example) and accurate surveillance and reporting. The regulatory and legal regimes have come under scrutiny due to the counterfeiting of drugs, both TCM remedies and cancer treatment drugs like Herceptin. Investigations 'exposing more than a thousand counterfeiting dens' producing US$315 million dollars in fake drugs were completed in 2011 (*Xinhua*, 24 November 2011). Food safety, a long-standing problem and one that has affected Hong Kong since the 1970s because the majority of food is imported from the mainland, continues unabated. Hong Kong monitoring continues to show high levels of heavy metals in shellfish, vegetables and fruits. The infamous tainted milk powder scandals (in 2008, 300,000 children on the mainland fell ill due to melamine contaminated milk powder) and 100 tonnes of the melamine-tainted milk powder was seized in 2010 (MacPherson 2008: 43–45; *South China Morning Post*, 22 August 2010, 3 March 2011).

Three processes have been identified as critical to solving imbalances in the system: 'market failures and insufficient government stewardship, inequities in the social determinants of health, and erosion of public perceptions of fairness and trust' (Tang *et al.* 2008: 1,496). This has been addressed partly by requiring that all individuals have health insurance in 2010, an infusion of government funds to redress inequalities in access to health care, technical, biomedical and epidemiological improvements such as the creation of a centres of disease control (CDC) in 2002 to achieve a 'Healthy China' in 2020.

## Comparative health care scenarios

Although China's geographic and demographic size and variability differentiates it from Hong Kong, they share a common ethnic and cultural heritage that defies borders. Divergence from the trajectory of socioeconomic policies from 1949 to 1978–1979 and the concerted commitment to adjust and reform its top-down command socialist system made possible the reintegration of Hong Kong. The agreed framework of 'one country, two systems' enshrined in the Basic Law has guaranteed that Hong Kong people can retain their 'capitalist system and lifestyle for 50 years'. From a demographic, epidemiological and public health perspective this raises many questions that must be resolved including not only when, but if, these disparities will deter or preserve the political commitment to an acceptable reintegration.

Hong Kong's epidemiological transition from CDs as the greatest cause of death, to NCDs by the late 1960s, was accomplished by a number of factors foremost of which were the commitment to child and maternal health, childhood vaccination for preventable CDs, ongoing surveillance and epidemiological expertise and a public health policy that rested on 'two pillars' – the private sector and the public – that ensured that the economically disadvantaged had access to free or low cost medical care. Economic growth, a low tax regime, individual and economic freedoms protected by law, and limited government sustained the system, and life expectancy ranks eighth in the world and infant mortality is the sixth lowest, despite the fact that Hong Kong continues to top league tables as having the highest income disparity (measured by the Gini coefficient) worldwide; although this ranking has been questioned since the income redistributive effect of social benefits, taxation policy and the change in household size had not been factored in (Economic Analysis Division 2007). Although a recent topic for actionable concern by government, legislators and civic groups (Henrad 2011), what is missed is that health status has dramatically and consistently improved, not declined, since the post-war period when Hong Kong was faced with providing a home for millions of mainland refugees seeking a better life.

Complacency about infectious disease control and the health care system was shattered, first in 1997, with the emergence of the highly virulent avian influenza (H5N1), first reported in Guangdong chicken farms, a major supplier to Hong Kong. The government took extraordinary steps to arrest the spread by culling 1.5 million chickens in the territory and stopping mainland imports. Lack of cooperation, transparency and surveillance capacity by the mainland over the aetiology of the virus strained cross-border relations. In 2003, SARS (acute respiratory syndrome), an emerging highly transmissible coronavirus, was globalized through Hong Kong, killing 300 people locally and 900 people worldwide. Again, the lack of transparency and denial of information from the mainland, where the disease originated, was damaging to China's reputation internationally and exposed the lack of competency in infectious diseases control. It was a wake-up call to Hong Kong that having transitioned to NCDs, and all that entailed for refining health policy and objectives, was not a unidirectional process. Vigilance in addressing the established and newly emerging CDs could not be relegated to benign neglect (MacPherson 2008: 39–49).

As multidimensional and complex as the epidemiological and demographic transitions are, the sociopolitical aspects and their cultural ramifications have to be factored in. One controversial issue that affects health care and population is the number of mainland women entering Hong Kong to give birth because of the high standards for maternal and infant care, but primarily because their children will have the right of abode in the city. In 2010, 40,000 babies were born to mainlanders out of 88,500 births and 80 per cent were not married to Hong Kong men. The strain on maternity care and hospital beds (often denying beds to local mothers-to-be) has prompted cross-border measures to crack down on illegal middleman agencies who arrange for mainland women to stay in Hong Kong, the blacklisting of pregnant women who travel frequently across the border and requiring ante-natal check-ups by local obstetricians and delivery booking certificates of public and private hospitals to try and cap the deliveries to 35,000 per year (*South China Morning Post*, 31 December 2011). One study has shown that mainland children who are taken back to China, when they return to Hong Kong do not do as well academically and in job status as children who stay in Hong Kong where there is no difference in academic attainment with the local population. The controversy escalated when a local newspaper published a broadside (funded by donations) calling mainlanders 'locusts' that 'eat' up medical resources and welfare benefits and 'refuse to follow our rules and order'. The ad opined, 'Are you willing for Hong Kong to spend one million Hong Kong Dollars every 18 minutes to raise children born to mainland parents?' Furthermore the ad said, 'Hong Kong people do not want Hong Kong to become mainland China'. A Beijing university professor, Kong Qingdong, countered by calling Hong Kong people 'bastards' and 'running dogs of the British government' (*Pingguo ribao*, 1 February 2012; *South China Morning Post*, 1 February 2012). Weibo internet blogs in Shanghai picked up the ad with a twist; calling the influx of migrant workers or 'outsiders' (who have lost their *hukou* and *danwei* welfare benefits and have to fall back on city resources) as 'locusts' where the city spends four million yuan to subsidize them and 'we have to endure you coming and ruining our culture' (*China Daily*, 3 February 2011).

The Hong Kong government supported 'One-way' permit scheme allows 55,000 people to migrate to Hong Kong every year. Eligible born children are a source of population growth in Hong Kong. This may offset the deficit in the working age population as Hong Kong's population ages. In fact, 93 per cent of Hong Kong's demographic growth comes from newly arrived mainlanders. Demographers and urban planners have estimated that Hong Kong can accommodate 8.3 to 8.79 million people in 2031 in the compact city model that now prevails. Thus in-migration will have to be controlled beyond the 1997 agreement, unless Hong Kong and Shenzhen (the first special economic zone created on the border between Hong Kong and Guangdong) merge into a mega-urban region (Kwan and Leung 2011: 18–21; MacPherson 1997: 279–286; Census and Statistics HKSAR 2007). A recent agreement was signed between the Shenzhen municipal government and the University of Hong Kong's medical school with the cooperation of both health departments, to open the Binhai hospital to provide cutting-edge medical research, treatment and medical staff training. The hospital that was opened in 2011 will also provide treatment for the 61,900 Hong Kong people who reside there. Medical emergency fees will be paid by the Hong Kong government and an agreement was reached between the two authorities to facilitate cross-border, ambulance services (*Shenzhen ribao*, 7 November 2011).

China has made some progress in addressing the lack of transparency concerning the outbreaks of newly emerging diseases such as SARS and avian influenza that had a deadly impact on Hong Kong and the world. However, epidemiological information, transparency and public health measures to arrest the spread of CDs leave much to be desired. With the transition to NCDs and an ageing population, a 'double disease burden' will challenge the government and society on all fronts. A debate is needed over the nature and role of government and the priorities of the state that has through its polices over the years framed the context in which, on the one hand, improvements to health and longevity are documentable, but so are disparities in health care delivery and financing between developed and underdeveloped regions, the urban rural divide, the 'floating population', demographic imbalances due to fertility control and social customs that favour males over females (Alcorn and Bao 2011: 1539–1340). Recently, a new draft law on senior citizens 'which requires people to visit their aging parents to help fulfill their emotional and spiritual life' speaks not only to a demographic and cultural shift but also to a top-down approach that improved preventive primary care delivered within communities and increasing the number of care homes and beds available (there are 38,000 care facilities which works out to 15 beds for every 1,000 seniors) to treat the unwell would be a better policy choice (*China Daily*, 10 January 2011).

No matter how abstract the theoretical literature is concerning the health transitions at the macro level of analysis, it is at the micro level where the transitions are felt, and public policy needs to be flexible and adjust to local needs and develop the competency to deal with new obligations attendant to the economy of public health, the implementation of public health agendas and the contingent consequences that these health transitions pose. China needs to continue to commit to the openness, politically, socially and economically, that will improve and enhance the health of the population, and Hong Kong is willing to share its expertise and experience to bring this to fruition.

## References

Alcorn, T. and Bao, B.B. (2011) 'China's Fertility Policy Persists, Despite Debate', *The Lancet*, 378(9802): 1539–1540.

Banister, J. (2004) 'Shortage of Girls in China Today', *Journal of Population Research*, 21(1): 19–45.

Bauhinia Foundation Research Centre Health Care Study Group (2007) 'Development and Financing Hong Kong's Future Health Care: Report on Preliminary Findings', Hong Kong, LC Paper No. CB (2)2460/06-07(01).

Census and Statistics HKSAR (2007) 'Population Projections 2007–2036'. Online, available at: www.statistics.gov.hk/publications/stats_statreport/population/B1120015032007 XXXB0202.pdf.

Centre for Health Protection (2005) *Tackling Obesity, its Causes, the Plight and Preventive Actions*, Hong Kong: Central Health Education Unit, Centre of Health Protection, Department of Health, the Government of the Hong Kong SAR.

Centre for Health Protection (2007) 'Hypertension', Department of Health, Government of the Hong Kong SAR. Online, available at: www.chp.gov.hk/en/content/9/25/60. html.

Centre for Health Protection (2011) *Special Preventive Programme*, Hong Kong: Department of Health, the Government of the Hong Kong SAR.

Centre for Health Protection (2012) 'Cerebrovascular Disease', Department of Health, Government of the Hong Kong SAR. Online, available at: www.chp.gov.hk/en/ content/9/25.html.

Chan, B.S., Tsang, M.W., Lee, V.W. and Lee, K.K. (2007) 'Cost of Type 2 Diabetes

Mellitus in Hong Kong Chinese', *International Journal of Clinical Pharmacology and Therapeutics*, 45(8): 455–468.

Chan, C. (2008) 'Childhood Obesity and Adverse Health Effects in Hong Kong', *Obesity Review*, Suppl. 1: 87–90.

Chan, N.N., King, A.P.S. and Chan, J.C.N. (2005) 'Metabolic Syndrome and Type 2 Diabetes: The Hong Kong Perspective', *Clinical Biochemistry Review*, 26(3): 51–57.

Chan, W.K., Chung, T.S., Lau, B.S.T., Law, H.T., Yeung, A.K.M. and Wong, C.H.Y. (2006) 'Management of Hypertension by Private Doctors in Hong Kong', *Hong Kong Medical Journal*, 12(2): 115–118.

Chao, J., Chang, E. and Ko, S. (2010) 'Hepatitis B and Liver Cancer Knowledge and Practices among Healthcare and Public Health Professionals in China: A Cross-sectional Study', *BMC Public Health*, 10(98): 1–11.

Cheng, K.K., Day, N.E., Duffy, S.W., Lam, T.H., Fox, M. and Wong, J. (1992) 'Pickled Vegetables in the Aetiology of Oesophageal Cancer in Hong Kong Chinese', *Lancet*, 339(8805): 1314–1318.

Cook, I. and Drummer, T. (2004) 'Changing Health in China: Re-evaluating the Epidemiological Transition Model', *Health Policy*, 67(3): 329–343.

Digby, K.H. (1951) 'Nasopharyngeal Carcinoma', *Annals of the Royal College of Surgeons*, 4(9 October): 253–265.

Dimond, E.G. (1971) 'Medical Education and Care in People's Republic of China', *JAMA*, 218(10): 1552–1557.

Director of Medical and Health Services (1963–1964) *Annual Departmental Report*, Hong Kong: Hong Kong Government Printer.

Economic Analysis Division, Financial Services Sector Office, Hong Kong SAR Government (2007) 'Analysis of Income Disparity in Hong Kong', 16 March. Online, available at: www.legco.gov.hk/yr06–07/english/fc/fc/papers/fc0301fc-46-e.pdf.

French, P. and Crabbe, M. (2010) *Fat China: How Expanding Waistlines are Changing a Nation*, London: Anthem Books.

Frenk, J. and Charon, F. (1991) 'International Health in Transition', *Asia Pacific Journal of Public Health*, 5(2): 170–175.

Fu, F.H. and Hao, X. (2003) 'The Prevalence of Coronary Heart Disease Risk Factors of Hong Kong Secondary School Students', *Journal of Exercise Science and Fitness*, 1(1): 23–32.

Fu, F.H., Nie, J. and Tong, K. (2004) 'An Overview of Health Fitness of Hong Kong Children and Adults in the Past 20 Years (1984–2004): Part 2', *Journal of Exercise Science and Fitness*, 2(2): 64–78.

Gauld, R. and Gould, D. (2002) *The Hong Kong Health Sector: Development and Change*, Hong Kong: Chinese University Press.

Harpham, T. and Stephens, C. (1991) 'Urbanization and Health in Developing Countries', *World Health Statistical Quarterly*, 44(2): 62–69.

Henrad, V. (2011) *Income Inequality and Public Expenditure on Social Policy in Hong Kong*, Hong Kong: Civic Exchange.

'The Hong Kong Cancer Fund' (1993) *The Hong Kong Practitioner*, 15(11): 2861–2863.

Hsieh, P. and Hsieh, Y. (2011) 'Impact of Liver Diseases on the Development of Type 2 Diabetes Mellitus', *Journal of Gastroenterology*, 17(48): 5240–5245.

Huang, K. (1972) 'Infectious and Parasitic Diseases', in Quinn, J. R. (ed.) *Medicine and Public Health in the People's Republic of China*, Washington, DC: US Government Printing Office, 239–262.

Ji, J., Pan, E., Li, J., Chen, J., Cao, J., Sun, D., Lu, S., Chen, S., Gu, D., Duan, X., Wu, X.

and Huang, J. (2011) 'Classical Risk Factors of Cardiovascular Disease among Chinese Steel Workers: A Prospective Cohort Study for 20 Years', *BMC Public Health*, 11(497): 1–8.

Khoo, R. (1965) 'Editorial: Cancer in Hong Kong', *Bulletin of the Hong Kong Chinese Medical Association*, 17(1): 23–24.

King, H. (1972) 'Cancer Research Organization and Preventive Programs', in Quinn, J.R. (ed.) *Medicine and Public Health in the People's Republic of China*, Washington, DC: US Government Printing Office, 263–288.

Ko, G.T.C. (2008) 'The Cost of Obesity in Hong Kong', *Obesity Reviews*, 9 March Suppl. 1: 74–77.

Ko, G.T.C. (2010) 'Obesity in Hong Kong: Risk and Burden', *Hong Kong Medical Bulletin*, 15(2): 9–11.

Ko, G.T.C. and Tang, J.S.F. (2007) 'Metabolic Syndrome in the Hong Kong Community: The United Christian Nethersole Community Health Service Primary Healthcare Programme 2001–2002', *Singapore Medical Journal*, 48(12): 1111–1116.

Ko, G.T.C., Chan, J.C.N., Chan, A.W.Y., Wong, P.T.S., Hui, S.S.C., Tong, S.D.Y., Ng, S.M., Chow, F. and Chan, C.L.W. (2007) 'Association between Sleeping Hours, Working Hours and Obesity in Hong Kong Chinese: The "Better Health for a Better Hong Kong" Health Promotion Campaign', *International Journal of Obesity*, 31(2): 254–260.

Kwan, D. and Leung, E. (2011) 'Vital Statistics in 2010', *Public Health and Epidemiology Bulletin*, 20(2): 15–30.

Lao, X., Zhang, Y., Wong, M., Xu, H., Nie, S., Ma, W., Thomas, G. and Yu, I. (2012) 'The Prevalence of Metabolic Syndrome and Cardiovascular Risk Factors in Adults in Southern China', *BMC Public Health*, 12(64) doi:10.1186/1471-2458-12-64.

Lee, S.C., Pu, Y.B., Chow, C.C., Yeung, V.T., Ko, G.T., So, W.Y., Li, J.K., Chan, W.B., Ma, R.C., Critchley, J.A., Cockram, C.S. and Chan, J.C. (2000) 'Diabetes in Hong Kong Chinese: Evidence for Familial Clustering and Parental Effects', *Diabetes Care*, 23(9): 1365–1368.

Li, G. (2010) *Nutrition Policies in China*, Beijing: Ministry of Health.

Li, J. and Wang, H. (2010) 'The Poor Control of Hypertension in China', *African Journal of Biotechnology*, 9(48): 8241–8242.

Li, J., Kang, L.N. and Qiao, Y.L. (2011) 'Review of the Cervical Cancer Disease Burden in Mainland China', *Asian Pacific Journal of Cancer Prevention*, 12(5): 1149–1153.

Lin, N., Tang, J. and Ismael, H. (2000) 'Study on Environmental Etiology of High Incidence Areas of Liver Cancer in China', *World Journal of Gastroenterology*, 6(4): 572–576.

Liu, E. and Yue, S.Y. (1998) *Health Care Expenditure and Financing in Hong Kong*, Hong Kong: Provisional Legislative Council Secretariat.

McGhee, S.M., So, J.C. and Thomas, G.N. (2009) 'Explaining Coronary Heart Disease Trends in Hong Kong: Creating a Model for Policy and Planning', *Hong Kong Medical Journal*, 15(1): 22–25, Suppl. 2, February.

MacPherson, K.L. (1997) 'The City and the State: Historical Reflections on Hong Kong's Identity in Transition, 1997 and Beyond', *Cities*, 14(5): 279–286.

MacPherson, K.L. (1987) *A Wilderness of Marshes: The Origins of Public Health in Shanghai, 1843–1893*, London: Oxford University Press.

MacPherson, K.L. (2008) 'Invisible Borders: Hong Kong, China and the Imperatives of Public Health', in M. J. Lewis and MacPherson K. L. (eds) *Public Health in Asia and the Pacific: Historical and Comparative Perspectives*, London: Routledge, 10–54.

Medical and Sanitary Reports (1936) *Administrative Reports*, Hong Kong.

Millman, A., Tang, D. and Perera, F. (2008) 'Air Pollution Threatens the Health of Children in China', *Pediatrics*, 122(8): 620–628.

Omran, A. (1971) 'The Epidemiological Transition: A Theory of the Epidemiology of Population Change', *Milbank Memorial Fund Quarterly*, 49(4) (Part 1): 509–538.

Orleans, L. (1972) 'Population Dynamics', in Quinn, J. R. (ed.) *Medicine and Public Health in the People's Republic of China*, Washington, DC: US Government Printing Office, 191–210.

Ping, Z., Dai, M., Chen, W. and Li, N. (2010) 'Cancer Trends in China', *Japanese Journal of Clinical Oncology*, 40(4): 281–285.

Preston, S. (1975) 'The Changing Relation between Mortality and Level of Economic Development', *Population Studies*, 29(2): 231–248.

Reynolds, T.A. and Tierney, L.M. (2004) 'Medical Education in Modern China', *JAMA*, 291(17): 2,141.

Rifkin, S.B. (1972) 'Health Care for Rural Areas', in Quinn, J. R. (ed.) *Medicine and Public Health in the People's Republic of China*, Washington, DC: US Government Printing Office, 137–150.

Scharping, T. (2002) *Birth Control in China 1949–2000: Population Policy and Demographic Development*, London: Routledge.

Selwyn-Clarke, P.S. (1975) *Footprints: The Memoirs of Sir Selwyn-Clarke*, Hong Kong: Sino-American Publishers.

Surveillance and Epidemiological Branch, Centre for Health Protection (2004) *Topical Health Report No. 4: Prevention and Screening of Cervical Cancer*, Hong Kong: Government of the Hong Kong SAR.

Tang, S., Meng, C. Chen, L., Bekedam, H., Evans, T. and Whitehead, M. (2008) 'Tackling the Challenges to Health Equity in China', *Lancet*, 372(9648): 1493–1509.

Thompson, W.S. (1929) 'Population', *American Journal of Sociology*, 34(6): 959–975.

Vallin, J. and Meslé, F. (2004) 'Convergence and Divergence in Mortality: A New Approach to Health Transitions', *Demographic Research*, 2(2): 11–44.

Wang, R. (2009) 'Heart Disease China's No. 1 Killer', *China Daily*, 21 April.

Wang, S., Patricio, M. and Langenbrunner, J. (2011) *Toward a Healthy and Harmonious Life in China: Stemming the Rising Tide of Non-communicable Diseases*, Geneva: World Bank Report Number 62318-CN.

Watson, A. (2009) 'Social Security for China's Migrant Workers: Providing for Old Age', *Current Chinese Affairs*, 38(4): 85–115.

Watts, J. (2008) 'China's Environmental Health Challenges', *Lancet*, 372(9648): 1451–1452.

WHO (2009) Global Tuberculosis Control. Country Profile: China 2009, 4. Online, available at: www.who.int/tb/publications/global_report/2009/pdf/chn.

Wilkinson, R. (2005) *The Impact of Inequality: How to Make Sick Societies Healthier*, New York: The Free Press.

Wong, C., Lo, V. and Tang, K. (2006) *China's Urban Health Reform: From State Protection to Individual Responsibility*, Lanham, MD: Lexington Books.

Woodward, D., Drager, N., Beaglehole, R. and Lipson, D. (2001) 'Globalization and Health: A Framework for Analysis and Action', *Bulletin of the World Health Organization*, 79(9): 875–881.

World Bank (1993) *World Development Report 1993: Investing in Health*, Oxford: Oxford University Press.

World Bank (2011) World Development Indicators Database Updated. Online, available at: http://data.worldbank.org/news/wdi2012-database-updated.

Wong, K.C. and Wu, L.T. (1936, 2nd edn) *History of Chinese Medicine*, Tientsin: Tientsin Press.

Xu, B., Rimpelä, A., Järvelin, M. and Nieminen, M. (1994) 'Sex Differences of Infant and Child Mortality in China', *Scandinavian Journal of Public Health*, 22(4): 242–248.

Yang, G., Kong, L., Zhao, W., Zhai, Y., Chen, L. and Kaplan, J. (2008) 'Emergence of Chronic Non-communicable Diseases in China', *Lancet*, 372(9650): 1,697–1,705.

Yang, W., Lu, J., Weng, J., Jia, W., Ji, L., Xiao, J., Shan, Z., Liu, J., Tian, J., Ji, Q., Zhu, D., Ge, J., Lin, L., Chen, L., Guo, X., Zhao, Z., Li, Q., Zhou, Z., Shan, G. and He, J., for the China National Diabetes and Metabolic Disorders Study Group (2010) 'Prevalence of Diabetes among Men and Women in China', *New England Journal of Medicine*, 362(12): 1090–1101.

Yeh, S.D.J. and Chow, B.F. (1972) 'Nutrition', in Quinn, J.R. (ed.) *Medicine and Public Health in the People's Republic of China*, Washington, DC: US Department of Health.

Yeoh, E.K. (1984) 'Editorial. Hepatitis B Vaccine: A Vaccine for the Prevention of Liver Cancer', *Bulletin of the Journal of the Hong Kong Medical Association*, 36(September): 17–20.

Yeoh, E. K. (1986) 'Editorial: Prevention of Primary Liver Cancer', *Journal of Hong Kong Medical Association*, 38(4): 155–156.

Yip, K.C. (1995) *Health and National Reconstruction in Nationalist China*, Ann Arbor, MI: Association for Asian Studies.

Zhang, Y.X. and Elvin, M. (1998) 'Tuberculosis and Environment in Modern China', in M. Elvin and T.J. Liu (eds) *Sediments of Time: Environment and Society in Chinese History*, Cambridge: Cambridge University Press, 520–544.

Zhao, P., Dai, M., Chen W. and Li, N. (2010) 'Cancer Trends in China', *Japanese Journal of Oncology*, 40(4): 281–285.

# 4 Health transition and the rising threat of chronic non-communicable diseases in India

*Sailesh Mohan and K. Srinath Reddy*

## Introduction

Since India attained independence in 1947, the country has witnessed remarkable progress in the health status of its population. In addition, notable progress in economic and social development has taken place, which has also in no small measure contributed to the improvements in health. However, many challenges remain including wide social inequalities that impede further progress. Over the past few decades Indian society has experienced major transitions that have impacted on health. Profound changes have occurred in economic development, nutritional status, fertility and mortality rates and, consequently, the disease profile has undergone changes. Although substantial progress has been achieved in controlling communicable diseases, they still contribute significantly to the national disease burden. Concomitantly, India has witnessed the emergence and accelerated rise of chronic non-communicable diseases (NCDs) resulting in a double burden of pre- and post-transitional diseases. In this chapter, we review these transitions and their contribution to the rising burden of NCDs in India.

## Major transitions in recent decades

### Demographic transition

One of the major transitions in India has been demographic, characterised by a shift from high to low fertility and mortality rates. During the twentieth century the population increased nearly fourfold from 238 million in 1901 to 1,027 million in 2001 (Haub and Sharma 2006: 4–10). Significant falls in crude death (25.1 per 1,000 population in 1951 to 7.6 in 2005) and birth (40.8 per 1,000 population in 1951 to 23.8 in 2005) rates have occurred. Annual population growth has been over 2 per cent and, given the sluggish decline in birth rates, the population has increased exponentially and is projected to increase to 1,400 million by 2026 ('Demographic Transition' 2010: 7–24). This has been accompanied by considerable increases in life expectancy at birth, which has risen from 33 years when India became an independent nation to 64 years currently ('Demographic Transition' 2010: 7–24; Adlakha 1997: 1–2). However, population growth, declines in birth and death rates and advances in life expectancy are not uniform. There are huge within-country differences with certain states such as Kerala and Tamil Nadu being in the advanced stages of this transition with birth rates at replacement levels or lower, increased longevity and a higher proportion of the aged, but other states like Uttar Pradesh and Bihar have comparatively high birth rates and low life expectancy. Further, the overall proportion of the aged (≥60 years) in the total population is expected to increase from 6.9 per cent (70.7 million) in 2001 to 12.4 per cent (173.2 million) in 2026 (Census of India 2001). This has a direct, accelerating influence on NCDs, with more people living to older ages and consequently being exposed to detrimental risk factors (such as tobacco use, unhealthy diets and physical inactivity) for longer periods, developing clinical disease (such as cardiovascular disease, diabetes, cancers) and suffering varying degrees of disability or indeed ultimately dying from an NCD. This has enormous implications for public health and healthcare costs. Not surprisingly, states in advanced stages of this transition have reported a higher NCD burden.

### Epidemiological transition

Against the backdrop of the above demographic changes, improvements in population control, sanitation, control of communicable diseases and societal development, the mortality and disease patterns have changed. Declines in morbidity and mortality from communicable diseases have been accompanied by a gradual shift to, and rise in the prevalence of, chronic non-communicable diseases (NCDs) such as cardiovascular disease (CVD), diabetes, chronic obstructive pulmonary disease (COPD), cancers and injuries. It is estimated that currently NCDs account for 53 per cent of the total mortality and 44 per cent of disability adjusted life years (DALYs) lost in India with projections indicating a further rise to 67 per cent of total mortality by 2030 (see Figure 4.1) CVD is the major contributor to this burden and accounts for 52 per cent of NCD-associated mortality and 29 per cent of total mortality (Prabhakaran and Ajay [in press]).

Available data indicate that the epidemiological transition is well underway in many states. However, as is the case with the demographic transition, there are wide within-country differences with certain states at the advanced end of the spectrum while others are progressing less rapidly. A case in point is the southern state of Kerala which has achieved remarkable reductions in fertility and mortality as well as notable improvements in health indicators including life expectancy at birth; these exceed those of many developing countries and are comparable to those of some developed countries (Haub and Sharma 2006: 4–10; Thankappan and Valiathan 1998: 1274–1275). However, recent reports indicate a very high prevalence of NCDs and their risk factors. Prevalence of diabetes was 16 per cent, hypertension 33 per cent, hypercholesterolemia 57 per cent, overweight 31 per cent and tobacco use 28 per cent (Thankappan *et al.* 2010: 53–63). This large burden is reflected in the patterns of mortality as well. Even in rural areas of the state, diseases of the circulatory system account for up to 40 per cent of total mortality, a figure close to that of urban Chennai where 39

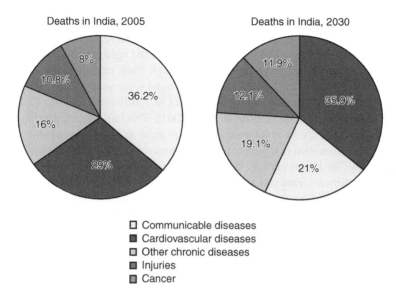

*Figure 4.1* Cause specific mortality in India (source: adapted from Prabhakaran and Ajay [in press]).

per cent of all deaths were attributable to CVDs (Soman *et al.* 2011: 898; Gajalakshmi and Peto 2004: 47). In another rural setting in Andhra Pradesh, CVDs were reported to be responsible for 32 per cent of all deaths with injuries accounting for 13 per cent; this is indicative of the profound changes in the disease profile that are sweeping across the country (Joshi *et al.* 2006: 1522–1529). These are harbingers of what the rest of the Indian states will likely experience as they move further along the pathway of the epidemiological transition.

### Socioeconomic transition

India has experienced rapid urbanisation in recent years as a result of population growth as well as an increased pace of economic development. The urban population has risen from 17 per cent in 1950–1951 to 28 per cent in 2001, and is projected to increase to 38 per cent by 2026; thereby accounting for nearly two-thirds of the population increase up to 2026 (Haub and Sharma 2006: 4–10; Census of India 2001; 'India: Urban Poverty Report' 2009). This has been associated with industrialisation, modernisation and increased utilisation of technology, and with unplanned expansion of cities into adjoining areas and increased within-country migration from rural to urban areas. In addition, it has placed increased demands on existing urban infrastructure, services and public spaces, leading to increases in the disease burden (including increased susceptibility to NCD risks such as tobacco, alcohol, unhealthy diet and physical inactivity). Prevalence of such risk factors is higher in urban than rural areas. Urbanisation had also led to increases in the number of automobiles and associated road traffic accidents and injuries. This process is not uniform nationally, with South India urbanising more speedily than the rest of the country (Census of India 2001; 'India: Urban Poverty Report' 2009; UNDP 2009). One of the chief drivers of urbanisation is migration from rural to urban locations (as well as from urban to urban for economic reasons). As people migrate from rural areas, they experience improvement in their standard of living but also adverse lifestyle and environmental influences concerning diet and behaviours that predispose them to NCDs. Evidence of this is emerging as rural migrants are reportedly reducing levels of physical activity, increasing intake of dietary fat and becoming more obese and prone to diabetes (Ebrahim *et al.* 2010: e1000268).

Further, reports also reveal the reversal of the social gradient whereby the poor suffer increased vulnerability to NCD risks and disease, a situation similar to that observed in developed countries that already have undergone health transitions. Risk factors which are initially high among the higher socioeconomic classes percolate down to lower classes gradually, and the lower classes then bear the brunt of the disease and risk burden. Data from India from certain settings provide clear evidence for this reversal (see Table 4.1). In a large, multisite, national study of industrial population, tobacco use (56.6 per cent versus 12.5 per cent) and hypertension (33.8 per cent versus 22.7 per cent) were significantly higher in the low education group than the high education group (Reddy *et al.* 2007: 16263–16268). In contrast, those with high education and located in highly urbanised areas had a lower prevalence of tobacco use, hypertension, overweight and diabetes than those with low education. A recent survey in

*Table 4.1* Prevalence of cardiovascular risk factors by educational status in an industrial population (%)

| Risk factor | ES I | ES II | ES III | ES IV | P value for trend |
|---|---|---|---|---|---|
| *Tobacco use* | | | | | |
| Men | 19.8 | 26.5 | 40.2 | 77.3 | <0.001 |
| Women | 1.2 | 1.6 | 2.7 | 42.1 | <0.001 |
| *Hypertension* | | | | | |
| Men | 27.2 | 29.9 | 28.6 | 32.6 | 0.05 |
| Women | 15.3 | 18.4 | 23.8 | 34.7 | <0.001 |
| *Overweight* | | | | | |
| Men | 37.0 | 33.1 | 30.4 | 9.1 | <0.001 |
| Women | 39.3 | 37.4 | 41.5 | 22.9 | <0.001 |
| *Diabetes* | | | | | |
| Men | 8.4 | 10.4 | 13.3 | 7.6 | 0.08 |
| Women | 4.2 | 4.8 | 9.8 | 11.2 | 0.01 |

Source: adapted from Reddy *et al.* 2007: 16265.

Notes
ES I: post graduate; ES II: graduate; ES III: secondary or high school; ES IV: primary or illiterate.

Kerala reported one of the highest diabetes prevalence rates (14.6 per cent) so far in a rural setting (Vijayakumar *et al.* 2009: 563–567). Even among the urban poor in North India, high rates of obesity (14 per cent), dyslipidaemia (27 per cent) and diabetes (10.3 per cent) have been reported (Misra *et al.* 2001: 1722–1729). Furthermore, a recent study from Chandigarh and Haryana found most CVD risk factors to be similar among those residing in urban and rural areas, indicating the increased vulnerability of the poor (Kar *et al.* 2010: 206–209). These data likely reflect the varying degrees of epidemiological transition that India is experiencing.

Concomitant with urbanisation, the liberalisation of the Indian economy in the early 1990s and resultant globalisation has increased transnational trade, exposure to Western lifestyles and food habits, and aggressive advertising that promote unhealthy lifestyles conducive to the rise of NCDs.

### *Nutritional transition*

One of the major determinants of the rising burden of NCDs is unhealthy diet. In consonance with other above transitions, a nutritional transition, characterised by increased consumption of energy-dense, nutrient-deficient diets, high in refined carbohydrates, saturated fats, sugars and salt, with lower amounts of fibre as well as processed foods in place of traditional diets that are high in complex carbohydrates and low in fat, is occurring (Popkin 2003: 581–597). Despite little discernible change in the per capita calorie consumption in India, notable increases in edible oil and fat intake have been reported in both rural and urban areas (Kulkarni and Gaiha n.d.). Oil intake increased from 18 g per person daily in 1990–1992 to 27 g per person daily in 2003–2005 while fat intake rose from 41 to 52 g per person daily during the same period (Prabhakaran and Ajay [in press]). Furthermore, high income groups are reported to consume 32 per cent of their energy intake from fat while their low income counterparts consume only 17 per cent, underlining a socioeconomic differential (Shetty 2002: 175–182). Although national data on individual fat and oil intake is limited, aggregate consumption data indicate an increasing trend in edible oil consumption,which has risen from 9.7 million tons in 2000–2001 to 14.3 million tons in 2007–2008, with a high proportion of unhealthy oils high in saturated and transfats (Prabhakaran and Ajay [in press]). Over the past decades, considerable improvements in the nutritional status have taken place, as indicated by the reduction in undernutrition, with the percentage of adults with a body mass index under 18.5 declining from 56 per cent to 33 per cent in men and 52 per cent to 36 per cent in women between 1975 and 2005 (Deaton and Dreze 2009: 42–65). However, undernutrition continues to be a major challenge, with close to 50 per cent of Indian children being underweight. Now, this has been compounded by the parallel rise of overweight and obesity in certain groups, resulting in overnutrition and a twin burden (Wang *et al.* 2009: 456–474). This has serious implications for NCDs, given that low birth weight and early childhood undernutrition in interaction with environmental and genetic influences increase the risk of CVD and diabetes in adulthood; thus producing a transgenerational effect on population health (Smith 2007: 216–226).

## Risk factor and disease burden: some trends

### *Tobacco use*

India is the second largest producer and the third largest consumer of tobacco in the world and is home to over 240 million tobacco users (Reddy and Gupta 2004: 72). Not surprisingly tobacco use is a leading cause of premature, NCD-associated death and disability, and a growing public health challenge. It currently causes nearly one million deaths, the poor being disproportionately affected with over half of these deaths occurring among illiterate adults (Jha *et al.* 2008: 1137–1147). Significantly, 70 per cent of these deaths are in the 30–69 year age group, which is the most economically productive segment of the population. Tobacco is used in myriad ways with bidis, cigarettes and smokeless (chewing) forms being the most common. Projections indicate that nearly 13 per cent of all deaths in India are tobacco related. Notably, 50 per cent of cancers among men, 20 per cent of cancers among women and 90 per cent of oral cancers are attributable to tobacco use. Further, over 80 per cent of COPD among men, 60 per cent of heart diseases in those less than 40 years of age and 53 per cent of myocardial infarctions among urban men are also attributed to tobacco use. In addition, smoking contributes to nearly half of tuberculosis deaths among men. In terms of numbers, nearly 154,000 cases of cancers, 4.2 million cases of heart disease and 3.7 million cases of COPD were also due to tobacco. The economic cost of treating these three, major tobacco-related diseases is colossal and in 1999 was estimated to be 277.6 billion rupees, which is substantially more than the revenue received by the government from tobacco sales (Reddy and Gupta 2004: 1–3; Jha *et al.* 2008: 1137–1147; Rastogi *et al.* 2005: 356–358)

Many small, sub-national studies have reported on tobacco use, but data from national surveys are available only from the 1990s. The latest National Family Health Survey (NFHS-3 of 2005–2006) indicates that currently 57 per cent men and 10.8 per cent women use some form of tobacco. Thirty-three per cent of men smoke and 37 per cent chew while 1.4 per cent women smoke and 8.4 per cent chew (International Institute for Population Sciences 2007: 432–434). Compared to the NFHS-2 of 1998–1999 in which 47 per cent men and 14 per cent women used some tobacco, there has been an increase among men, particularly at younger ages and in urban areas (Thankappan and Mini 2008: 2842–2843). In addition, there are huge, interstate and socioeconomic variations, with many states having a prevalence of over 60 per cent tobacco use, the poor using more tobacco and rural areas having a higher prevalence than urban areas (Reddy and Gupta 2004: 49–56).

Disconcertingly, tobacco use is also increasing among the youth which portends a huge NCD burden in the future. Findings of the Global Youth Tobacco Survey (GYTS) among 13–15 year old school children indicated that 17.5 per cent were current tobacco users. There were wide interstate variations, with Nagaland having the highest (62.8 per cent) and Goa the lowest (3.3 per cent) prevalence of current tobacco use (Reddy and Gupta 2004: 1–3). Another study reported higher tobacco use among sixth-grade students in comparison to eighth-grade students; this is perhaps indicative of a shift in age of initiation to the tobacco habit and its increased use among youth (Reddy *et al.* 2006a: 589–594).

### Overweight and obesity

Although tremendous progress has been made in reducing undernutrition, India currently faces the twin burden of under- and overnutrition, underlining the need for nutritional policies that promote not only adequate but appropriate nutrition. Large national surveys provide an indication of the time trends, particularly among women. The NHFS-3 reported that 36 per cent women in reproductive age group (15–49 years) have a BMI of <18.5 indicating undernutrition; a slight improvement (33 per cent) over NFHS-2. In contrast, 10 per cent were over-weight and 3 per cent obese, a marginal increase compared to that in the NFHS-2. Among men, 8 per cent were overweight and 1 per cent obese (Wang *et al.* 2009: 456–474; International Institute for Population Sciences 2007: 309). A time trend for men cannot be determined as they were not assessed in NFHS-2. In general, women in urban areas with higher educational and income levels were more likely to be overweight or obese. The highest rates were observed in the epidemiologically and nutritionally advanced states of Punjab, Kerala and Delhi, which, incidentally, also have higher rates of NCD risk and disease burden (Gupta *et al.* 2006: 291–300; International Institute for Population Sciences 2007: 307). The Jaipur Heart Watch studies demonstrated an increasing trend in overweight/obesity among urban men (21.1 per cent in 1994 to 50.9 per cent in 2005) as well as in women (15.7 per cent in 1994 to 57.7 per cent in 2005) (Gupta and Gupta 2009: 349–355). More worrying is the increasing trend of overweight and obesity among schoolchildren in various urban areas, as indicated by different, local sample studies (Bhardwaj *et al.* 2008: 172–175; Wang *et al.* 2009: 456–474). This foreshadows a huge, future increase in obesity-related NCDs, particularly hypertension and diabetes.

Further, Indians have a lesser BMI than Caucasian populations and increase in body weight, even within the ideal levels of BMI, confers a higher risk of CVD and diabetes. At equivalent BMI, they also have a significantly higher visceral obesity than Caucasians. Based on these facts, lower normal BMI cut-off value for overweight ($>23\,kg/m^2$) and obesity ($>27.5\,kg/m^2$) have been suggested for identification of individuals and determination of the risk status (Ramachandran *et al.* 2010: 408–418).

### Physical inactivity

Population-based data on physical inactivity levels are sparse in India. The World Health Survey, the only national level survey thus far, found that 29 per cent of the adult population had inadequate physical activity levels. One-quarter of men (24 per cent) and one-third of women (34 per cent) had inadequate physical activity levels (defined as one to 149 minutes of activity in the week before the survey). It was higher in urban than rural people and increased in those aged 45 years or more with over half of them being inadequately active (International Institute for Population Sciences 2006: 44).

Given the rapid urbanisation, increased motorisation, mechanisation and sedentarism at workplaces, further increases are likely, particularly among the working age groups, so predisposing this segment of society to premature NCDs.

## High blood pressure

India has a large number of hypertensives with projections indicating nearly a doubling from 118 million in 2000 to 213 million by 2025. Hypertension prevalence in adults is between 20 and 40 per cent in urban areas and 12 and 17 per cent in rural areas (Reddy *et al.* 2005: 1744–1749). A meta-analysis reported 25 per cent prevalence among urban adults and 10 per cent among rural adults (Gupta 2004: 73–78). A large survey across ten industries covering all major regions of India reported a prevalence of 28 per cent in those aged 20 to 69 years (Reddy *et al.* 2006b: 461–469). The Indian Council of Medical Research (ICMR) estimates that 16 per cent of ischemic heart disease, 21 per cent of peripheral vascular disease, 24 per cent of acute myocardial infarctions and 29 per cent of strokes in India could be attributable to high blood pressure (Shah *et al.* n.d.). National data are unavailable, but many sub-national studies have reported increases in hypertension across the country (Gupta 2004: 73–78). It is worth noting between 1942 and 1997, the mean systolic blood pressure has increased from 120 mmHg to 130 mmHg, particularly among 40 to 49 year old, urban men (World Health Organization 2004: 28). Population time trends in national prevalence are unavailable but well conducted cross-sectional studies such as the Jaipur Heart Watch from Western India provide evidence of an increase over time; and this likely indicates the pattern of increase in the country as a whole. In the period, 1993–2005, a significant increase was observed both among men and women. Age-adjusted prevalence increased in men from 29 to 45 per cent and in women 22 to 38 per cent (Gupta and Gupta 2009: 349–355). Studies from other regions also point to an increasing burden of hypertension (Thankappan *et al.* 2006: 28–33; Gupta *et al.* 2008: 16–26). Furthermore, detection, management and control rates are sub-optimal. Various reports indicate that only about 30 per cent of people with hypertension are detected, less than half of those diagnosed take anti-hypertensives and only half of them have their blood pressure treated and controlled (Prabhakaran and Ajay [in press]). Notably, once hypertension-related CVD occurs, the use of evidence-based, secondary prevention therapies is also very low in primary and secondary care, leading to a large and increasing burden of avoidable and premature mortality (Sharma *et al.* 2009: 1007–1014; Mendis *et al.* 2005: 820–829; Joshi *et al.* 2009: 1950–1955).

### Coronary heart disease (CHD) and stroke

The prevalence of CHD ranges from 6.6 to 12.7 per cent in urban and 2.1 to 4.3 per cent in rural India among those aged 20 years or older. Prevalence has increased almost four times in rural areas and six times in urban areas over the last 40 years. It is estimated that there are currently 30 million CHD patients, with 14 million residing in rural and 16 million in urban areas. But these are likely underestimates given that epidemiological surveys do not include those with asymptomatic CHD (Reddy *et al.* 2005: 1744–1749).

The age-adjusted, stroke prevalence is reported to be between 334 and 424 per 100,000 population in urban India and 244 and 262 per 100,000 population in rural India and has increased in both during the past few decades (Gupta *et al.* 2008: 16–26). Population-based, stroke data are limited and most estimates are largely from small hospital-based studies, making assessment of secular trends difficult. The age-adjusted incidence rate of stroke in urban studies has increased from 13 per 100,000 persons per year in 1970 to 105 in 2001 and 145 in 2005, indicating an upward trend which is in consonance with the increased burden of its major risk factors like hypertension and smoking. In addition, the 30-day case fatality rate is reported to be 41 per cent, which is much higher than that in developed countries (17 to 33 per cent) (Mishra and Khadilkar 2010: 28–32; Das *et al.* 2007: 906–910).

In comparison to other countries, CVD in India is distinguished by earlier onset and premature mortality, higher case fatality rate of CVD-related complications and manifestation of clinical disease at lower risk factor thresholds, particularly with overweight and obesity. CVD disproportionately affects the young in India with 52 per cent of deaths occurring under the age of 70 compared to just 23 per cent in Western countries (Ghaffar *et al.* 2004: 807–810). The most recent data from a rural setting in an advanced stage of the epidemiological transition reveal that 60 per cent and 40 per cent of CHD deaths and 40 per cent and 20 per cent of stroke deaths, in men and women respectively, occurred in those under 65 years, underlining how devastating CVD is from a societal perspective (Soman *et al.* 2011). Consequently, the country suffers a very high loss in potential productive years of life because of premature CVD deaths among those aged 35 to 64 years: 9.2 million years lost in 2000 and 17.9 million years expected to be lost in 2030 (Reddy 2007: 1370–1372). In addition, CVD and diabetes entail a huge economic burden with the projected foregone national income during the period, 2005–2015, estimated to be more than $200 billion ('Preventing Chronic Diseases' 2005).

### Diabetes

Diabetes prevalence has been increasing rapidly, with the country being often labelled as the 'diabetes capital' of the world. Currently there are about 51 million people with diabetes, a figure that is projected to increase to 87 million by the year 2025 (*IDF Diabetes Atlas* 2009). Available data indicate a prevalence varying from 5 to 15 per cent in urban and 2 to 5 per cent in rural areas. In addition, between 9 and 30 per cent of Indians have impaired glucose tolerance (IGT), a likely indicator of further future increases in the disease burden. Moreover, diabetes-related complications are a major contributor to morbidity and mortality: for instance, CHD prevalence is considerably higher among diabetics and those with IGT (21.4 per cent and 14.9 per cent) compared to non-diabetics (9.1 per cent). Similarly, the prevalence of peripheral vascular disease is also higher among diabetics than among non-diabetics (6.3 per cent versus 2.7 per cent). Microvascular complications such as diabetic retinopathy, overt nephropathy and microalbuminuria affect 17.6 per cent, 2.2 per cent and 26.9 per cent of Indians respectively. Southern states have a higher prevalence compared to the rest of India and recent data indicate that in certain settings a reversal of the social gradient is occurring with those in lower social classes experiencing an increasing burden. Well-designed, repeat surveys in Chennai provide evidence of the increasing trend, particularly in urban areas. The prevalence increased from 8.3 per cent in 1989 to 11.6 per cent in 1995, and to 13.9 per cent in 2000, and this marked an increase of 70 per cent, with a shift in the age of onset of diabetes within a relatively short time span (Mohan *et al.* 2007: 217–230; Ramachandran *et al.* 1997: 232–237).

The escalation in the diabetes burden means high healthcare costs for the individual besides contributing to foregone national income: thus, in 2010 the annual, median, direct cost per diabetic individual was reported to be US$525, and the annual total cost of diabetes care in India was estimated to be US$32 billion, underlying the huge economic impact NCDs such as diabetes have on households as well as the national economy (Tharkar *et al.* 2010: 334–340).

## Cancer

Cancer prevalence in India is estimated to be around 2.5 million persons. About 800,000 new cases of cancer occur each year with this figure projected to increase to one million by 2016. The mortality is also expected to rise from about 550,000 deaths currently to 670,000 by 2016 (Prabhakaran and Ajay [in press]; 'Disease Burden in India' n.d.: 4). As already mentioned, tobacco use is one of the main risk factors. In addition, dietary, reproductive and sexual practices account for 20 to 30 per cent of cancers (Varghese n.d.: 49–59). The age-standardised rates are 96.4 per 100,000 in men and 88.2 in women (Bobba and Khan 2003: 93–96). The most common cancers in men are those of the oral cavity, oesophagus and lung. The chief cancer sites in women are the cervix, breast and ovaries (apart from tobacco-related ones). Data from the National Cancer Registry Program show increasing trends between 1982 and 1990 for breast, gallbladder and thyroid cancers and non-Hodgkin's lymphoma in women and for the cancers of oesophagus, prostate, mouth and non-Hodgkin's lymphoma in men (Satyanarayana and Asthana 2008: 35–44). Early detection and management is sub-optimal with more than 75 per cent of cancer patients presenting and seeking care when already in advanced stages of the disease, thereby reducing likelihood of positive treatment outcomes (Varghese n.d.: 49–59).

### Chronic obstructive pulmonary disease (COPD)

COPD is more common in men (5 per cent) than in women (2.7 per cent) aged 30 years and over, with the prevalence being higher among smokers. From available data, it appears that there has not been much discernible change since the 1970s when prevalence was reported to be 4.2 per cent in men and 2.7 per cent in women (Murthy and Sastry n.d.: 264–274). However, most studies are limited in size and scope, and national data on both prevalence and associated mortality are not available, making inference concerning time trends difficult. The number of COPD patients is estimated to increase from 13 million in 1996 to 22 million by 2016 with many likely requiring hospitalisation and with significant financial implications for individuals and the healthcare system. These numbers may increase further given the high exposure to indoor air pollution through lack of clean fuels for the vast majority of the rural population (Murthy and Sastry n.d.: 264–274; Jindal *et al.* 2006: 23–29).

### Road traffic accidents and injuries

Given the high levels of urbanisation, population growth and economic development, there have been phenomenal increases in motorisation in India. Automobile production has increased prodigiously and during the period, 1981–2004, the number of vehicles rose nearly 14 times from 5.1 million to 73 million and it continues to increase each year. This has had a cascading impact on road traffic, accident-related deaths which doubled (50,700 to 110,000) and injuries which quadrupled (109,100 to 465,282) between 1991 and 2005; and it is now among the leading causes of death and disability in the productive age group, 15–44 years. The estimated annual mortality rate was 20.9 per 100,000 population for all ages in 2002 (Gururaj 2008: 14–20). The majority of victims are men, often belonging to poorer strata of society, and they are usually pedestrians, motorcyclists or bicyclists. States with rapid and higher motorisation rates have greater numbers of related injuries and deaths. Public transport systems are grossly inadequate and deaths due to accidents are projected to increase by 147 per cent by 2020 (Kopits and Cropper 2005: 169–178).

## Limitations in NCD data-gathering mechanisms

There is a paucity of nationally representative and standardised data for most NCD risk factors and diseases in India. Most available data are from small, local or regional sample studies many of which have methodological limitations and variations in methods of measurement and diagnostic criteria. Prospective data which would enable ascertainment of disease incidence and more accurate estimation of the associated disease and risk factor burden are largely absent. Given the diversity of the population, the disease profiles and the varied health transitions that are occurring, large nationally representative studies and surveillance mechanisms to measure and monitor trends of NCDs and their risks on a regular systematic basis are warranted; so that adequate and appropriate public health action can be initiated. Some recent endeavours such as the multi-site, sentinel, CVD surveillance in industrial populations, the ICMR-initiated, NCD risk factor surveillance, the Government of India's Integrated Disease Surveillance Project and CARRS (Center for Cardio-metabolic Risk Reduction in South Asia) surveillance study initiated by the Public Health Foundation of India are encouraging and they are expected to provide reliable data that can aid in framing an appropriate public health response to the escalating burden of NCDs.

## Recent responses

Because of the lack of adequate data and the rapidity of changes, it took a long while for the health transition that was occurring in India to be understood. In addition, NCDs were perceived by both policymakers and public health professionals as largely a problem of the urban rich (Reddy 2007: 1370–1372). However, both policymakers and the public health community now better understand this transition as a result of emerging information as well as advocacy efforts directed at prevention and control of NCDs. Well-conducted analyses and studies that provide projections of current and future disease burdens, and the huge economic impact that NCDs will have on India's economy and healthcare system, have further enhanced understanding of this epidemic and underlined the importance of dealing with it through initiation of appropriate programmes and policies. Recently, the Indian Government has launched the National Programme for Prevention and Control of Cancer, Diabetes, Cardiovascular Diseases and Stroke. This aims to provide (a) assessment of risk factors, early diagnosis and appropriate disease management for high risk groups, and (b) health promotion for the general population (Reddy 2007: 1370–1372; National Programme for Prevention and Control of Cancer, Diabetes, Cardiovascular Diseases and Stroke 2010). It is expected to be integrated into the healthcare system, which is still oriented to providing acute care and dealing with communicable diseases and reproductive health. Further, legislative efforts to control tobacco use have led to India being a signatory to the Framework Convention on Tobacco Control and the implementation of the National Tobacco Control Act. This Act provides for smoking bans in public and work places, bans on advertisements, prohibition of sales to minors, regulating the contents of tobacco products and graphical warnings. These efforts, encompassing both public health and clinical approaches, will provide a strong impetus for prevention and control of NCDs and reduce associated morbidity, mortality and economic costs in the future.

## References

Adlakha, A. (1997) 'Population Trends: India'. US Department of Commerce, Economics and Statistics Administration. Bureau of the Census. Online, available at: www.census. gov/ipc/prod/ib-9701.pdf (accessed 26 July 2010).

Bhardwaj, S., Misra, A., Khurana, L., Gulati, S., Shah, P. and Vikram, N.K. (2008) 'Childhood Obesity in Asian Indians: A Burgeoning Cause of Insulin Resistance, Diabetes and Sub-clinical Inflammation', *Asia Pacific Journal of Clinical Nutrition*, 17: 172–175.

Bobba, R. and Khan, Y. (2003) 'Cancer in India: An Overview'. Online, available at: www.pharm-olam.com/pdfs/Cancer%20in%20India.pdf (accessed 11 July 2010).

Census of India 2001. 'Population Projections for India and States 2001–2026', Report of Technical Group on Population Projections Constituted by National Commission of Population. Online, available at: http://nrhm-mis.nic.in/UI/Public%20Periodic/Population_Projection_Report_2006.pdf (accessed 8 July 2010).

Das, S.K., Banerjee, T.K., Biswas, A., Roy, T., Raut, D.K., Mukherjee, C.S., Chaudhuri, A., Hazra, A. and Roy, J. (2007) 'A Prospective Community-based Study of Stroke in Kolkata, India', *Stroke*, 38: 906–910.

Deaton, A. and Drèze, J. (2009) 'Nutrition in India: Facts and Interpretations 2008', *Economic and Political Weekly*, XLIV: 42–65.

'Demographic Transition' (n.d.). Online, available at: http://wcd.nic.in/research/nti1947/2.Demographic%20transition.pdf (accessed 30 July 2010).

'Disease Burden in India. Estimation and Causal Analysis' (n.d.) NCMH Background Papers. Online, available at: www.whoindia.org/LinkFiles/Commision_on_Macroeconomic_and_Health_Bg_P2_Burden_of_Disease_Estimations_and_Casual_analysis.pdf (accessed 10 July 2010).

Ebrahim, S., Kinra, S., Bowen, L., Andersen, E., Ben-Shlomo, Y., Lyngdoh, T., Ramakrishnan, L., Ahuja, R.C., Joshi, P., Das, S.M., Mohan, M., Davey Smith, G., Prabhakaran, D. and Reddy, K.S. (2010) 'Indian Migration Study Group. The Effect of Rural-to-Urban Migration on Obesity and Diabetes in India: A Cross-sectional Study', *PLoS Medicine*, 7: e1000268. doi:10.1371/journal.pmed.1000268.

Gajalakshmi, V. and Peto, R. (2004) 'Verbal Autopsy of 80 000 Adult Deaths in Tamilnadu, South India', *BMC Public Health*, 4: 47.

Ghaffar, A., Reddy, K.S. and Singhi, M. (2004) 'Burden of Non Communicable Diseases in South Asia', *BMJ*, 328: 807–810.

Gupta, R. (2004) 'Trends in Hypertension Epidemiology in India', *Journal of Human Hypertension*, 18: 73–78.

Gupta, R. and Gupta, V.P. (2009) 'Hypertension Epidemiology in India: Lessons from Jaipur Heart Watch', *Current Science*, 97: 349–355.

Gupta, R., Joshi, P., Mohan, V., Reddy, K.S. and Yusuf, S. (2008) 'Epidemiology and Causation of Coronary Heart Disease and Stroke in India', *Heart*, 94: 16–26.

Gupta, R., Misra, A., Pais, P., Rastogi, P. and Gupta, V.P. (2006) 'Correlation of Regional Cardiovascular Disease Mortality in India with Lifestyle and Nutritional Factors', *International Journal of Cardiology*, 108: 291–300.

Gururaj, G. (2008) 'Road Traffic Deaths, Injuries and Disabilities in India: Current Scenario', *National Medical Journal of India*, 21: 14–20.

Haub, C. and Sharma, O.P. (2006) 'India's Population Reality: Reconciling Change and Tradition', *Population Bulletin*, 61: 4–10. Online, available at: www.prb.org/pdf06/61.3IndiasPopulationReality_Eng.pdf (accessed 30 July 2010).

*IDF Diabetes Atlas* (2009) 4th edn. Online, available at: www.diabetesatlas.org/ (accessed 20 July 2010).

'India: Urban Poverty Report 2009 Factsheet'. Online, available at: http://data.undp.org.in/poverty_reduction/Factsheet_IUPR_09a.pdf (accessed 5 July 2010).

International Institute for Population Sciences, World Health Organization (2006) (WHO)-India-WR Office. *World Health Survey, 2003*. Mumbai: IIPS.

International Institute for Population Sciences (2007) Macro International. *National Family Health Survey (NFHS-3) 2005–06*, Mumbai: IIPS.

Jha, P., Jacob, B., Gajalakshmi, V., Gupta, P.C., Dhingra, N., Kumar, R., Sinha, D.N., Dikshit, R.P., Parida, D.K., Kamadod, R., Boreham, J. and Peto, R. (2008) 'A Nationally Representative Case-control Study of Smoking and Death in India', *New England Journal of Medicine*, 358: 1137–1147.

Jindal, S.K., Aggarwal, A.N., Chaudhry, K., Chhabra, S.K., D'Souza, G.A., Gupta, D., Katiyar, S.K., Kumar, R., Shah, B. and Vijayan, V.K. (2006) 'Asthma Epidemiology Study Group: A Multicentric Study on Epidemiology of Chronic Obstructive Pulmonary Disease and its Relationship with Tobacco Smoking and Environmental Tobacco Smoke Exposure', *Indian Journal Chest Disease and Allied Sciences*, 48: 23–29.

Joshi, R., Cardona, M., Iyengar, S., Sukumar, A., Raju, C.R., Raju, K.R., Raju, K., Reddy, K.S., Lopez, A. and Neal, B. (2006) 'Chronic Diseases Now a Leading Cause of Death in Rural India: Mortality Data from the Andhra Pradesh Rural Health Initiative', *International Journal of Epidemiology*, 35: 1522–1529.

Joshi, R., Chow, C.K., Raju, P.K., Raju, R., Reddy, K.S., Macmahon, S., Lopez, A.D. and Neal, B. (2009) 'Fatal and Nonfatal Cardiovascular Disease and the Use of Therapies for Secondary Prevention in a Rural Region of India', *Circulation*, 119: 1950–1955.

Kar, S.S., Thaku, J.S., Virdi, N.K., Jain, S. and Kumar, R. (2010) 'Risk Factors for Cardiovascular Diseases: Is the Social Gradient Reversing in Northern India?' *National Medical Journal of India*, 23: 206–209.

Kopits, E. and Cropper, M. (2005) 'Traffic Fatalities and Economic Growth', *Accident Analysis and Prevention*, 37: 169–178.

Kulkarni, V.S. and Gaiha, R. (n.d.) 'India in Transition: Dietary Transition in India'. Online, available at: http://casi.ssc.upenn.edu/iit/kulkarnigaiha (accessed 7 August 2010).

Mendis, S., Abegunde, D., Yusuf, S., Ebrahim, S., Shaper, G., Ghannem, H. and Shengelia, B. (2005) 'WHO Study on Prevention of Recurrences of Myocardial Infarction and Stroke (WHO-PREMISE)', *Bulletin of the World Health Organization*, 83: 820–829.

Mishra, N.K. and Khadilkar, S.V. (2010) 'Stroke Program for India', *Annals of Indian Academy of Neurology*, 13: 28–32.

Misra, A., Pandey, R.M., Devi, J.R., Sharma, R., Vikram, N.K. and Khanna, N. (2001) 'High Prevalence of Diabetes, Obesity and Dyslipidaemia in Urban Slum Population in Northern India', *International Journal of Obesity and Related Metabolic Disorders*, 25: 1722–1729.

Mohan, V., Sandeep, S., Deepa, R., Shah, B. and Varghese, C. (2007) 'Epidemiology of Type 2 Diabetes: Indian Scenario', *Indian Journal of Medical Research*, 125: 217–230.

Murthy, K.J.R. and Sastry, J.G. (n.d.) 'Economic Burden of Chronic Obstructive Pulmonary Disease', NCMH Background Papers. Online, available at: www.whoindia.org/LinkFiles/Commision_on_Macroeconomic_and_Health_Bg_P2_Economic_burden_of_chronic_obstructive_pulmonary_disease.pdf (accessed 15 July 2010).

'National Programme for Prevention and Control of Cancer, Diabetes, Cardiovascular Diseases and Stroke (NPCDCS) approved' (2010) Press Information Bureau, Government of India, Press Release 8 July. Online, available at: http://pib.nic.in/release/release.asp?relid=63087&kwd= (accessed 10 August 2010).

Popkin, B.M. (2003) 'The Nutrition Transition in the Developing World', *Development Policy Review*, 21: 581–597.

Prabhakaran, D. and Ajay, V.S. (in press) 'Non-Communicable Diseases in India: A Perspective', World Bank Background Paper on Non-Communicable Diseases in India.

'Preventing Chronic Diseases: A Vital Investment' (2005) World Health Organization, Geneva. Online, available at: www.who.int/chp/chronic_disease_report/full_report.pdf (accessed 25 July 2010).

Ramachandran, A., Ma, R.C. and Snehalatha, C. (2010) 'Diabetes in Asia', *Lancet*, 375: 408–418.

Ramachandran, A., Snehalatha, C., Latha, E., Vijay, V. and Viswanathan, M. (1997) 'Rising Prevalence of NIDDM in an Urban Population in India', *Diabetologia*, 40: 232–237.

Rastogi, T., Jha, P., Reddy, K.S., Prabhakaran, D., Spiegelman, D., Stampfer, M.J., Willett, W.C. and Ascherio, A. (2005) 'Bidi and Cigarette Smoking and Risk of Acute Myocardial Infarction among Males in Urban India', *Tobacco Control*, 14: 356–358.

Reddy, K.S. (2007) 'India Wakes up to the Threat of Cardiovascular Diseases', *Journal of the American College of Cardiology*, 50: 1370–1372.

Reddy, K.S. and Gupta, P.C. (eds) (2004) *Report on Tobacco Control in India*, New Delhi: Ministry of Health and Family Welfare.

Reddy, K.S., Perry, C.L., Stigler, M.H. and Arora, M. (2006a) 'Differences in Tobacco Use among Young People in Urban India by Sex, Socioeconomic Status, Age, and School Grade: Assessment of Baseline Survey Data', *Lancet*, 367: 589–594.

Reddy, K.S., Prabhakaran, D., Chaturvedi, V., Jeemon, P., Thankappan, K.R., Ramakrishnan, L., Mohan, B.V., Pandav, C.S., Ahmed, F.U., Joshi, P.P., Meera, R., Amin, R.B., Ahuja, R.C., Das, M.S. and Jaison, T.M. (2006b) 'Methods for Establishing a Surveillance System for Cardiovascular Diseases in Indian Industrial Populations', *Bulletin of the World Health Organization*, 84: 461–469.

Reddy, K.S., Prabhakaran, D., Jeemon, P., Thankappan, K.R., Joshi, P., Chaturvedi, V., Ramakrishnan, L. and Ahmed, F. (2007) 'Educational Status and Cardiovascular Risk Profile in Indians', *Proceedings of the National Academy of Sciences USA*, 104: 16263–16268.

Reddy, K.S., Shah, B., Varghese, C. and Ramadoss, A. (2005) 'Responding to the Threat of Chronic Diseases in India', *Lancet*, 366: 1744–1749.

Satyanarayana, L. and Asthana, S. (2008) 'Life Time Risk for Development of Ten Major Cancers in India and its Trends over the Years 1982 to 2000', *Indian Journal of Medical Sciences*, 62: 35–44.

Shah, B., Kumar, N., Menon, G.R., Khurana, S. and Kumar, H. (n.d.) 'Assessment of Burden of Non-Communicable Diseases', Indian Council of Medical Research, New Delhi. Online, available at: www.whoindia.org/EN/Section20/Section306_1025.htm (accessed 10 August 2010).

Sharma, K.K., Gupta, R., Agrawal, A., Roy, S., Kasliwal, A., Bana, A., Tongia, R.K. and Deedwania, P.C. (2009) 'Low Use of Statins and Other Coronary Secondary Prevention Therapies in Primary and Secondary Care in India', *Vascular Health and Risk Management*, 5: 1007–1014.

Shetty, P.S. (2002) 'Nutrition Transition in India', *Public Health Nutrition*, 5: 175–182.

Smith, G.D. (2007) 'Life-course Approaches to Inequalities in Adult Chronic Disease Risk', *Proceedings of the Nutrition Society*, 66: 216–236.

Soman, C.R., Kutty, V.R., Safraj, S., Vijayakumar, K., Rajamohanan, K. and Ajayan, K. (2011) 'All-Cause Mortality and Cardiovascular Mortality in Kerala State of India: Results From a 5-Year Follow-up of 161 942 Rural Community Dwelling Adults', *Asia Pacific Journal of Public Health*, 23: 896–903.

Thankappan, K.R. and Mini, G.K. (2008) 'Case-control Study of Smoking and Death in India', *New England Journal of Medicine*, 358: 2842–2843.

Thankappan, K.R. and Valiathan, M.S. (1998) 'Health at Low Cost: The Kerala Model', *Lancet*, 351: 1274–1275.

Thankappan, K.R., Shah, B., Mathur, P., Sarma, P.S., Srinivas, G., Mini, G.K., Daivadanam, M., Soman, B. and Vasan, R.S. (2010) 'Risk Factor Profile for Chronic Non-Communicable Diseases: Results of a Community-based Study in Kerala, India', *Indian Journal of Medical Research*, 131: 53–63.

Thankappan, K.R., Sivasankaran, S., Sarma, P.S., Mini, G., Khader, S.A., Padmanabhan, P. and Vasan, R. (2006) 'Prevalence-Correlates-Awareness-Treatment and Control of Hypertension in Kumarakom, Kerala: Baseline Results of a Community-based Intervention Program', *Indian Heart Journal*, 58: 28–33.

Tharkar, S., Devarajan, A., Kumpatla, S. and Viswanathan, V. (2010) 'The Socioeconomics of Diabetes from a Developing Country: A Population based Cost of Illness Study', *Diabetes Research and Clinical Practice*, 89: 334–340.

UNDP, Ministry of Housing and Urban Poverty Alleviation (2009) 'India: Urban Poverty Report', Oxford University Press. Online, available at: www.undp.org.in/sites/default/files/INDIA-URBAN-POVERTY-REPORT-2009.pdf (accessed 1 August 2010).

Varghese, C. (n.d.) 'Cancer Prevention and Control in India'. Online, available at: http://mohfw.nic.in/pg56to67.pdf (accessed 10 July 2010).

Vijayakumar, G., Arun, R. and Kutty, V.R. (2009) 'High Prevalence of Type 2 Diabetes Mellitus and Other Metabolic Disorders in Rural Central Kerala', *Journal of Association of Physicians of India*, 57: 563–567.

Wang, Y., Chen, H.J., Shaikh, S. and Mathur, P. (2009) 'Is Obesity Becoming a Public Health Problem in India? Examine the Shift from Under- to Overnutrition Problems Over Time', *Obesity Reviews*, 10: 456–474.

World Health Organization (2004) *The Atlas of Heart Disease and Stroke*, Geneva: World Health Organization.

# 5 The double disease burden in Asia and the Pacific

## Japan and its diseases

*Mahito Fukuda*

## Introduction

If longevity is viewed as a general indicator of health, then Japan, the nation with the world's highest life expectancy, might be considered the healthiest place on earth. In the interest of maintaining health and longevity, the Japanese have traditionally paid considerable attention to the welfare and soundness of the body. At the same time, sometimes steadily, at other times in dramatic leaps attending broader historical events, there has been considerable change. Of course, the history of health in Japan is not entirely divorced from the history of other countries in the Asia-Pacific region, or in the world for that matter, from the influence of ancient Chinese health practices to the dramatic impact of Western style medicine in the nineteenth century, then on into the era of globalization with its own pressing health issues. Nevertheless, the story of health in Japan is substantially different from those of most of its Asian neighbours. Many health advances came earlier and were more quickly integrated into Japanese culture than elsewhere; it does not today have the same double burden of both poverty- and wealth-related diseases, or at least to the same extent.

However, this is not to say that everything is well. In a sense, Japan's very success, as marked by its citizens' renowned longevity, has been and remains the source of some of its potentially most crippling problems. There has been a marked historical inversion, from a traditional regime of high fertility and high mortality to one of low fertility and low mortality and this has brought with it urgent demographically driven issues, most notably those associated with a rapidly ageing population. Meanwhile, as will be discussed later in this chapter, its remarkable economic progress has been bought at the cost of environment- and lifestyle-related diseases. In addition, since the country has been in recession for well over a decade, all of the above now exist in the context of considerable economic uncertainty and stress.

I cannot hope to provide here an exhaustive history of health and medicine in Japan, but in the pages that follow an attempt will be made to sketch some of the key points of modern cultural change, events that can be said to have played an especially important role in bringing about the health situation of the country today. From there I would like to examine the crucial issues that have emerged in contemporary Japan around the subjects of health and medical care. It is hoped that marking points at which Japan diverges from its neighbours, as well as those areas in which it shares some common ground with them, will help in a small way towards our creation of a complex, nuanced picture of health issues in the region.

## Historical background: traditional Edo to Westernized Meiji

Historically, Japanese healthcare was heavily influenced by Chinese medicine, transmitted through Korea, beginning in the fifth century, when it adopted the Chinese medical system as well as its botanical knowledge and herbal medicines, some aspects of which are still used today. Tea drinking became feverishly fashionable among the ruling classes as well as commoners following the teaching of the Zen religious sect from the end of the twelfth century. A tradition of eating only vegetables, derived from Buddhism, was dominant in Japanese society from its introduction to Japan in the sixth century till the end of the Edo Era (1603–1868). However, with more than two centuries of isolation policy (1633–1858) under the Edo Shogunate, public health concepts such as those being developed in European countries were not familiar to the pre-modern Japanese.

Nevertheless, the Japanese people placed value on living a long life. They were consequently keen to maintain their good health, and although scientifically founded ideas about nutrition were not available, they followed Chinese tradition in having an awareness of the value of certain foods and beverages, even pure water. The idea of a health regimen (*yojo*) was common in the culture, embracing such issues as exercising the body, sleeping in suitable conditions, thinking appropriately, even having sexual intercourse the right way. As for hygiene, the picture is not so clear: there was no science of hygiene and in some respects conditions were certainly unhygienic, yet the Japanese could sometimes exhibit a certain degree of scrupulousness concerning personal cleanliness. Throughout the long Edo period there was little change in health practices due to the dominance of traditional Chinese medicine. The main guardians of health were almost all Chinese doctors, who put much emphasis on health practices based on the idea of *Ki* (Chi) and the lessons of *Shoukanron* (*The Discussion on Fevers*); this is considered the first complete clinical textbook, written by Zhang Zhongjing and published in the third century AD. Chinese acupuncture, moxibustion and massage were very popular among ordinary people as ways to maintain physical and mental health.

Both birth rates and death rates are believed to have been low in Japan through the seventeenth and eighteenth centuries, an unusual phenomenon for a pre-industrial society, but it would account for Japan's stable, or only very gradually increasing, population in that period (Hanley and Yamamura 1977: 317). The low death rate was due to some degree to the fact that because its isolation policy and its geographic location restricted interaction with the outside world, the country was relatively safe from pandemics of cholera and other communicable diseases taking terrible tolls elsewhere. Japan was hardly some Shangri-la of health, however. Despite the abovementioned concern with certain health practices among Chinese medical practitioners and some of the general populace, even in the late Edo period the average Japanese often lived in insanitary living conditions; many suffered from malnutrition due to agricultural shortfalls and the policies of an oppressive political regime; there was no public health system and neither preventive nor prophylactic medicine; religious or superstitious beliefs held sway among a good number of the people. The situation would soon change considerably, however, in terms of both healthcare and disease.

Before Japan ended its self-imposed isolation policy in the middle of the nineteenth century it had actually allowed limited intercourse with the outside world for some time through designated trade ports on its west coast, namely Dejima in Nagasaki and Hirado. It was through these limited channels that Western science, including Western medicine, was first introduced to Japan, particularly through what was called *Rangaku* (Dutch education), extending through much of the nineteenth century. Despite the fact that other foreigners were able to visit Nagasaki, such as the Chinese and some Germans passing themselves off as Dutch, the Dutch were the only Europeans who were allowed to come, stay in Japan and trade with the Japanese. They not only engaged in trading goods but were also responsible for introducing Western culture, including medical knowledge. A number of books on pharmacology and anatomy were translated from Dutch, German and Latin into Japanese, but such knowledge was available only to a very limited and elite group and cannot be said to have permeated the culture.

It was only when, under military and political duress, Japan finally opened its doors to the outside world in 1854 that information as well as technology, some of it medical, began to move more freely about the country, although even then many citizens were too poor to consult a doctor or receive medicine. That would be a serious problem, because the foreigners brought with them not just gifts of knowledge but serious infectious diseases. In the early years of the Meiji Era (1868–1912), infectious diseases had a devastating impact. Dysentery, cholera, typhoid, typhus and smallpox were among the most virulent diseases, with a combined death toll exceeding more than 100,000 people (see Table 5.1). The average Japanese lifespan at this time was actually reduced.

At the same time, all sorts of Western ideas came into Japan, including medical practice and education. A fierce struggle ensued between traditional Chinese medicine and the newly imported Western style theory and practices. With the establishment of the Medical System (*Isei*) in the Fifth Year of Meiji (1873), only those who had received Western medical training could obtain a medical licence to practise. The shift from Chinese traditional medicine to the newly introduced Western medicine influenced the whole course of science and the attitudes of the people towards diseases and medical practices.

Western medicine was officially adopted by the new government and it became dominant throughout Japan under government orders. Traditional medicine was brusquely cast aside as old-fashioned. Western doctors were invited to

*Table 5.1* Number of patients and deaths from infectious diseases, 1876–1899

| Meiji | Year | Cholera | | Dysentry | | Typhoid | | Smallpox | |
|---|---|---|---|---|---|---|---|---|---|
| | | Patients | Deaths | Patients | Deaths | Patients | Deaths | Patients | Deaths |
| 9 | 1876 | – | | 976 | 76 | 869 | 108 | 318 | 145 |
| 10 | 1877 | 13,816 | 8,027 | 349 | 38 | 1,964 | 141 | 3,441 | 653 |
| 11 | 1878 | 902 | 275 | 1,078 | 181 | 4,092 | 558 | 2,896 | 685 |
| 12 | 1879 | 162,637 | 105,786 | 8,167 | 1,477 | 10,652 | 2,530 | 4,799 | 1,295 |
| 13 | 1880 | 1,580 | 618 | 5,047 | 1,305 | 17,140 | 4,177 | 3,415 | 1,731 |
| 14 | 1881 | 9,389 | 6,237 | 6,827 | 1,802 | 16,999 | 4,203 | 342 | 34 |
| 15 | 1882 | 51,631 | 33,784 | 4,330 | 1,313 | 17,308 | 5,231 | 1,106 | 197 |
| 16 | 1883 | 669 | 434 | 20,172 | 5,066 | 18,769 | 5,043 | 1,271 | 295 |
| 17 | 1884 | 904 | 417 | 22,702 | 6,036 | 23,279 | 5,969 | 1,703 | 410 |
| 18 | 1885 | 13,824 | 9,329 | 47,307 | 10,690 | 29,504 | 6,672 | 12,759 | 3,329 |
| 19 | 1886 | 155,923 | 108,405 | 24,326 | 6,839 | 66,224 | 13,807 | 73,337 | 18,678 |
| 20 | 1887 | 1,228 | 654 | 16,147 | 4,257 | 47,449 | 9,813 | 39,779 | 9,967 |
| 21 | 1888 | 811 | 410 | 26,815 | 6,576 | 43,600 | 9,211 | 4,052 | 853 |
| 22 | 1889 | 751 | 431 | 22,873 | 5,970 | 35,849 | 8,623 | 1,324 | 328 |
| 23 | 1890 | 46,019 | 35,227 | 42,633 | 8,706 | 34,736 | 8,464 | 296 | 25 |
| 24 | 1891 | 11,142 | 7,760 | 46,358 | 11,208 | 43,967 | 9,614 | 3,608 | 721 |
| 25 | 1892 | 874 | 497 | 70,842 | 16,844 | 35,636 | 8,529 | 33,779 | 8,409 |
| 26 | 1893 | 633 | 364 | 167,305 | 41,284 | 34,069 | 8,183 | 41,898 | 11,852 |
| 27 | 1894 | 546 | 314 | 155,140 | 38,094 | 36,667 | 8,054 | 12,418 | 3,342 |
| 28 | 1895 | 55,154 | 40,154 | 52,711 | 12,959 | 37,015 | 8,401 | 1,284 | 268 |
| 29 | 1896 | 1,481 | 907 | 85,876 | 22,356 | 42,505 | 9,174 | 10,704 | 3,388 |
| 30 | 1897 | 894 | 488 | 91,077 | 23,763 | 26,998 | 5,697 | 41,946 | 12,276 |
| 31 | 1898 | 655 | 374 | 90,976 | 22,392 | 25,297 | 5,697 | 1,752 | 362 |
| 32 | 1899 | 829 | 487 | 108,713 | 23,763 | 27,673 | 6,452 | 1,215 | 245 |

Source: Kosheisho Imukyoku 1976: 544–545.

take up temporary positions in Japan as *Oyatoi Gaikokujin Kyoshi* (hired foreign teachers) to create medical schools at the newly built Japanese universities, and students were also sent abroad to study in Western countries such as Germany, Britain and France in order to acquire the latest medical knowledge and techniques. The European influence was so strong, in fact, that from the Meiji period through to the end of the Second World War, German was a mandatory foreign language for Japanese students of medicine. Patient medical cards in Japanese teaching hospitals were even written in German. In 1875, the Law Concerning the National Qualification Examination of Medical Doctors was promulgated. Training was professionalized according to a biomedical model of disease formed in the West, and Chinese-style herbalists were required to become licensed medical doctors in order to practise.

Under the influence of Western style modernization, the daily life of the average Japanese changed rapidly from the Meiji Era in ways that would have an important impact on public health. The introduction of innovations such as vaccines brought improvement in the average life expectancy. The idea of hygiene changed from a focus on a personal regimen to public health, from personal welfare to the welfare of the masses. The water supply and drainage systems improved immensely. The first water purification plant was built in Yokohama by a British engineer, Henry Spencer Palmer (1838–1893), who later had a second one constructed in Hakodate and then many others in different cities. A water drainage system was introduced under the planning of a British public health engineer William Kinninmond Burton (1856–1899). In 1877, Burton was invited by the Meiji Government to become the first Professor of Sanitary Engineering and a lecturer in Rivers, Docks and Harbours at the Imperial University of Tokyo. Later he became Resident Engineer to the London Sanitary Protection Association.

As mentioned at the outset, a thorough survey of modern Japanese medical history is beyond the scope of this chapter, but an understanding of the cultural changes wrought by intensified interaction with foreigners, by diseases, and by responses to them may be served by examining specific examples of public health issues. One such instance concerns the problem that arose around syphilis, a major sexually transmitted disease.

According to a noted physician, Sugita Genpaku (1733–1817) in the Edo Era, a staggering 700 to 800 out of 1,000 patients had syphilis, which was a difficult condition to cure in those days and would continue to be a serious public health issue well into the Meiji Era. Christian missionaries naturally had much to say about this, including one James Curtis Hepburn (1815–1911), who remarked in his journals that it seemed to be 'one of the hereditary sins of the Japanese people' (Hepburn 1955: 126). A Dutch doctor, Johannes Lijdius Catharinus Pompe van Meerdervoort (1829–1908), generally known as Pompe, proposed to the Shogunate government the abolition of prostitution and the introduction of a medical examination for syphilis as early as 1857 but his suggestion was bitterly rejected. Under his guidance, though, many Japanese doctors learned how to examine venereal disease by direct inspection of the genital organs, especially of prostitutes.

Significantly, the first official examination was carried out in Inasa, Nagasaki, in 1860 for the purpose of preventing the disease from being transmitted to Russian frigate crews. It was far from being a simply domestic issue, then. Through the widespread use of prostitutes by foreigners ashore in Japan it became an international issue in a sense and, more to the point, a military concern. It is no surprise that the first collective countermeasures were sought and implemented by the Western battalions stationed in Japan. The French battalion stationed in Yokosuka near Yokohama was the first, in 1867, to undertake systematic venereal disease examinations, focusing on prostitutes servicing French crews, under the guidance of the French army doctor, Paul Amédée Ludovic Savatier (1830–1891).

In 1868, the British battalion stationed in Yokohama likewise came to realize how serious the problem was. The navy surgeon, George Bruce Newton (1829–1871) petitioned the Edo government to conduct genital examinations of prostitutes in the area, a proposal that again met great resistance. He finally succeeded in instituting methods for examining syphilis patients and in establishing the first Lock Hospital, an institution designed especially for the treatment of VD,[1] in September 1868. Other such hospitals were set up in the port cities of Hyogo (Kobe) and Nagasaki in succeeding years in a concerted effort to combat a disease that had become a critical matter for both military and civilian populations.

In part due to the concerns of the British army and navy, the Contagious Diseases Act had been passed in Britain in 1864 as the VD problem was intensifying. The aim was to secure the health of soldiers and officers of the Imperial Army and Navy as well as factory workers. Resistance to this campaign from the Edo government was quite strong, but it paled in comparison to the reaction from the prostitutes. Having never been examined in any way before, the women considered such treatment a gross intrusion and embarrassment. The idea of medical examinations was not prevalent in Japan at that time nor was the idea of 'infectiousness' familiar to the Japanese; similarly, notions of medication and prevention were unfamiliar. The entire conceptualization of disease was in more than one sense 'foreign' in a time and place when diseases still tended to be accepted as fate or as a curse born of the immoral deeds of ancestors.[2]

Nonetheless, it would be a mistake to conclude that the considerable resistance to the new measures – notably stronger than in Europe – was entirely due to ignorance and pre-modern attitudes. First, these policies, which were extraordinarily invasive of both individual privacy and national sovereignty, were being led by the military, which would have given them an especially aggressive tenor. Moreover, the Japanese, who had not at the time established politically, let alone psychologically, a modern sense of the nation state, did not accede as readily as Europeans might have to the assumption that the practical imperatives of the armed forces and captains of industry must be granted absolute priority.

Another important medical problem, and a useful historical narrative in terms of elucidating the changing concepts of disease and health along with the cultural climate of the time, concerns beriberi (*kakke*). Many people were suffering from this disease, yet medicine was not able to conclusively establish the cause. Bacteriology was in the process of being recognized within medical circles as well as by the general public. The miasmatic theory retained a profound influence upon medical thought, while there were still superstitiously inclined citizens who regarded the disease as a form of divine punishment.

Dr Takaki Kanehiro (1849–1920), a navy physician, maintained that nutritional deficiency was responsible for beriberi (considered endemic to Japan), a serious problem on warships that thus affected naval efficiency. Takaki knew that beriberi was not common in Western navies.[3] He also noticed that Japanese naval officers, whose diet consisted of various types of vegetables and meat, rarely suffered from the disease. On the other hand, it was common among ordinary crewmen, whose diet consisted almost exclusively of white rice.

In 1883 Takaki learned of a very high incidence of beriberi among cadets on a nine-month training mission from Japan to Hawaii: 169 of the 376 men onboard developed the disease and 25 died. Adopting a statistical approach responsible for earlier breakthroughs in Western medical history, combined with his nutritional hypothesis, Takaki undertook an experiment with an improved diet for seamen that included more meat, milk, bread and vegetables. This succeeded in reducing the number of beriberi cases and convinced Naval Headquarters that poor diet was the prime factor. Through nutritional changes, the disease was soon eliminated from the fleet.

It is significant, however, that here too there was resistance despite demonstrable progress, and this time from within the military and educational establishments. Although Takaki clearly established that the cause was nutritional (what we now know as Vitamin B1 deficiency), this conflicted with the prevailing opinion among medical scientists that beriberi was an infectious or hereditary disease. Indeed, the Imperial Japanese Army, dominated by doctors from Tokyo Imperial University, persisted in the belief that it was an infectious disease caused by an unidentified bacillus; they maintained that only laboratory-based data, not statistics, could be regarded as legitimate scientific evidence. For decades they refused to implement a remedy. In the Russo-Japanese War (1904–1905), 211,600 soldiers suffered from beriberi and 27,000 died, compared to 47,000 deaths in combat.

Apart from an institutional conservatism which is not unique to Japan but has long had a peculiar sway there, the main impediment in this case was conceptual: the notion of vitamins had not yet been developed. Dr Suzuki Umetaro (1874–1943) discovered the new material and named it *Oryzanin* in 1910. Two years later it was given the now more well-known name 'vitamin', coined from Latin by a Polish biochemist, Kazimierz Funk (1884–1967). It is noteworthy that Takaki's success occurred ten years before Christiaan Eijkman (1858–1930), working in Batavia in Indonesia, advanced his theory that beriberi was caused by a nutritional deficiency; his later identification of vitamin B1 as the key factor earned him the 1929 Nobel Prize in Physiology and Medicine. What is clear from all this, from Takaki through to Suzuki, is that Japanese medical science was becoming a force in its own right. In the long run, the commitment to training of doctors and researchers would allow the Japanese as a people to wrest back control of their health.

There is little question, though, that the impact of systematic Western intervention in health was enormous and the degree and speed of social change was such that some Japanese were naturally disconcerted. In developing its own health system and institutions, there were of course mistakes. At first, medical measures and hygiene policy-making were the responsibility of the Interior Ministry along with the police forces. When cholera epidemics occurred, police would lay siege to the area, closing off houses with picket lines and cleansing the area with a thoroughness and severity deemed appropriate given the gravity of the matter. This kind of response generated a general fear and a reluctance to cooperate among the ordinary people, which in turn led to low levels of reporting of infectious diseases. A survey conducted as late as 1940 showed that only 22,827 cases of TB were reported nationally when the number of deaths was 153,154, whereas in England and Wales, 71,745 cases were reported with 38,173 deaths and in Prussia, 44,051 cases with 21,400 deaths (Kondo 1948: 217).

The formation of the Ministry of Health in the Third Year of Showa (1928) marked a general shift in the course of public health measures in Japan. Policy-making became the domain of specialized public health officials, trained in combating diseases and applying prophylactic measures.

A total of 1,300 designated health centres (*Hokenjo*) were constructed throughout the country, with the primary aim of addressing communicable diseases, especially tuberculosis, the number one cause of mortality at the time. Because of low levels of reporting, it was believed that for each recognized TB sufferer there were at least ten more among the ordinary people.[4] Ishikawa Prefecture was the primary locale addressing the tuberculosis problem in the early years of Showa because its TB death and morbidity rates were the highest in Japan, a consequence of the Prefecture's inadequate facilities and countermeasures against the disease. There were insufficient beds available for TB patients and preventive measures were simply inadequate. For example, the number of TB patients was 6,140 and the number of beds in hospitals in Kanazawa City was just 80 in 1944. The number of beds per 100 TB patients was 1.3, whereas in Tokyo the number was 16.2 beds per 100 patients (Ishikawa Prefecture 1936: 44) The measures brought to bear by the central government were:

- propaganda – picture card shows, movies and leaflets on health issues;
- increasing the number of hospitals;
- forming a group of itinerant medical check-up workers;
- increasing the number of healthcare centres and workers;
- enlightenment through health education in elementary schools;
- building up a reporting system among doctors, schools and families.

The network of health centres set up by the Ministry of Health functioned to investigate and monitor the health of the public and to give advice to patients and their families about how to combat diseases. This new network was actually very efficient not only in controlling TB, but also in improving the general health of the public. It was responsible for the quality of the water supply, food, collecting garbage and so forth. The infant mortality rate was lowered dramatically, which contributed to a marked improvement in life expectancy at birth. Through the medical centres and general education, new medical ideas and more sophisticated notions of hygiene gradually permeated the society. These, along with certain long-held traditions such as bathing everyday in order to cleanse the body in Japan's humid climate, would lead eventually to the hyper-hygienic society of today.

## Health in contemporary Japan

Modernization, including urbanization and industrialization, continued apace in Japan through the early twentieth century, although resources were increasingly directed towards militarist and imperialist enterprises that placed a strain on a nation still building infrastructure and national wealth. The military adventures took a severe toll, not only in terms of deaths and injuries on the battlefield, and the devastation in the Second World War resulting from Allied bombing, but the general health of the populace. As a result of consecutive wars, the people experienced relatively poor health, with a high incidence of tuberculosis and diseases related to malnutrition.

It is well known that following the Second World War Japan made extraordinary progress in economic development. Attending this, and continuing the advances that had been underway for decades before the war, the health of the populace enjoyed a rapid improvement under the leadership of governmental health institutions and financed by economic expansion. The stronger and more confident economic environment, constant improvements in medical services and technology, as well as changes in the diet and lifestyle of the people, brought significant positive results, reflected in a lower death rate and a higher birth rate than before.

Medical education continued to develop along Western lines, with doctors being required to undertake considerable study in order to succeed in the stringent national qualification examinations. A national health system emerged under an 'insurance for all' policy, to the point where today it is compulsory for all citizens to be enrolled in an insurance programme. There are two main complementary systems: *Kokumin Kenkō Hoken* (National Health Insurance) is generally for self-employed people and students, while *Kenkō-Hoken* ([Social] Health Insurance) is typically for corporate employees. Patients are able to choose doctors, clinics or hospitals freely, and to a certain extent their fees are covered by their insurance. Those who cannot afford to pay such fees are covered by the *Seikatsu Hogo Ho* (Life Protection Law) which among other things guarantees medical expenses are covered.

This is not to say that the Japanese approach to health has become entirely beholden to the West. Old customs and manners are still preserved even among many young people. Today people who become ill in Japan have a number of options. Apart from visiting a Western style doctor, a person may seek the assistance of traditional healers such as herbalists, masseurs, moxibustionists and acupuncturists. He or she may visit a priest or send a family member in his or her place. Chemical and herbal over-the-counter medications from the East and West are readily available and numerous traditional folk remedies are still shared. *Onsen* (hot spring baths) remain a very conspicuous part of the culture as a place for curing ailments as well as bodily and mental regeneration.

Generally speaking, then, people's health, as well as the range of their healthcare options, improved enormously through the twentieth century. The innovations in public health, along with a private concern with healthcare among citizens, led to Japan having the world's highest life expectancy at birth today: 85.6 years for females and 80.5 for males. However, in somewhat the same way as coming out of isolation in the middle of the nineteenth century brought both revolutionary health improvement and devastating catastrophes of communicable disease, so have the economic and health successes of the twentieth century brought with them serious negative consequences, particularly in the form of the rise of non-communicable diseases.

It should be noted that Japan's 'economic miracle' of rapid industrialization has sometimes been achieved at the expense of the natural environment, which may provide salutary lessons for Asian neighbours now undergoing speedy economic transformation. Many of the environmental repercussions are not immediately apparent, and may take decades or even centuries to emerge into the public consciousness. In other cases, the effects are more readily discerned, if rather too late, because the impact upon humans living in that environment is severe. There are two conspicuous examples in post-War Japanese history which are illustrative of the fact that regardless of medical technology and techniques, humans are inextricably connected to and dependent upon the health of their environment.

The first case, Minamata disease, refers to the outbreak of neurological disorders caused by ethyl mercury in industrial wastewater released into Minamato Bay by the Chisso Corporation from 1956 until 1973. The main symptoms are a narrowing of the field of vision, debilitating effects upon speech and hearing, psychological illness and paralysis. The other egregious case was Yokkaichi Zensoku (asthma), which was caused primarily by sulfur oxide in gases released by petroleum refineries in Yokkaichi city in Mie Prefecture from 1960 to 1972. This produced severe cases of chronic obstructive pulmonary disease, chronic bronchitis, pulmonary emphysema and bronchial asthma. Due in part to the seriously debilitating effects of these industrially sourced diseases, the Japanese government decided eventually to implement Air Pollution Control Laws in 1968, limiting exhaust from factories. In both of these cases the government was incredibly slow in instituting effective measures and promulgating laws limiting the activity of the factories contaminating the environment. It was not until well into the 1970s that non-governmental organizations formed to combat effectively such disasters and to help protect the health of the general public.

In many cases, determining the impact of industry upon the health of the environment and humans is more complicated since the effects may be not only slowly progressive but indirect and/or may be lost within a welter of other possible contributing factors. The collection and analysis of medical statistics have played an important role in this regard, both in discerning specific local instances of certain health problems and in identifying broad national trends. Statistics also allow the national and regional governments to determine health policy effectiveness and future strategies. For over a century Japan's various government agencies have devoted considerable resources to the recording of health data that pinpoint key problems and historical trends. From the beginning of the census in 1899, pneumonia, bronchitis, tuberculosis and gastroenteritis were the major causes of death in Japan, but their impact receded from around 1950. With medical treatment improving in those areas, cerebrovascular disease became the primary cause of mortality (see Table 5.2).

A clear picture of the most serious health issues in contemporary Japan is provided by the Ministry of Health and Welfare. The major causes of mortality as of 2000 were as follow:

- Malignant tumour (295,484 deaths; 235.2 per 100,000 population; 30.7% of total deaths)
- Cardiovascular disease (146,741; 116.8; 15.3%)
- Cerebrovascular disease (132,529; 105.5; 13.8%)
- Pneumonia (86,938; 69.2; 9.0%)
- Injuries (39,484; 31.4; 4.1%)
- Suicide (30,251; 24.1; 3.1%)
- Decrepitude (senility) (21,213; 16.9; 2.2%)
      (Jinko Tokei Shiryo (Population Statistical Databook) 2010: 5–21)

Below are figures for 2008. Of a total of 1.142 million deaths, malignant tumours (cancers) were by a considerable margin the major cause of death. In fact, this has been the case since 1981, but now the number is twice as high as that of cardiovascular disease:

- Malignant tumor (342,963 deaths; 272.3 per 100,000 population; 30.0% of total deaths)
- Cardiovascular disease (181,928; 144.4; 15.9%)
- Cerebrovascular disease (127,023; 100.9; 11.1%)
- Pneumonia (115,317; 91.6; 10.1%)
- Injuries (38,153; 30.3; 3.3%)
- Suicide (30,229; 24.0; 2.6%)
- Decrepitude (senility) (35,975; 28.6; 3.1%)
      (Jinko Tokei Shiryo (Population Statistical Databook) 2010: 5–21)

So cancer, having increased sharply over the past half century, is now responsible for nearly one-third of deaths. The number of deaths as well as mortality rates in 2005 were around four times what they were half a century earlier. Overall, 32,670 males and 31,758 females died from some form of cancer in 1950 (a mortality rate of 77.7 per 100,000 population), whereas the figures were 196,603 males and 129,338 females (a mortality rate of 260.4 per 100,000) in 2005. One of the key cancers is lung cancer and the recorded death toll stood at 789 males and 330 females (1.35 per 100,000) in 1950, but by 2005 it had soared to 45,189 males and 16,874 females (49.95 per 100,000), a nearly 40-fold increase over a half century. Today, in general, about half of men and one-third of women will suffer from cancer in their lifetime.

While the number of deaths and the mortality rate of stomach cancer rose somewhat over this period, those for lung cancer show a 60-fold increase for men and a 37-fold increase for women. The core reasons cited for the overall increase in cancer deaths are:

- population concentration in the urban areas where the air is polluted due to heavy traffic and exhaust from houses and other buildings;
- toxic and otherwise harmful fumes from industrial areas;
- certain chemical compounds used in the workplace and domestic environments;
- tobacco smoking, especially in relation to the incidence of lung cancer.

A silent epidemic of sexually transmitted diseases (chlamydia, genital herpes, gonorrhoea and human papillomavirus) is spreading among the nation's sexually active young. AIDS cases in the past decade have reached a level that has confounded and alarmed the health establishment in Japan. The first HIV case was reported in 1979 and the first AIDS case in 1985. By 2010, totals recorded were 12,050 for HIV and 5,542 for AIDS. These figures include 1,439 haemophiliac patients who were infected with HIV due to the use of contaminated blood products imported from the United States (AIDS Yobo Joho Net 2010: Table 5.2) and are not high compared to those in other countries, but the morbidity rate has been increasing rapidly among the young, especially males under 35 years. A survey by UNAIDS showed that only 17.2 per cent of Japanese believed that the government was executing effective countermeasures against HIV/AIDS, whereas the figures were 70 per cent in Senegal, 59.6 per cent in the United States, 54.8 per cent in China, 51.5 per cent in the United Kingdom and 40.3 per cent in India (Sidibé 2010: 5).

Despite this apparent concern, and perhaps because the number of AIDS cases remains relatively small by international standards, it tends to be widely believed within Japan that HIV/AIDS is not a serious problem. Therefore, although AIDS education is mandatory in schools, most Japanese are largely indifferent to the issue. At the same time, there remains a social stigma attached to the disease which is inhibiting effective countermeasures. These varied and sometimes conflicting factors make it difficult to predict what will happen next to Japan. Suffice to say, however, that given that Asia, relatively unaffected by the problem until the 1990s, now has nearly 4.7 million people with either HIV or AIDS, this is not a problem that Japan or its neighbours can ignore.

*Table 5.2*  Causes of death (per 100,000 population)

| | No. 1 | | No. 2 | | No. 3 | | No. 4 | | No. 5 | | No. 6 | | No. 7 | | No. 8 | | No. 9 | | No. 10 | |
|---|---|---|---|---|---|---|---|---|---|---|---|---|---|---|---|---|---|---|---|---|
| | Cause | Death rate | Cause | Death rate | Cause | Death rate | Cause | Death rate | Cause | Death rate | Cause | Death rate | Cause | Death rate | Cause | Death rate | Cause | Death rate | Cause | Death rate |
| 1899 | P & B | 206.1 | CEVD | 170.5 | TB | 155.7 | G | 149.7 | D | 127.2 | — | — | — | — | — | — | — | — | — | — |
| 1900 | P & B | 226.1 | CEVD | 163.7 | CEVD | 159.2 | G | 133.8 | D | 131 | — | — | — | — | — | — | — | — | — | — |
| 1905 | P & B | 247.4 | TB | 206 | CEVD | 163.4 | D | 139.9 | G | 137.2 | — | — | — | — | — | — | — | — | — | — |
| 1910 | P & B | 262 | TB | 230.2 | G | 213.4 | CEVD | 131.9 | D | 120.2 | — | — | — | — | — | — | — | — | — | — |
| 1915 | P & B | 261.1 | TB | 223.7 | TB | 219.7 | CEVD | 128.8 | D | 112.5 | — | — | — | — | — | — | — | — | — | — |
| 1920 | P & B | 408 | G | 254.2 | TB | 223.7 | Influenza | 193.7 | CEVD | 157.6 | — | — | — | — | — | — | — | — | — | — |
| 1925 | P & B | 275.6 | G | 238.2 | TB | 194.1 | CEVD | 161.2 | D | 117.3 | — | — | — | — | — | — | — | — | — | — |
| 1930 | G | 221.4 | P & B | 200.1 | TB | 185.6 | CEVD | 162.8 | D | 118.8 | — | — | — | — | — | — | — | — | — | — |
| 1935 | TB | 190.8 | P & B | 186.7 | G | 173.2 | CEVD | 165.4 | D | 114 | — | — | — | — | — | — | — | — | — | — |
| 1940 | TB | 212.9 | P & B | 185.8 | CEVD | 177.7 | G | 159.2 | D | 124.5 | — | — | — | — | — | — | — | — | — | — |
| 1947 | TB | 187.2 | P & B | 174.8 | G | 136.8 | CEVD | 129.4 | D | 100.3 | — | — | — | — | — | — | — | — | — | — |
| 1948 | TB | 179.9 | CEVD | 117.9 | G | 109.9 | P & B | 98.6 | D | 79.5 | — | — | — | — | — | — | — | — | — | — |
| 1949 | TB | 168.9 | CEVD | 122.6 | G | 100 | G | 92.6 | D | 80.2 | — | — | — | — | — | — | — | — | — | — |
| 1950 | TB | 146.4 | CEVD | 127.1 | P & B | 93.2 | G | 82.4 | MT | 77.4 | D | 70.2 | CVD | 64.2 | NBD | 62.2 | A | 39.5 | Nephritis | 32.4 |
| 1951 | CEVD | 125.2 | TB | 110.3 | P & B | 82.2 | MT | 78.5 | D | 70.7 | D | 67.7 | CVD | 63.6 | NBD | 56 | A | 37.8 | Nephritis | 29.2 |
| 1952 | CEVD | 128.5 | TB | 82.2 | MT | 80.9 | D | 69.3 | P & B | 67.1 | CVD | 61.3 | G | 53.1 | NBD | 47.3 | A | 36.4 | Nephritis | 25.8 |
| 1953 | CEVD | 133.7 | MT | 82.2 | D | 77.6 | P & B | 71.3 | TB | 66.5 | CVD | 64.9 | G | 46.1 | NBD | 42.1 | A | 39.3 | Nephritis | 23.2 |
| 1954 | CEVD | 132.4 | MT | 85.3 | D | 69.5 | TB | 62.4 | CVD | 60.2 | A | 54.7 | A | 39.4 | G | 39 | NBD | 36.2 | Suicide | 23.4 |
| 1955 | CEVD | 136.1 | MT | 87.1 | D | 67.1 | D | 60.9 | TB | 52.3 | P & B | 48.3 | A | 37.3 | G | 31.7 | NBD | 31.4 | Suicide | 25.2 |
| 1956 | CEVD | 148.4 | MT | 90.7 | D | 75.8 | CVD | 66 | TB | 48.6 | P & B | 48.4 | A | 36.8 | NBD | 30.5 | G | 30 | Suicide | 24.5 |
| 1957 | CEVD | 151.7 | MT | 91.3 | D | 80.5 | CVD | 73.1 | P & B | 59.2 | TB | 46.9 | A | 37.9 | NBD | 26.4 | G | 25.7 | Suicide | 24.3 |
| 1958 | CEVD | 148.6 | MT | 95.5 | CVD | 64.8 | CVD | 55.5 | P & B | 47.6 | TB | 39.4 | A | 38.9 | Suicide | 25.7 | G | 25.1 | NBD | 23.4 |
| 1959 | CEVD | 153.7 | MT | 98.2 | CVD | 67.7 | D | 56.7 | P & B | 45.2 | A | 44.8 | TB | 35.5 | G | 23.3 | Suicide | 22.7 | NBD | 21 |
| 1960 | CEVD | 160.7 | MT | 100.4 | CVD | 73.2 | D | 58 | P & B | 49.3 | A | 41.7 | TB | 34.2 | Suicide | 21.6 | G | 21.2 | NBD | 18.5 |
| 1961 | CEVD | 165.4 | MT | 102.3 | CVD | 72.1 | D | 58.2 | A | 44.1 | P & B | 41.6 | TB | 29.6 | Suicide | 19.6 | G | 19.5 | NBD | 17.4 |
| 1962 | CEVD | 169.4 | MT | 103.2 | CVD | 76.2 | D | 57.5 | P & B | 45 | A | 40.3 | TB | 29.3 | HBP | 18.4 | G | 18 | Suicide | 17.6 |
| 1963 | CEVD | 171.4 | MT | 105.5 | CVD | 70.4 | D | 50.4 | A | 41.3 | P & B | 33.2 | TB | 24.2 | HBP | 18.2 | Suicide | 16.1 | G | 16.1 |
| 1964 | CEVD | 171.7 | MT | 107.3 | CVD | 70.3 | D | 48.4 | A | 41.6 | P & B | 32.1 | TB | 23.6 | HBP | 18.7 | Suicide | 15.1 | G | 14.6 |
| 1965 | CEVD | 175.8 | MT | 108.4 | CVD | 77 | D | 50 | A | 40.9 | P & B | 37.3 | TB | 22.8 | HBP | 19.3 | Suicide | 14.7 | G | 12.9 |
| 1966 | CEVD | 173.8 | MT | 110.9 | CVD | 71.9 | D | 44.6 | A | 43 | P & B | 28.2 | TB | 20.3 | HBP | 18.6 | Suicide | 15.2 | G | 11.3 |
| 1967 | CEVD | 173.1 | MT | 113 | CVD | 75.7 | D | 43.3 | A | 41.9 | P & B | 28.7 | TB | 18.3 | TB | 17.8 | Suicide | 14.2 | NBD | 11.4 |
| 1968 | CEVD | 173.5 | MT | 114.6 | CVD | 80.2 | A | 40.2 | D | 39.4 | P & B | 31.8 | HBP | 17.9 | TB | 16.8 | Suicide | 14.5 | Cirrhosis | 11.2 |
| 1969 | CEVD | 174.4 | MT | 116.2 | CVD | 81.7 | A | 42.2 | D | 37.1 | P & B | 31.6 | HBP | 17 | TB | 16.1 | Suicide | 14.5 | Cirrhosis | 11.8 |
| 1970 | CEVD | 175.8 | MT | 116.3 | CVD | 86.7 | A | 42.5 | D | 38.1 | P & B | 34.1 | HBP | 17.7 | TB | 15.4 | Suicide | 15.3 | Cirrhosis | 12.5 |
| 1971 | CEVD | 169.6 | MT | 117.7 | CVD | 82 | A | 40.7 | D | 34 | P & B | 28.4 | HBP | 16.7 | Suicide | 15.6 | TB | 13 | Cirrhosis | 12.5 |
| 1972 | CEVD | 166.7 | MT | 120.4 | CVD | 81.2 | A | 40.1 | D | 30.8 | P & B | 28.1 | Suicide | 17 | HBP | 16.5 | Cirrhosis | 12.8 | TB | 11.9 |
| 1973 | CEVD | 166.9 | MT | 121.2 | CVD | 87.3 | A | 37.2 | P & B | 31.3 | D | 30.9 | HBP | 17.5 | Suicide | 17.4 | Cirrhosis | 13.2 | TB | 11.1 |

| Year | 1 | 2 | 3 | 4 | 5 | 6 | 7 | 8 | 9 | 10 |
|---|---|---|---|---|---|---|---|---|---|---|
| 1974 | CEVD 163 | MT 122.2 | CVD 89.8 | A 33 | P & B 32.6 | D 29.7 | HBP 18.4 | Suicide 17.5 | Cirrhosis 13.4 | TB 10.4 |
| 1975 | CEVD 156.7 | MT 122.6 | CVD 89.2 | P & B 33.7 | A 30.3 | D 26.9 | HBP 18 | HBP 17.8 | Cirrhosis 13.6 | TB 9.5 |
| 1976 | CEVD 154.5 | MT 125.3 | CVD 92.2 | P & B 32.6 | A 28 | D 26.4 | HBP 17.6 | Suicide 17.6 | Cirrhosis 13.8 | TB 8.5 |
| 1977 | CEVD 149.8 | MT 128.4 | CVD 91.2 | P & B 28.6 | A 26.7 | D 25 | Suicide 17.9 | HBP 16.4 | Cirrhosis 13.6 | Diabetes 8.4 |
| 1978 | CEVD 146.2 | MT 131.3 | CVD 93.3 | P & B 30.3 | A 26.2 | D 24.4 | Suicide 17.6 | HBP 14.2 | HBP 14 | Diabetes 8.5 |
| 1979 | CEVD 137.7 | MT 135.7 | CVD 96.9 | P & B 28.5 | A 25.5 | D 25.3 | Suicide 18 | CHD 14.2 | HBP 13.7 | Nephritis 8 |
| 1980 | CEVD 139.5 | MT 139.1 | CVD 106.2 | P & B 33.7 | A 27.6 | D 25.1 | Suicide 17.7 | CHD 14.2 | HBP 13 | Nephritis 8.8 |
| 1981 | MT 142 | CEVD 134.3 | CVD 107.5 | P & B 33.7 | D 25.5 | A 24.8 | Suicide 17.1 | CHD 17.1 | HBP 13.7 | Nephritis 9.1 |
| 1982 | MT 144.2 | CEVD 144.3 | CVD 106.7 | P & B 35 | D 24.7 | A 23.3 | Suicide 17.5 | CHD 17.5 | Nephritis 11.7 | Nephritis 9.7 |
| 1983 | MT 148.3 | CEVD 125 | CVD 111.3 | P & B 39.3 | A 25 | D 24.7 | Suicide 21 | CHD 14.1 | Nephritis 11.3 | Nephritis 10.3 |
| 1984 | MT 152.5 | CEVD 112.8 | CVD 113.9 | P & B 37.6 | A 24.6 | D 24.1 | Suicide 19.4 | CHD 14.2 | Nephritis 10.9 | Nephritis 10.6 |
| 1985 | MT 156.1 | CVD 117.2 | CEVD 112.2 | P & B 42.7 | A 24.6 | D 23.1 | Suicide 21.2 | CHD 14.3 | Nephritis 11.2 | HBP 10.6 |
| 1986 | MT 158.5 | CVD 117.3 | CEVD 106.9 | P & B 43.9 | A 23.7 | D 22.2 | Suicide 19.6 | CHD 14 | CHD 11.6 | HBP 9.7 |
| 1987 | MT 164.2 | CVD 117.9 | CEVD 101.7 | P & B 44.9 | A 23.2 | D 20.8 | Suicide 18.7 | CHD 13.7 | CHD 11.8 | HBP 8.8 |
| 1988 | MT 168.4 | CVD 118.4 | CEVD 105.5 | P & B 51.6 | A 24.8 | D 21.6 | Suicide 17.3 | CHD 13.9 | CHD 13 | HBP 8.4 |
| 1989 | MT 173.6 | CVD 129.4 | CEVD 98.5 | P & B 52.7 | A 25.4 | D 19.4 | Suicide 16.4 | CHD 13.6 | CHD 13.4 | Diabetes 7.6 |
| 1990 | MT 177.2 | CVD 128.1 | CEVD 99.4 | P & B 60.7 | A 26.2 | D 19.7 | Suicide 16.1 | Nephritis 14 | RF 13.7 | Diabetes 7.7 |
| 1991 | MT 181.7 | CVD 134.8 | CEVD 96.2 | P & B 62 | A 26.9 | D 18.8 | Suicide 16.9 | Nephritis 13.8 | RF 13.7 | Diabetes 7.8 |
| 1992 | MT 187.8 | CVD 137.2 | CEVD 95.6 | P & B 65 | A 28.1 | D 18.9 | Suicide 16.6 | Nephritis 14.8 | HD 13.8 | Diabetes 8 |
| 1993 | MT 190.4 | CVD 142.2 | CEVD 96 | P & B 70.6 | A 28 | D 18.7 | Suicide 16.9 | Nephritis 14.9 | HD 13.6 | Diabetes 8.3 |
| 1994 | MT 196.4 | CVD 145.6 | CEVD 96.9 | P & B 72.4 | A 29.1 | D 18.9 | Suicide 15.1 | Nephritis 15.1 | HD 13.3 | Diabetes 8.8 |
| 1995 | MT 211.6 | CVD 128.6 | CEVD 112 | Pneumonia 64.1 | A 36.5 | Suicide 17.3 | D 17.2 | HD 13.7 | HD 13 | Diabetes 11.4 |
| 1996 | MT 217.5 | CEVD 117.9 | CVD 110.8 | Pneumonia 56.9 | A 31.4 | Suicide 17.8 | D 16.7 | HD 13.2 | HD 13.3 | Diabetes 10.3 |
| 1997 | MT 220.4 | CEVD 112.6 | CVD 111 | Pneumonia 63.1 | A 31.1 | Suicide 18.8 | D 17.2 | RF 13.3 | HD 12.9 | Diabetes 9.9 |
| 1998 | MT 226.7 | CVD 112.2 | CEVD 110 | Pneumonia 63.8 | A 31.1 | Suicide 25.4 | D 17.1 | RF 13.3 | HD 10 | Diabetes 10 |
| 1999 | MT 231.6 | CVD 114.3 | CEVD 110.8 | Pneumonia 74.9 | A 32 | Suicide 25 | D 18.2 | RF 14.1 | HD 13.2 | CLD 10.4 |
| 2000 | MT 235.2 | CVD 120.4 | CEVD 105.5 | Pneumonia 69.2 | A 31.4 | Suicide 24.1 | D 16.9 | RF 13.7 | HD 12.8 | CLD 10.2 |
| 2001 | MT 238.8 | CVD 116.8 | CEVD 104.7 | Pneumonia 67.8 | A 31.4 | Suicide 23.3 | D 17.6 | RF 14 | HD 12.6 | CLD 10.4 |
| 2002 | MT 241.7 | CVD 117.8 | CEVD 103.4 | Pneumonia 69.4 | A 30.7 | Suicide 23.8 | D 18 | RF 14.4 | HD 12.3 | CLD 10.3 |
| 2003 | MT 245.4 | CVD 121 | CEVD 104.7 | Pneumonia 75.3 | A 30.7 | Suicide 25.5 | D 18.6 | RF 14.9 | HD 12.5 | CLD 10.8 |
| 2004 | MT 253.9 | CVD 126.5 | CEVD 102.3 | Pneumonia 75.7 | A 30.3 | Suicide 24 | D 19.1 | RF 15.2 | HD 12.6 | CLD 10.7 |
| 2005 | MT 258.3 | CVD 126.5 | CEVD 105.3 | Pneumonia 85 | A 31.6 | Suicide 24.2 | D 20.9 | RF 16.3 | HD 13 | CLD 11.4 |
| 2006 | MT 261 | CVD 137.2 | CEVD 101.7 | Pneumonia 85 | A 30.3 | Suicide 23.7 | D 22 | RF 16.8 | HD 12.9 | CLD 11.4 |
| 2007 | MT 266.9 | CVD 137.2 | CEVD 100.8 | Pneumonia 87.4 | A 30.1 | Suicide 24.4 | D 24.4 | RF 17.2 | HD 12.8 | CLD 11.8 |
| 2008 | MT 272.3 | CVD 144.4 | CEVD 100.9 | Pneumonia 91.6 | A 30.3 | D 28.6 | Suicide 24 | RF 17.9 | HD 12.9 | CLD 12.3 |

Source: Koseisho Imukyoku 1976: 564–567.

Notes

A = accident; CEVD = cerebrovascular disease; CHD = chronic hepatic disease; CLD = chronic lung disease; CVD = cardiovascular disease; D = decrepitude (senility); G = gastroenteritis; HBP = high blood pressure; HD = hepatic disease; MT = malignant tumour (cancer); NBD = newborn baby disease; P & B = pneumonia and bronchitis; RF = renal failure.

Overall, Japan's national profile of major diseases has changed dramatically from acute infections such as smallpox, cholera, dysentery and typhoid, through chronic infections such as tuberculosis, to what have come to be termed 'lifestyle-based diseases like diabetes, cardiovascular disease and cancers. It should be remarked that the increase in this last group of diseases is to some degree a consequence of the success in preventing, treating or eradicating those infections which were formerly the major causes of mortality. Nevertheless, there are clearly other factors involved (such as those listed above), even if in many cases, especially where cancer is concerned, causal connections have not as yet been precisely determined.

A commonly cited factor in 'advanced industrialized countries' and now, as other chapters in this book show, in developing countries, is changes in eating habits. These have been very pronounced in Japan. While traditional food containing mostly rice, seafood and various vegetables has not been discarded, it has ceded ground to Western-style meals with large quantities of meat, dairy products and bread. One effect of the altered nutritional balance, perhaps especially the increased intake of protein and calcium, is that the average height of a Japanese person rose from 158.9 cm in 1899 to 168.5 cm in 2007. It does demonstrate in very concrete terms that lifestyles – perhaps above all, eating styles – have changed dramatically.

As in so many countries, the intake of saturated fats, overeating and irregular eating (Japan is a world leader in convenience store innovation and automated food and drink technology) are having health consequences. At the same time that Japanese are eating more, and with less regularity, they are on the whole exercising less. As citizens of one of the world's most technologically advanced nations, many tend to work in sedentary jobs (often for long hours), indulge in hi-tech, low-exercise, leisure pursuits and take advantage of extraordinary levels of convenience.

The rapid increase in the number of those suffering from problems such as obesity, cardiovascular disease, certain forms of cancer and diabetes is readily understandable in this context. The change is apparent in the constantly increasing body mass index (BMI), a factor known to relate to the development of insulin resistance, impaired glucose tolerance and diabetes (Kawamori 2000: 226). The number of diabetic patients was 30,000 in 1970, 6.9 million in 1998 and is 10.8 million in 2010. It is estimated that more than 12 million Japanese are hyperglycaemic and the number is increasing among the young. Cardiovascular diseases remain a constant concern of medical professionals. 'Increases in levels of risk factors' especially in cholesterol and blood pressure, 'appear to account for a substantial amount of the age-related increase in coronary heart disease' (Sasayama 2008: 2,669).

Quite predictably, there has been an intensification of discussion around the subject. The fact that BMI has taken on popular cultural currency would seem to indicate a greater level of awareness. 'Metabo', a Japanese abbreviation of 'metabolic syndrome', has very recently become a common term in Japan's popular media. As in some other countries, the self-monitoring propensity of the educated middle class, of which Japan has a good number, has produced a para-doxical and self-perpetuating economics of personal health. Modern 'evils' of ill health brought about through media-supported habits of consumption are con-fronted by the neo-liberal individual through the consumption of health-supporting products and services. Health-conscious people are increasingly likely to purchase medicines and dietary supplements to enhance their wellbeing. Fitness clubs, yoga clubs and jogging are enormously popular among a certain demographic, often following Western trends. Meanwhile, and paradoxically, due to vested interests in the tobacco industry and a degree of cultural and insti-tutional inertia, smoking, which remains one of the largest public health issues, taking more than 100,000 lives per annum and accounting for almost one in ten deaths (*Daily Yomiuri*, 8 September 2008), is being addressed more slowly in Japan than in other advanced countries.

The living environment for many people is far from ideal. In 1970, 33.9 per cent of the population lived in the three urban areas of Tokyo, Osaka and Nagoya. By 2000, the figure had risen to 48.7 per cent (Nihon Tokei Kyokai 2005: 37). Japanese cities typically have a high population density, and the atmosphere, despite ongoing reform projects, is often far from desirable. Indus-trial and car fumes, food additives, home detergents and solvents as well as many other chemical compounds encountered by citizens in their daily lives are likely to be important factors in various ailments.

There are less tangible elements, however. In popular discourse, the Japanese characterize the present period in their long history as the 'stress *jidai*', (the era of stress). It is extremely difficult to assess to what extent that pervasive sense of stress contributes to the lifestyle diseases. While the precise relations between stress and cardiovascular disease or cancer have yet to be clearly delineated, it is generally accepted that there are indeed connections, both direct and indirect. If stress contributes to poor eating or drinking habits or to smoking, for example, then it is a causal factor for various diseases. Much of the stress relates to the economic situation. Japan's economy peaked and then collapsed in the 1990s. A generation is now entering adulthood which, while it enjoys unprecedented com-forts and amusements, has known nothing but bad economic news and faces a very uncertain future in terms of employment. Social commentators often remark upon the passing of the 'corporate socialism' of life-long employment, age-determined promotions and generous retirement packages that fostered the famous loyalty of Japanese labourers and 'salarymen' to their company. Much of that collapsed with the stock market and under the influence of economic reforms driven by global competition. '*Ristra*', restructuring or downsizing, has been instrumental in creating a large population of homeless, mostly middle-aged men.

Over the past decade Japan's suicide rate, typically related to some form of stress, has become an increasingly important and widely reported health issue. For over a decade the number of suicides has exceeded 30,000 per year and reached 32,845 in 2009. Between 1977 and 1995 it was the seventh major cause of death, between 1996 and 2007 it ranked sixth and it is now the most common cause of death among men aged 20–44 years and women aged 15–34 (see Table 5.2). This overall rate is significantly higher than in all but a few nations and nowhere matched by any of the other leading industrialized countries, being two-and-a-half to three times higher than that of the United States or Britain. Certainly stress is a factor here, but the picture is somewhat complicated, as indicated by a recent article in Britain's *Guardian* newspaper (Chambers 2010: 3).

This elevated suicide rate is the result of a complex interplay between health-care provision, social attitudes, cultural influences and economic factors. Yuzo Kato, Director of the Tokyo Suicide Prevention Centre, argues: 'The most common factor behind suicide in Japan is depression caused by a failure to cope with [social pressure] either because of poverty or the demands of work.' The stockmarket crash in 1997 precipitated business failures, loss of savings and unemployment. In 1998 the Japanese suicide total rose by 35 per cent (Chambers 2010: 1).

Economics is undeniably a factor. First, a phenomenon called *karoshi* or death by overwork is being driven not simply by an over-commitment to one's profession but by the anxieties attending the increasing presence of global market competition, and some suicides are driven by the same economic environment. The social attitudes are influential. There is a tendency to regard the unemployed as largely responsible for their own predicament, and a belief among a good number of people that suicide is a noble act, especially if it secures an insurance payout that erases debts and/or provides security for the remaining family.

Healthcare provision itself is a primary driving force of suicide in Japan. The medical system itself is stressed and ailing. In 2007, 49 per cent of medical expenses were covered by health insurance, 14.4 per cent by the patients themselves and 36.6 per cent was covered by the municipality and the central government. The total was 33 trillion Yen (around US$330 million) in 2007, whereas in 1995 it was 26 trillion Yen (US$260 million). This means that expenses had increased by an average of 60 billion Yen (US$6 million) per year in a country which in the past decade has had near zero inflation. Despite its long history, the national health system is believed to be deteriorating. One reason for this is that developments in medicine and medical technology have caused medical costs to rise sharply. However, it should be pointed out that doctors have not necessarily benefited. In Japan doctors earn an average of 2.8 times more than the average wage earner. In France it is 3.5 times, in the United Kingdom 5.4 times, in the United States 5.7 times and in Canada 7.1 times (Nihon Tokei Kyokai 2005: 146).

Another major factor is demographic, and this returns us to the issue of achievements in healthcare contributing to current problems. Growing life expectancy is increasing the nation's medical expenses: for example, over two million people (about 10 per cent of those over 65 years) now suffer from Alzheimer's disease and this is expected to increase, along with other geriatric diseases. If there is a double disease burden in Japan this may well be it. Not only is the number of geriatric disorders increasing with the ageing population, but because this is happening at the same time as a partly economically driven decline in the birth rate, the ratio between the number of working people and retirees is generating financial stress for the health system. In 1990, there were 5.9 people of working age for each retiree, and in 2000, 3.9. By 2025, that number is expected to fall to 2.1. With fewer workers paying tax, government revenue will fall at the same time that pensions and healthcare costs rise. For the average Japanese of any age this basic mathematical and demographic dilemma must itself be a cause of anxiety. In short, for a culture which places so much emphasis on *anzen anshin* (security and peace of mind), Japan is indeed in a stressful historical period.

## Conclusion

Japan's journey through modern times has been characterized by horrifying disasters and spectacular achievements. Yet, overall, the nation has made substantial progress, not least of all in health. Pushed into radical change by the reforming zeal of foreigners and driven, too, by the diseases those foreigners brought with them, Japan has striven hard to assume control of its own destiny through healthcare. Because it underwent modernization relatively early, it is not faced with quite the same double burden of disease with which its neighbours are now wrestling. Yet there are clearly some very serious issues to be addressed: there is the rise to prominence of a new range of lifestyle-related diseases, a protracted weakness of the economy that threatens the provision of healthcare, a demographic collision, as its much vaunted longevity faces off against a declining population. All of this is happening at a time when, under the imperatives of globalization, the nation is being pushed into opening its doors still further to the outside world. However, it would be a mistake to assume that Japan, wracked with stresses, is doomed. As the earlier part of this brief modern history demonstrates, Japan has a record of responding to crises with vigorous determination.

## Notes

1 The London Lock Hospital, the first venereal disease clinic in London, was opened by William Bromfield (1713–1792) in January 1747 and it closed in 1953 (Williams 1995: 1–3).
2 One of the most surprising – to some people, odd – things which happened during the Meiji Era occured amid the cholera-related protests which arose among ordinary people fearing the fierce infectiousness of the disease. Some people actually became frightened of electric poles simply because the Japanese term '*densen*' is a homonym meaning both electric line and infection. More and more people were caught up in the misconception and the government had to take measures to prevent the unacceptable behaviour arising from it.
3 Scurvy was once a very feared disease among seafarers and it was James Lind (1716–1794), a British naval surgeon, who thought citrus fruits such as lemon and lime would decrease its incidence. The British navy was very conscious of seamen's health and pursued other measures such as ventilation and the regular washing of bodies and clothing to help secure the health of crews.

4 This was not just a Japanese problem. It was consistent with results gained in the Framingham Community Health and Tuberculosis Demonstration conducted in Framingham, Massachusetts between 1917 and 1923, with the support of the Metropolitan Insurance Company; nearly 15 per cent of the Company's subscribers had died from TB (Armstrong 2005: 1183–1187; Matson 1924: 1243–1247).

## References

AIDS Yobo Joho Net (2010) *The Number of HIV/AIDS Patients in Japan as of 27 June 2010*, Table 2, AIDS Prevention Information Network. Online, available at: http://api-net.jfap.or.jp/status/2010/1008/hyo_02.pdf (accessed 6 September 2010).

Armstrong, D.B. (2005) 'Community Health and Tuberculosis', *International Journal of Epidemiology*, 34(6): 1183–1187.

Chambers, A. (2010) 'Japan: Ending the Culture of the "Honourable" Suicide', *Guardian*. Online, available at: www.guardian.co.uk/commentisfree/2010/aug/03/japan-honourable-suicide-rate (accessed 3 August 2010).

Fukuda, M. (1995) *Kekkaku no Bunkashi (A Cultural History of Tuberculosis)*, Nagoya: Nagoya University Press.

Hanley, S.B. and Yamamura, K. (1977) *Economic and Demographic Change in Pre-Industrial Japan, 1600–1868*, Princeton, NJ: Princeton University Press.

Hepburn, J.C. (1955) *The Letters of Dr. J. C. Hepburn*, Tokyo: Toshinbo Shobo.

Ishikawa Prefecture (1936) *Ishikawaken ni okeru Kekkaku no jokyo to Shisetsu (The Conditions of Kekkaku and Health Institution)*, Kanazawa: Ishikawa Prefecture.

Jinko Tokei Shiryo (Population Statistical Databook) (2010) National Institute of Population and Social Security Research. Online, available at: www.ipss.go.jp/syoushika/tohkei/Popular/P_Detail2010.asp (accessed 2 September 2010).

Kawamori, R. (2000) 'Diabetes Trends in Japan', International Symposium, EASD, Israel, September.

Kondo, K. (1948) *Kekkaku no Yobo to sono Taisaku (Tuberculosis and its Prophylaxis and Countermeasures)*, Tokyo: Nanzando Publishing Company.

Kosei-Rodosho (Ministry of Health, Labour and Welfare) (2010) Jinko Dotai Tokei (Vital Statics), Trends in Leading Causes of Death, Tokyo. Online, available at: www.mhlw.go.jp/english/database/db-hw/populate/pop1-t1.html (accessed 9 September 2010).

Koseisho Imukyoku (Medical Bureau, Ministry of Health and Welfare) (1976) *Isei Hyakunen – Shi (One Hundred Years' History of the Medical System)*, Tokyo: Gyosei Publishing Co.

Matson, R.C. (1924) 'The Framingham Health and Tuberculosis Demonstration: Community Prevention, Control, and Treatment of Diseases, as Carried out at Framingham, Massachusetts, U.S.A.', *Lancet*, 26(24): 1243.

Nihon Tokei Kyokai (2005) *Tokei de miru Nihon (Japan seen from Statistical Data)*, Tokyo: Japan Statistical Society.

Sasayama, S. (2008) 'Heart Disease in Asia', *Circulation*, 118: 2669–2671.

Sidibé, M. (2010) 'The Benchmark: Japan', Special Report, UNAIDS. Online, available at: http://api-net.jfap.or.jp/status/pdf/The%20Benchmark%20Japan.pdf (accessed 2 October 2010).

Williams, D.I. (1995) *The London Lock: A Charitable Hospital for Venereal Disease: 1746–1952*, London: Royal Society of Medicine Press.

# 6 Challenges of, and responses to, the double disease burden in Korea

*In-sok Yeo*

## Introduction

Korea dramatically changed after World War II, the Korean War (1950–1953) and the political division of the country into the Republic of Korea in the south and the Democratic People's Republic in the north.[1] Change affected every domain of Korean society and this was reflected in the patterns of diseases. The control of acute communicable diseases (CDs) such as cholera, typhoid fever and Japanese encephalitis were urgent problems of public health in the following decades. With rapid economic development in the 1970s, the incidence of CDs began to decline (in particular controlling parasitic diseases was remarkably successful) and as life expectancy increased, chronic diseases such as cardiovascular disease, cancer and diabetes became the new health problems. However, chronic infectious diseases such as tuberculosis still remain one of the major health problems in Korea. Malaria re-emerged after an absence of 20 years and Korea faces newly emerging, globalized, infectious diseases such as avian and swine flu. This chapter will discuss the shift of disease patterns during the past 60 years focusing on tuberculosis, malaria, HIV/AIDS, cancer and diabetes. Although each disease has its own record, they are related at a deeper level reflecting the underlying changes which characterize the dynamics of Korean society. Given that a disease, its incidence and control is not determined by biological factors alone, but by social, economic, cultural and environmental factors as well, its health burden should be analyzed from multiple perspectives.

## Challenge of communicable diseases

Throughout human history CDs posed a major threat to human lives until quite recently. Koreans, too, suffered from the heavy burden of CDs at least until the 1960s. In particular, the years of political instability that followed the end of the World War II and the Korean War, saw frequent outbreaks of acute CDs such as typhoid fever, cholera, smallpox and Japanese encephalitis.

Typhoid fever was the most common enteric disease in Korea. There were 11,287 cases of typhoid reported in 1946, 8,250 cases in 1947 and 4,996 cases in 1948 in South Korea alone (Choi 1949: 31). Despite extensive vaccinations, the numbers did not drop significantly. Although cholera may have been the most deadly, acute communicable disease in the nineteenth and twentieth centuries, there were no recorded outbreaks of cholera from 1920 to 1945 in Korea. But in the summer of 1946, an epidemic of cholera occurred due to the massive repatriation of Koreans from Manchuria. By December 1946, 15,748 cases of cholera were reported with 10,191 deaths, a mortality rate of 64 percent. Smallpox, another deadly disease of the past, reached epidemic proportions in 1946 and 20,810 cases were reported in all provinces except Seoul, until December 1948 when an outbreak occurred in the city. The number of reported cases totaled 596 with 202 deaths, a mortality rate of 35.6 percent (Choi 1949: 33). Japanese B encephalitis was first reported in 1946 and it was followed by an epidemic outbreak in August, 1949. The reported cases reached as many as 5,616 with 2,797 deaths, a mortality rate of 50 percent.

The control program against CDs was not effective due to the inadequate production of vaccines and serum. After Liberation, the National Institute for Prevention of Infectious Diseases was established in 1945, and its major task was to produce various vaccines and serum for prevention and diagnosis of a variety of CDs. However, despite its efforts to meet the full demand, the production was far below what was necessary on account of lack of resources for mass production. Another reason was the lack of proper facilities for isolation and quarantine of patients. There were fewer than 400 beds for acute communicable disease patients in South Korea and adequate measures for quarantine were hampered because of the large population returning to Korea from China, Japan and other countries after World War II. Establishing systems for controlling CDs were about to be made when the Korean War broke out.

The Korean War (1950–1953) provided a favorable environment for the outbreaks of various CDs. In particular, an outbreak of typhus fever occurred in 1951 with 32,211 reported civilian cases alone. In the same year there was a massive epidemic of smallpox, and 43,123 cases were reported, with 11,530 deaths. Korean hemorrhagic fever was first reported in 1951 among UN soldiers. Besides the above mentioned diseases, the year 1951 saw unprecedented massive epidemics of other CDs such as dysentery (9,004 cases) and typhoid fever (81,575 cases). Such a phenomenon can be explained by the presence of a large drifting population in the early years of the war and worsening conditions of hygiene and nutrition. The situation improved from 1952 thanks to the stabilization of the war front and massive efforts for prevention and treatment.

## Epidemiological transition

Korean society underwent a significant epidemiological transition related to a demographic shift, economic growth, improved nutrition, a rise in life expectancy and a change in the causes of death (Kim 1982: 52). The transition took place over 20 years after the Korean War. The critical period of transition in each domain does not exactly coincide, but each transition falls into the period between 1955 and 1975. Indeed, the occurrence of acute CDs began to drop dramatically after 1955 due to the use of antibiotics, pesticides and the effect of massive immunization (Han and Kim 1987: 237). Despite the sporadic outbreaks of CDs in the 1960s and extending into 1970, the scale and severity of the outbreaks fell far below those before and during the Korean War: for example, there were 414 cases of cholera reported in 1964, 1,538 in 1969, 206 in 1970 and 145 in 1980, respectively. Before 1970, between 3,000 and 5,000 cases of typhoid fever were reported annually, but the number declined abruptly thereafter, with 300–500 cases a year reported. The last reported case of smallpox was in 1960 (Lim 2005: 118). This change in disease patterns was closely related to the socioeconomic transition.

The demographic transition began with the population increasing by 16.2 percent over a five-year period between 1955 and 1960; probably the result of a typical, postwar baby boom. The growth dropped to 2.7 percent by 1966, an outcome of active family planning launched in 1961. There was also a change in the population structure. The proportion of the population under the age of 15 was over 40 percent before 1970, reaching 42 percent in 1970. It declined abruptly over the next ten years and fell to 34 percent in 1980 and 16.8 percent in 2009. The proportion of the population over 65 years was 3.3 percent in 1955 and it tripled over the next 50 years, reaching 10.7 percent in 2009. The infant mortality rate dropped from 93.2 per 1,000 live births in 1965 to 4.1 in 2009. Economic stability and growth helped to accelerate urbanization after the war. In 1955, 24.5 percent of the Korean population lived in urban areas, but this almost doubled over the next 20 years, reaching 56.9 percent in 1980 and 80.3 percent in 2005. Economic growth also increased the supply of and access to food and, after 1969, a transition from under-nutrition to over-nutrition became manifest. Life expectancy increased steadfastly from 51 years in 1955 to 79.4 in 2010 with no specific period of abrupt transition. With regard to the causes of death, infections ranked first in the 1920s and remained within the fifth rank (that is, one of five main causes of death) until 1965. Then it fell below the fifth rank in 1979 ranking tenth after 1990. The relative contribution of CDs to aggregate mortality gradually decreased: 18.2 percent in 1942, 14.8 percent in 1965, 9.7 percent in 1974, 5.4 percent in 1980, 3.4 percent in 1990, 2.5 percent in 2000 and 2.2 percent in 2003.

## Challenge of chronic non-communicable diseases: cancer and diabetes

In Korea, CDs ceased to be a major, life-threatening factor by the 1960s and non-communicable diseases (NCDs) such as circulatory diseases and neoplasms began to take their place from the 1970s (Kim 1989: 173). Rapid economic development in the 1970s and subsequent changes of lifestyle such as high caloric intake and less physical activity created new types of health problems.

The rise in life expectancy increased the chances of developing cancer. Indeed, cancer is the primary cause of mortality. In Korea, 360,000 people currently suffer from cancer and each year approximately 130,000 persons are diagnosed with cancer. Deaths due to cancer account for 27.6 percent of all deaths in 2007. Considering the magnitude of the rising incidence of and the cost of treatment, cancer is without doubt one of the most pressing health problems. The increase in cancer patients is related to the aging of the population. In response, the Korean government created the Cancer Control Division within the Ministry of Health and Welfare in 2000 and the National Cancer Center was founded in the same year to carry out research, improve patient care, and promote education and medical training. The Cancer Control Act was passed in 2003 and in 2006 a comprehensive, second-term cancer control plan for the next ten years was introduced.

Although cancer is the most feared disease, some other chronic diseases are no less damaging and burdensome. In particular, diabetes is an illness which is becoming one of the most disastrous diseases in the world. The number of diabetics is increasing year by year and is expected to reach 333 million world-wide by 2025. The cost of treatment will be huge. In Korea, about 20 percent of the national health insurance budget is being expended for treatment and control of diabetes and related diseases (Kim and Choi 2009: 126). Life expectancy may decline for the first time in 200 years because of diabetes.

Traditionally, diabetes was regarded as an illness of the rich and of developed countries. However, recently, the incidence of diabetes has been rising in under-developed countries including Asian countries. The recent sudden increase of diabetics in Korea is related to a great change in Koreans' lifestyle. The prevalence rate of diabetes reached 4.85 percent (~2.2 million people) in 2006. What is more alarming in Korea is the increased number of deaths due to diabetes: 10.8 per 100,000 persons in 1985, 28.8 in 1990 and 33.7 in 2000. The number reached 35.3 in 2003 the highest prevalence among OECD nations; more than double the OECD average (Research Institute for Healthcare Policy 2007: 11).

The characteristic features of diabetes in Korea are a very low rate of insulin dependent diabetes (type 1) but a relatively high rate of non-insulin-dependent diabetes (type 2). More than 90 percent are presumed to have type 2 diabetes. To explain type 2 diabetes, the thrifty phenotype hypothesis has been proposed. The main point of this hypothesis is that poor nutrition in fetal and early infant life prevents development of insulin-secreting, pancreatic cells and creates susceptibility to type 2 diabetes in later life (Hales and Baker 1992: 595).

This hypothesis can partly explain the high rate of type 2 diabetes in Koreans. Most patients who are over age 50 tend to have suffered from under-nutrition in early life and then were exposed to over-nutrition. But the effect of this nutritional transition may not be so critical in the Korean case (Lee *et al.* 2002: 197–203). Compared to other ethnic groups, the rate of obesity in type 2 diabetes patients is not so high among Koreans. The rate of the non-obese among type 2 diabetics is reportedly twice as high as obese type 2 diabetes patients (Huh *et al.* 1992: 63). Various hypotheses have been proposed to explain the phenomenon, but no definite explanation has been established. With regard to the high mortality due to the complications of diabetes among Koreans, it is important to see the problem in terms of health disparities (Peek 2007: 56). Diabetes is a disease that requires life-long care and control. It means that besides individual responsibility, accessibility to a supportive health care system is a crucial factor. The patient's level of education and socioeconomic status affects knowledge of the disease and accessibility to effective treatment.

Compared to other diseases, both policy and public health programs have treated diabetes as a lesser priority. Historically, CDs with high mortality were considered the main diseases to be controlled and prevented and public health systems were first created to reduce their impact on society. One can expect, at least theoretically, to eradicate CDs by vaccination or drug therapy, whether it is tuberculosis or even AIDS. However the prevention and treatment of NCDs and, in particular, diabetes do not fit this paradigm. We are faced with a totally different situation with diabetes.

First of all, diabetes is a non-curable disease. The main purpose of control is to maintain blood sugar levels as close to normal as possible, thus preventing complications from developing. Of foremost importance in controlling diabetes is education. It aims to modify lifestyle. Of course, education is important in the control of other diseases but it is only one of many modalities available for prevention and control.

This characteristic feature of diabetes control makes it difficult for the government to intervene. Lifestyle is regarded by many as a personal matter related to choice. The State has justified the CD control in terms of the hazard to society as a whole; and because CDs may form dangerous reservoirs for further outbreaks. But diabetes is not communicable. It is regarded as a prototypical personal disease. That is why the State has been reluctant to intervene.

However, the reason for government intervention is the estimated financial and social cost due to various complications of diabetes. In response to criticism from medical specialists, in 2007 the government launched a model project for controlling diabetes in Daegu, the third largest city in Korea with a population of 2.5 million. The project aims to cover the costs of all the diabetics in the city and to raise the rate of continued treatment.

While government initiatives play an essential role in control, the contribution of NGOs is also considerable: for example, the Korea Association of Diabetes, founded in 1995, actively engages in a variety of activities including educational programs such as open lectures and a diabetes camp for the diabetics and their families.

## New and re-emerging CDs: tuberculosis, malaria and HIV/AIDS

Despite the successful control of CDs in the late 1940s and 1950s, the overall CD burden was not reduced as expected. Tuberculosis persisted, malaria returned and HIV/AIDS made an appearance.

### *Tuberculosis*

Tuberculosis, a major health problem since the nineteenth century, despite great progress in diagnosis and treatment, remains problematical. During the first half of the twentieth century, tuberculosis was one of the main causes of death in Korea as was the case in many other countries: for example, the tuberculosis mortality rate increased from 18.5 per 100,000 to 71.7 between 1926 and 1941, a period marked by growing urbanization and war (Korean National Tuberculosis Society 1998: 249–252). The situation worsened from 1941 when Japan provoked World War II in the Pacific. A colony of Japan, Korea faced food shortages and malnutrition made the population more susceptible to tuberculosis. During the colonial period the Japanese policy on tuberculosis was restricted to opening several sanatoria and to community education. Production of BCG (bacille Calmette-Guerin) vaccine in Korea was possible from 1942 (*Maeil Daily*, 14 November 1942). In 1944, the colonial government planned a massive BCG vaccination campaign for factory workers, miners and students, but it was not carried out (*Maeil Daily*, 10 October 1944).

The Korean people faced further hardship with the outbreak of the Korean War and the division of the country. In the midst of the truce conference, the American Korean Foundation was created for rehabilitation of postwar Korea. Howard A. Rusk took charge of aid in education and public health. He had a particular interest in controlling tuberculosis. The National Center for Tuberculosis was established in 1954 thanks to the substantial aid from this Foundation. The center launched a nationwide project which included education for prevention, mass BCG vaccinations, a survey to ascertain the rate of prevalence and so on. Additional aid for tuberculosis control followed. A special clinic opened in 1954, with the help of the Church World Service, within the Severance Hospital in Seoul. The new, effective, triple-drug therapy – streptomycin, PAS (para-amino-salicyclic acid) and isoniazid – was provided free. Since the clinic was out-patient based, a special facility was urgently needed for patients requiring hospitalization. The US Eighth Army built a special hospital of 100 beds within the Severance Hospital in 1958.

Despite a shortage of funds, the Ministry of Health launched a five-year project for controlling tuberculosis in 1955, with the help of agencies such as WHO (World Health Organization), UNKRA (United Nations Korean Reconstruction Agency) and CAC (Civil Assistance Corp). The project's goals were to spread knowledge of tuberculosis, promote BCG vaccination and X-ray mass screening and establish an out-patient treatment system as well as train special personnel for tuberculosis control (Han 1955: 10–11). The project was quite successful. BCG vaccinations were administered to children aged five to seven years and the number of the vaccinated reached over 300,000 each year between 1955 and 1960. The accumulated number of X-ray mass screenings between 1955 and 1960 was 2.3 million. The first nationwide survey of tuberculosis was carried out in 1957 and 1958. The number of active cases was estimated to be about 1.6 million. The clinics of the National Center for Tuberculosis and the Severance Hospital were very successful. The government provided some financial aid to private sanatoria as creating new public wards was difficult due to lack of sufficient funds.

Even though much progress in tuberculosis control was made during the 1950s, the role of the Korean government was limited. Major efforts were made during the 1950s by several institutes supported by foreign aid organizations. The government began to take the initiative from the 1960s and it established a system of control through the network of public health centers. To set up effective control, reliable statistics were needed. Previous statistics were mostly obtained in a particular center and extrapolated to estimate the situation at the national level. The first nationwide survey was carried out in 1965 and from that time a survey was carried out every five years until 1995. The prevalence rate declined dramatically from 5.1 percent of the population in 1965 to 1.0 percent in 1995 (Korean National Tuberculosis Society 1998: 773). The number of active cases was reduced from 1.24 million in 1965 to 169,000 in 2005. However, the rate of decline slowed after 2000. Moreover, the number of new cases per year did not decline. Thus, the number increased from 31,503 cases in 2004 to 35,269 in 2005, and it remained at that level subsequently (Korea Center for Disease and Prevention 2010: 30). The most urgent problem in recent years, therefore, is its incidence and mortality rate. The incidence rate per 100,000 population reached 90 in 2009, the highest rate among 30 OECD countries. The mortality rate was ten per 100,000 people, which was also the highest rate among 30 OECD countries (Global Health Observatory Database). One of the alarming features is the increase of multi-drug-resistant cases, especially among people in their 20s and those aged over 60 years.

Alarmed by the gravity of the problem, the Korean government regarded the current tuberculosis situation as a public health crisis and prepared a plan to improve it. Called the 2030 plan for elimination of tuberculosis, it aims to lower the rate to one patient per 1,000,000 of the population by 2030. First of all, TBnet was set up as an integrated network system designed to manage tuberculosis patients and provide information on tuberculosis. In fact, it unified several nationwide systems such as the Korean Tuberculosis Surveillance System (KTBS), Tuberculosis Laboratory Management Information System (TBIS) and Tuberculosis Picture Archiving Communication System (TBPACS); they process disease notification, the inspection and the reading of chest X-rays respectively. Second, provision was made for expanding vaccination: babies less than one month old are vaccinated to boost immunity as well as to monitor and secure the stable production of BCG vaccine. Third, efforts are being made to enhance the treatment of patients the success of which largely depends on regular administration of drugs during the prescribed period. Each local public health center provides continuous follow-up of the registered patients and a 90 percent success rate in the public sector has followed. In contrast, in private institutions the rate remains about 50 percent due to the lack of active follow-up. A mixed public–private system has been established to enhance the rate in private institutions. In addition, the government runs two national hospitals that carry out specialized treatment and conduct clinical research. Their inpatients are those suffering from intractable tuberculosis.

Before closing the discussion on tuberculosis in Korea, something needs to be said about tuberculosis in North Korea. Although reliable statistics are not available, it is estimated that there are eight million tuberculosis patients there; about one-third of the whole population is afflicted with tuberculosis. A system for tuberculosis control was set up as early as 1947 and from the late 1960s to the mid-1970s, an effective system was in place. However, a disastrous flood in the 1990s combined with the long-term economic downturn aggravated the situation, and the number of patients escalated. The health authorities came to regard tuberculosis as the nation's primary public health problem. Proper control could not be maintained due to lack of medical resources. As a result, in 1997 the Ministry of Health asked for aid from the Eugene Bell Foundation, which had been pursuing humanitarian activities including tuberculosis control.

The foundation has made a great contribution to control. It distributes assistance 'packages' to a network of tuberculosis care centers and hospitals in the northwest part of the nation where one-third of the population lives. The packages comprise drugs, equipment for diagnosis, agricultural support for providing better nutrition, transport vehicles, and facilities and expendables for maintenance and repair of related equipment (Eugene Bell Foundation 2009: 10). Recently, MDR (multi-drug resistant) tuberculosis has emerged as a new problem, as is the case with other countries.

## *Malaria*

Controlling parasitic diseases was one of the main health issues in Korea, and it has successfully eradicated intestinal parasitic diseases which were extremely prevalent until the 1970s (Yeo 2008: 82). However, other problems such as zoonotic infections, imported parasitic diseases and malaria have come to the fore. In particular, special attention needs to be paid to the return of malaria from the mid-1990s for it reveals the close relationship between disease and ecological change.

Malaria is believed to have been endemic from ancient times. It appeared as early as the twelfth century, and according to the report of a missionary doctor who worked in Korea in the late nineteenth century, 'malaria is the most common cause of disease and "four-day ague" the most common complaint' (Allen and Heron 1886: 7). After Japan annexed Korea in 1910, the public health system was fundamentally changed. During the colonial period, acute infectious diseases such as cholera, typhoid fever, dysentery, typhus, scarlet fever, smallpox and paratyphoid fever were under special surveillance. Among chronic infectious diseases, tuberculosis and leprosy were placed under special control. In spite of its high prevalence, malaria did not receive much attention and no serious measures were taken.

Prior to 1945 vivax malaria was prevalent throughout the Korean peninsula, but with an uneven geographical distribution; with a higher incidence rate in mountainous areas than the large rice-growing regions (Ree 2000: 122). There was a slight decrease in incidence from the 1930s, and this seems to have continued during the 1940s. The situation became worse during and after the Korean War that lasted from 1950 to 1953. Several statistics illustrate this. Among 6,311 soldiers examined, 1,044 (16.5 percent) had febrile episodes due to malaria during six months in 1950 (Chun and Kim 1959: 63–66). Korean army medical records list 8,855 cases in 1953 and 5,741 in 1954 (Paik and Tsai 1963: 195). Foreign armies also became victims of malaria. Although US soldiers received weekly chloroquine chemoprophylaxis during the transmission season, 1,513 soldiers were reported to have been infected from July 1951 to November 1952 (Hankey *et al.* 1953: 958–988). Moreover, 152 (11 percent) of 1,350 Canadian veterans developed malaria in 1952 (Hale and Halpenny 1953: 444–448).

The incidence seems to have decreased a little after the war. However, there were still many endemic foci throughout the country. The mountainous north-eastern area had a high prevalence along with the northern part of Kyung-ki province near the Demilitarized Zone (DMZ). In order to cope with malaria the National Malaria Eradication Service (NMES) was launched in April 1959 as a joint project of the government of Korea and the UN/WHO Western Pacific Regional Office. A national study was carried out in 1960. Various methods such as the spleen survey, mass blood survey, passive case detection and active case detection were used to diagnose malaria. A total of 18,697 blood smears was collected randomly from 278 areas, and 212 cases (1.1 percent) were diagnosed positive for *P. vivax* (Paik *et al.* 1988: 55–66). The rate per 10,000 population was significantly higher in the north and northeastern areas (13.0) than in the south and southeastern areas of South Korea. Chloroquine administration and vector control by DDT were carried out. Thanks to these activities the prevalence began to decrease by the end of the 1960s. The decline was more dramatic during the 1970s. In 1970, 15,926 malaria cases were reported, and by 1980 they were down to zero. If you exclude the imported malaria cases, there was no indigenous case after 1984.

However, the situation began to change from 1993. In July 1993, a young soldier who was camping near the DMZ developed a fever which had a periodic pattern. He was diagnosed with vivax malaria. In the next year, 23 cases were reported and the number increased exponentially: 108 cases in 1995, 368 cases in 1996, 1,771 cases in 1997, 3,978 cases in 1998, 3,621 cases in 1999 and 4,142 cases in 2000. There was an epidemic outbreak during 1995–1998. The majority of the cases were soldiers. At the beginning of the outbreak more than 90 percent of the cases were soldiers and veterans who served near the northern part of Kyungki province; rate of infection of soldiers decreased and the proportion of civilian cases increased by 20–25 percent in 1997–1998.

At first, the outbreak was confined to Paju and Yonchon in Kyung-ki province, both of which are located within 10–15 km of the DMZ. The areas of re-emerging malaria began to expand southward. Some cases were also reported far from these areas. The majority of the cases were either recently discharged veterans who had served in the DMZ or in the vicinity of the DMZ, or civilians who had traveled to those areas, all of whom could be possible sources of secondary transmission.

Several hypotheses were proposed to explain the re-emergence of malaria. One possibility was a natural transmission from relapsed or long-term latent infection of indigenous cases in Paju area where malaria was highly prevalent in the past. The possibility was discarded as malaria was virtually eradicated in South Korea in 1979 and it seemed impossible for endemicity to be re-established in 1993 and 1994. The second possibility was malaria transmission by imported cases. This possibility is also hardly plausible since most of the reported patients had not traveled to foreign countries where malaria is prevalent. The third possibility, the most plausible, is the introduction of sporozoite-infected mosquitoes dispersed from North Korea to the South across the DMZ (Chai 1997: 728–733). Malaria was prevalent throughout the Korean peninsula before Korea was divided in 1945. Although we do not have detailed and reliable information on disease statistics in North Korea, it is presumed that malaria had persisted in North Korea even if with low endemicity. The situation seemed to have changed from 1993 when the first indigenous malaria case occurred in South Korea.

Ecological change in North Korea near the DMZ is presumed to be the cause of the re-emergence of malaria. Despite the lack of meteorological data on North Korea, we know that it suffered from unusual flooding from 1993 onward, especially during the summer season. The flood that devastated North Korea can not only be attributed to heavy rain, but also to the reckless deforestation carried out in the previous years. These floods seemed to have provided extensive breeding places for vector mosquitoes, *Anopheles sinensis*. Malaria epidemics might have started then. The species of vector mosquitoes, *Anopheles sinensis*, is highly zoophilic: 97.3 percent of female mosquitoes feed on cows and pigs. However, the floods decimated the cattle population whereas the mosquito reproduction increased due to the favorable natural conditions. As a result, most female vectors had no other choice than to feed on humans (Ree 1998: 399).

The Korean case shows that malaria epidemics return when environmental factors such as climatic, socio-ecological and political factors change in favor of vectors or parasites.

## HIV/AIDS

HIV/AIDS emerged as one of the world's major health problems from the 1980s, and it was in 1985 that the first HIV/AIDS case was identified in Korea. There was a sharp increase in the number of cases throughout the world from 1985 to 1995. Then there was a marked decrease and, from 2000, stabilization. In terms of the number of HIV/AIDS positives, Korea is relatively low in the international order, but the incidence has been increasing year by year and reached 797 in 2008.[2] The cumulative number of HIV positives in Korea has reached 5,323 of which 980 have died. Given that the actual number of HIV positives is ten times more than the official statistic, the situation is a cause for concern.

Most of the infected are male (91.7 percent) and sexual intercourse is the main route of infection (99 percent). Perinatal infection and infection by transfusion are negligible. Infection among those aged 20–40 years is 73.3 percent of the total. The number of newly infected teens rose from one or two cases to 20 in 2008. But it is probable that the more effective system of detection and reporting may be responsible for the increased number. In fact, the system of management in Korea is based on the classical model of controlling acute infectious diseases (Cho 2005: 111).

Concerning the system of detection and reporting, there is a controversy over the priority between the right of privacy and security of the whole society. Active detection, obligatory reporting and compulsory treatment characterized the initial 'Law for Prevention of AIDS' that was promulgated in 1987. The initial law was based on the idea of surveillance and control, an idea adopted by medical police of past centuries. For example, those who are suspected to be afflicted or are identified with high risk groups were made to undergo the test for AIDS against their will. The identity of the infected was listed and the local government which is in charge of the area where the infected dwelled was obliged to keep the list. In addition, it was stipulated that the itinerary of infected individuals was to be traced and reported. The patient could also be isolated and treated according to the order of the minister of health. The obligation of reporting was imposed upon doctors and employment of infected individuals was restricted.

In addition, foreigners who wished to reside for lengthy periods in Korea were obliged to submit a certificate of HIV negative status at the time of immigration. Those with no certificate were obliged to undergo testing within 72 hours of admission. Immigration of HIV positives is not allowed and foreigners known to be HIV positives become the object of compulsory deportation. The above articles reflect that the legislation on AIDS was based on the idea that AIDS is a disease spread by foreigners. According to the report of Ministry of Law, the number of foreigners expelled due to AIDS was 315 over the period of 1988 to 2004. Korea is one of the few countries that restricts admission and stipulates compulsory deportation of HIV positives at the same time. For example, in the United States and Japan, HIV positives are inadmissible to the country but not deportable. But in Korea, foreign workers who have contracted AIDS, tuberculosis, syphilis and hepatitis are to be deported.

The law was in fact highly discriminatory, violating human rights and privacy. In a sense, the law showed how social stigma of a disease could be institutionalized. Critical voices emerged against the law and in response major revisions were made in 2006, and those articles were abolished. A new article was created to prohibit discrimination of employment and the compulsory listing of HIV positive individuals. However, in spite of the introduction of 'anonymity' in examination and treatment, which is a significant change, the reporting system still remains discriminatory.

Despite progress at the institutional level in terms of controlling AIDS, there remains, widespread negative attitudes toward HIV positive individuals. According to the Korea Center for Disease Control (KCDC 2006), 41.5 per cent of the responders supported the isolation of HIV positives from the society (KCDC 2006: 44). This striking result reveals how strong the social prejudice and stigma of AIDS is in Korean society, which is attributable to a lack of correct knowledge and groundless fear about infectivity of HIV. This generalized fear and antipathy is often expressed by journals, television programmers and even in the National Assembly. The government is often criticized for being too mild or idle in controlling HIV positives. The main discontent of the critics is that the whereabouts of HIV positives is not traced properly. One member of the National Assembly expressed surprise at the number of 'the lost HIV positives' which numbered 103 in 2009, and demanded more 'active control' of the government (*Kukmin Ilbo*, 30 September 2009).

The episodes showing such prejudice are abundant. To take another example, an HIV positive individual had to be isolated in a prison because of the protest of the other inmates (*Daejon Daily*, 27 March 2007). Considering the fear and antipathy against HIV positives among prison inmates, the government attempted to designate one local prison for incarcerating them. However, the plan met with a violent opposition from the inhabitants of the region and as a result had to be abandoned. The above examples illustrate well that overcoming social prejudice is much more difficult than inducing an institutional change.

Recently, significant attempts to change the social perception of HIV positive individuals have been made and the Korean government, too, strives to keep up with such changes. The goals set by the Korean government for HIV/AIDS control are: preventing the spread of HIV/AIDS; adequate care and support for people living with HIV/AIDS; and minimizing adverse effects of HIV/AIDS on the society. Various measures are employed to achieve these goals. They include education and publicity for HIV prevention, voluntary counseling and testing of the susceptible for early diagnosis, care and support for those living with HIV/AIDS, encouraging condom use, education of personnel for qualified management of HIV/AIDS, and creating the Korea Advisory Committee on HIV/AIDS Prevention Program (KACPP) which deals with various related issues on HIV/AIDS (Hong 2005: 29–31): in particular, treatment is fully funded by the government and supplementary financial aid is given to the infected persons who are economically deprived. Medically, HIV/AIDS is treated as a chronic CD, however the problem of social discrimination remains to be solved. In terms of social perception and control policy, the classical model of controlling acute CD seems to apply here.

## Conclusion

Changes in the pattern of diseases coincide with the changes in Korean society that have accompanied sustained economic development over the past 60 years. The increase of chronic non-communicable diseases such as cancer and diabetes reflect the increase of life expectancy and undesirable changes that have come about in lifestyle. In addition, social and cultural factors, such as long working hours and frequent drinking accompanied with a heavy meal after work with colleagues, are considered to be partially responsible for the increase of many chronic NCDs.

Many infectious diseases that once were life-threatening declined dramatically or almost disappeared due to the development of public health interventions.

Nevertheless, some communicable diseases such as tuberculosis remain a major health problem and, we may add, even more so in North Korea since the 1990s. HIV/AIDS is a new infectious disease that suddenly appeared about 30 years ago and spread globally. HIV/AIDS is not just a medical problem but also a problem of social discrimination. Sometimes, ecological change brings about an unexpected outcome. The re-emergence of malaria in the central region of the Korean peninsula evokes ecological change as a factor of the utmost importance in viewing the profile of diseases. The increase of chronic NCDs such as cancer and diabetes reflect the increase of life expectancy and undesirable changes that have come about in lifestyle. The need for prevention of such diseases cannot be stressed too much for once developed the costs to the individual and society can be enormous. Therefore, a social program for healthy lifestyle, including diet and exercise, should be promoted by governmental policy in order to minimize the social burden due to these diseases.

The burden of acute communicable diseases and to some extent chronic CDs has been greatly reduced with the epidemiological transition during the past decades in Korea. However, it is highly questionable if the burden of disease as a whole has been reduced for the burden of chronic NCDs affects a growing proportion of the population. With regard to new or re-emerging CDs, the burden lies not only in the outcome of the disease itself, but also in the uncertainty about its overall impact. As was the case with HIV/AIDS, avian flu and, recently, swine flu, their appearance is largely unpredictable. Globalization of disease is not confined now to CDs. Chronic NCDs, too, are manifest in international patterns as can be seen in the recent explosive increase of diabetes both in developed and developing nations (Zimmet *et al.* 2001: 782). The age of globalization demands international cooperation in disease control more urgently than ever before.

## Notes

1 This chapter will primarily focus on South Korea because of the dearth of reliable data for the North Korean situation.
2 The source of statistics cited in this chapter is the Korean Statistical Information System (http://stat.cdc.go.kr/) if there is no special mention.

## References

Allen, H.N. and Heron, J.W. (1886) *First Annual Report of the Korean Government Hospital*, Yokohama: R. Meiklejohn.

Chai, J.I. (1997) 'Re-emerging Malaria', *Journal of Korean Medical Association*, 40: 728–733 (in Korean).

Cho, B.H. (2005) 'Social Impacts of HIV/AIDS in Korea', in *The Social and Economic Impacts of HIV/AIDS Infection in Korea*, Seoul: KCDC, 77–126.

Choi, C.C. (1949) *Public Health in Korea*, Seoul: Deputy Minister of Public Health and Welfare, American Military Government.

Chun, C.H. and Kim, J.J. (1959) 'Malaria in Korea', *Korean Medicine*, 2: 63–66 (in Korean).

Eugene Bell Foundation (2009) *Annual Report 2008*, Seoul: Eugene Bell Foundation.

Global Health Observatory Database. Online, available at: http://apps.who.int/ghodata?vid=510 (accessed 4 April 2011).

Hale, T.R. and Halpenny, G.W. (1953) 'Malaria in Korean Veterans', *Canadian Medical Association Journal*, 68: 444–448.

Hales, C.N. and Baker, D.J.P. (1992) 'Type 2 (Non-insulin-dependant) Diabetes Mellitus: The Thrifty Phenotype Hypothesis', *Diabetologia*, 35: 595–601.

Han, E.S. (1955) 'Countermeasures for Tuberculosis in 1955', *Bokounseke (The Health and Anti-Tuberculosis Monthly)*, 1(2): 10–11 (in Korean).

Han, S.B. and Kim, J.S. (1987) 'A Study on the Epidemiologic Trends of Reported Major Communicable Diseases in Korea', *Korean Journal of Epidemiology*, 9(2): 236–263 (in Korean).

Hankey, D.D., Jones, R., Coatney, G.R., Alving, A.S., Coker, W.G., Garrison, P.L. and Donovan, W.N. (1953) 'Korean Vivax Malaria I. Natural History and Response to Chloroquine', *American Journal of Tropical Medicine and Hygiene*, 2(6): 958–988.

Hong, S.G. (2005) 'Current Status and Policy of HIV/AIDS in Korea', in *The Social and Economic Impacts of HIV/AIDS Infection in Korea*, Seoul: KCDC, 27–31.

Huh, K.B., Lee, H.C., Kim, H.M., Cho, Y.W., Kim, Y.L., Lee, K.W., Lee, E.J., Lim, S.K., Kim, D.H. and Yoon, J.W. (1992) 'Immunogenetic and Nutritional Profile in Insulin-using Youth-onset Diabetics in Korea', *Diabetes Research and Clinical Practice*, 16(1): 63–70.

Kim, J.S. (1982) 'A Study of Epidemiologic Transition in Korea', *Korean Journal of Epidemiology*, 4(1): 52–89 (in Korean).

Kim, J.S. (1989) 'Perspective and Transition of Death Causes among Koreans', *Korean Journal of Epidemiology*, 11(2): 155–174 (in Korean).

Kim, S.G. and Choi, D.S. (2009) 'Epidemiology and Current Status of Diabetes in Korea', *Hanyang Medical Reviews*, 29(2): 122–129.

Korea Center for Disease Control (2006) *A Survey on Knowledge, Attitude, Belief and Behavior*, Seoul: KCDC.

Korea Center for Disease and Prevention (2010) *2009 Annual Report on the Notified Tuberculosis Patients in Korea*, Seoul: Korea Center for Disease and Prevention.

Korean Diabetes Association (2003) *Five Thousand Years of Diabetes*, Seoul: Korean Diabetes Association (in Korean).

Korean National Tuberculosis Society (1998) *A History of Tuberculosis in Korea*, Seoul: Korean National Tuberculosis Society (in Korean).

Korean Statistical Information System. Online, available at: http://stat.cdc.go.kr/ (accessed 4 March 2011).

Lee, M.J., Popkin, B.M. and Kim, S. (2002) 'The Unique Aspects of the Nutrition Transition in South Korea', *Public Health Nutrition*, 5(1A): 197–203.

Lim, H.S. (2005) 'Changing Patterns of Communicable Diseases in Korea' *Journal of Preventive Medicine and Public Health*, 38(2): 117–124 (in Korean).

Paik, Y.H., Ree, H.I. and Shim, J.C. (1988) 'Malaria in Korea', *Japanese Journal of Experimental Medicine*, 58: 55–66.

Paik, Y.H. and Tsai, F.C. (1963) 'A Note on the Epidemiology of Korean Vivax Malaria', *New Medicine Journal*, 6: 37–43 (in Korean).

Peek, M.E., Cargill, A. and Huang, E.S. (2007) 'Diabetes Health Disparities: A Systematic Review of Health Care Interventions', *Medical Care Research Review*, 64(5 Suppl.): S101–S156.

Ree, H.I. (1998) 'Can Malaria be Endemic in South Korea?' *Korean Journal of Infectious Diseases*, 30(4): 397–400.

Ree, H.I. (2000) 'Unstable Vivax Malaria in Korea', *Korean Journal of Parasitology* 38(3): 119–138.

Research Institute for Healthcare Policy (2007) *Analysis of the OECD Health Care Data 2007*, Seoul: Research Institute for Healthcare Policy (in Korean).

TBnet. Online, available at: http://tbnet.cdc.go.kr (accessed 4 March 2011).

Yeo, I. S. (2008) 'A History of Public Health in Korea', in M. J. Lewis and K. L. MacPherson (eds) *Public Health in Asia and the Pacific: Historical and Comparative Perspectives*, London: Routledge, 73–86.

Zimmet, P., Alberti, K.G. and Shaw, J. (2001) 'Global and Societal Implications of the Diabetes Epidemic', *Nature*, 414: 782–787.

# 7 Good health at low cost

## The Sri Lankan experience

*Margaret Jones and Amala de Silva*

In 1949 S.W.R.D. Bandaranaike, the Minister of Health for the newly independent nation of Sri Lanka,[1] declared his government's acceptance as a fundamental human right of the World Health Organization's (WHO) concept of health defined as 'a state of complete physical, mental and social well-being'. This declaration looked back to the colonial legacy which had seen the gradual establishment of a system of free health care for all and it confirmed that this policy would remain the basis of the health care system for the future. In turn, the 2007–2016 Health Master Plan (*Health and Shining Island in the 21st Century*) reiterated for the twenty-first century the Sri Lankan government's continuing commitment to '**providing basic health care free of cost** to the individual at the point of delivery, in State sector institutions' (bold in original) (Ministry of Healthcare and Nutrition 2009: 1). Sri Lanka, defined as a lower middle income country with a GDP per capita in 2008 of US$2014 (Central Bank of Sri Lanka 2009b: IV) is deemed an example of how a poor country can deliver good health care to its citizens at low cost, as evidenced by its inclusion as one of nine country case studies in the World Bank publication *Good Practices in Health Financing* (Fleisher *et al.* 2008: 3–8). This chapter first explores the development of Sri Lanka's exemplary health care system in the colonial and immediate post-colonial period. Second, it analyses the acute problems now challenging that system: can Sri Lanka continue to provide successful health care for its citizens given demographic transition and the double disease burden?

## Close to client, supply-side and social growth: the colonial legacy

Sri Lanka's health system is notable for the wide accessibility to allopathic medicine[2] available through an extensive network of hospitals, clinics, dispensaries and maternity homes. This is termed a supply-side, close to client care system (de Silva 2004: 427). This network of institutions was based initially in the colonial period on the provision of curative services – in particular on that most iconic symbol of Western medicine – the hospital.[3] Sri Lanka today has a range of curative institutions, from teaching hospitals with specialized services in the major towns to small outpatient-only rural clinics known as central dispensaries.

The origins of these curative services date back to the last quarter of the nine-teenth century when the presence of a large Indian immigrant labour force gave impetus to the spread of district hospitals and dispensaries to ensure the produc-tivity of that labour force but which at the same time acted as a catalyst for the expansion of government hospitals for the indigenous population. These hospi-tals dealt with the casualties of communicable diseases like malaria, hookworm, and respiratory and bowel infections – the major health threats up to the 1950s. They also served as care centres for the chronically ill, aged and indigent and maintained this dual role up to and beyond independence in 1948. The quality of the services offered varied widely from small rural hospitals of 6–12 beds to the Colombo General Hospital (GH) in the capital, the only teaching and research hospital in the island until 1962. Table 7.1 illustrates this growth of hospitals from the mid-nineteenth century through to the post-colonial period. What is noticeable in this table is the substantial increase in the 1940s and 1950s when numbers increased almost threefold.

From the 1920s this network of curative institutions was supplemented by preventive health care provision, initially through the establishment of health units. Inspired by the hookworm programme of the Rockefeller Foundation (RF) and modelled on those set up by the RF in the southern states of the US (Hewa 1995: 122–159; Jones 2004: 71–75), their primary purpose was preventive. The programme of work at the first unit at Kalutara in 1926, for instance, included health education, the organization of maternity and child welfare clinics, atten-tion to the sanitary work of the town, school medical inspections, setting up rou-tines in communicable diseases work and, last, an anopheline survey (Jones 2004: 73). This was the pattern of all future units; their significance lies in the impetus they gave to the progress of public health work in the island in the fol-lowing decades. After the catastrophic malaria epidemic of 1934–35 when an estimated 100,000 people lost their lives, the health units were remodelled and extended by the Malaria Control and Health Scheme, designed to provide an intensive general health scheme. It combined direct measures to treat sufferers

*Table 7.1* Number of government civil hospitals and inpatients treated for selected years

| Year | Hospitals | Inpatients treated |
| --- | --- | --- |
| 1867 | 17 | 9,371 |
| 1880 | 23 | 17,956 |
| 1890 | 33 | 24,970 |
| 1900 | 65 | 41,906 |
| 1910 | 72 | 61,457 |
| 1920 | 90 | 151,969 |
| 1930 | 102 | 208,464 |
| 1940 | 126 | 425,540 |
| 1950 | 232 | 846,000 |
| 1960 | 411 | 1,391,867 |

Source: Jones 2009: 16.

and control the vector with indirect methods designed to deal with the 'conditions of existence which aggravated the incidence of malaria'. This again included maternal, child welfare and school health work, general sanitary work and health education (Jones 2004: 203–204). Thus from the 1920s onwards preventive health care work formed an integral part of the health care system. This primary health care (PHC) provision, expanded yet further in the post-colonial period, presaged the WHO's Alma Ata Declaration on Primary Health Care in 1978.

The government's commitment to subsidizing the supply of health care also originated in the colonial period. Initially, the financing of both curative and preventive provision came from both private and public sources. Hospitals often began life as a result of group or individual philanthropy; hospitals such as the Kandy Hospital (1830s) and the De Soysa Maternity Hospital (1880) (Jones 2009: 36–40, 46–47). District hospitals in the plantation areas were partly funded by the planters until they were fully absorbed into government provision. It was intended that hospitals would charge fees for treatment but since these were means tested, treatment was virtually free to all. Health units, maternal and child welfare services, local hospitals were partly locally funded. However, ultimately what emerged was a publicly funded government service.[4] In 1950 free health care at the point of delivery as a right of citizenship was enshrined in law. As the medical director confidently claimed in that year, his department had assumed 'responsibility almost solely for the curative and preventive services of the entire country. Ours is truly a National Health Service' (Wickremesinghe 1950: 2).

This health care was delivered by a well-established medical profession which had taken shape early in the colonial period. The Colombo Medical School had been established in 1870. In 1876 the government instituted a scholarship scheme, which provided free training in Colombo but more significantly enabled the student to go to the United Kingdom and obtain post-graduate qualifications in medicine and surgery. This, the medical director argued, would be a 'valuable prize in inducing well-educated young men to join the medical class' and aid recruitment to the medical service (Kynsey 1876: 94). Government grants for training in the United Kingdom continued up to and after independence. In 1888 the Colombo Licentiate in Medicine and Surgery (LMS) was recognized by the General Medical Council of the United Kingdom. In practical terms this meant that Ceylon LMS holders could practise anywhere in the Empire and could undertake postgraduate study in the UK without having to repeat undergraduate courses.[5] In 1905 both college and doctors were given legal status with the passing of two ordinances – the incorporation of the Council of the Ceylon Medical College (Ordinance No. 3 1905) and the Medical Registration Ordinance (Ordinance No. 2 1905). For Sri Lanka's highly Westernized elite, medicine was an important avenue of upward social mobility. Thus, uniquely among British colonial medical services, the Sri Lankan service was staffed and run predominantly by Sri Lankans; 1936 saw the culmination of this process when a Sri Lankan became the director of the medical service. Sri Lankan doctors formed a self-confident and independent group in colonial society. They had power to exert pressure for the growth and development of medical services within their own community; and they also in a wider sense contributed to the development of a public service ethos.

However, the contributions of health care provision and the medical profession must be considered alongside other salient factors. First among these is the growth in literacy rates, in particular female literacy. Access to an education whether vernacular or English was limited in the nineteenth and early twentieth centuries, especially in the interior of the island, but a steady expansion in the availability of schools led to progressive increases in the literacy rate, notably by independence, female literacy rates were singularly high for a colony – 44 per cent in 1946 (Panditaratne and Selvanayagam 1973: 309).

In 1931, under the Donoughmore Constitution, Sri Lanka won virtual self-government and health care was under the control of a Sri Lankan Minister of Health. Universal suffrage meant that the provision of health services became an issue at the ballot box and health care was politicized. The dramatic increase of hospitals in the 1940s as illustrated in Table 7.1 is evidence of this process. Every State Council representative wanted a hospital in its constituency; it supposedly spoke of a genuine commitment to constituents, political acumen and modernity. An elected government not only gave a huge impetus to public spending on health care services; it also meant public money was found for other areas of social growth; such as education, rural reconstruction schemes and food subsidies. This growth of government intervention was such that Sri Lanka in the 1940s has been described as an 'embryo welfare state' (de Silva 1997: xxxii).

As Sri Lanka entered nationhood so its health profile changed. In the post-war period there was a dramatic fall in mortality; between 1946 and 1958 according to one estimate the crude death rate fell from 20.3 per 1,000 to 9.2. At the same time the infant mortality rate (IMR) fell from 141 per 1,000 live births to 64 and the maternal mortality rate (MMR) from 15.5 per 1,000 live births to 3.9. Such a fall, although based on somewhat dubious statistics, was too great to be merely a statistical artifact (Padley 1961: 2). The dominating factor in this dramatic fall was the control of malaria, and the other common communicable diseases (CDs). Death rates from the preventable diseases such as tuberculosis (TB), typhoid, respiratory disease and hookworm also fell quite dramatically. For instance, the death rate from TB fell from an average of 50 per 10,000 to below 20 by 1955, and typhoid from 12 per 100,000 in 1949 to two by 1958. However, as Dr Richard Padley, the WHO epidemiologist, pointed out in 1961, improvements in therapeutics 'lowered the death rate without necessarily affecting the level of morbidity' (Padley 1961: 2). Furthermore, the decline in death rates from CDs exposed the threat from non-communicable diseases (NCDs). As Dr J. Kahawita, the Director of Health Services, pointed out in 1955,

> the killers of a quarter of a century ago, cholera, plague, smallpox, malaria, pneumonia and typhoid – have now given way to cancer, degenerative diseases of the tissues of the heart and blood vessels, and to the chronic system diseases of strains and stresses of modern life.

(1955: 26)

Furthermore, the evidence of falling death rates and the improved therapeutics of Western medicine had the effect of increasing public confidence in its institutions at a time when expectations of what the state would provide in terms of welfare had been raised. Hence, the public demand for hospital services, for instance, increased. In 1955, for example, the Director of Health Services estimated that one in eight of the population had been at least once in a hospital (Kahawita 1955: 19).To illustrate this ongoing increase Padley calculated that in 1946 the number of in-patients treated in hospital was equivalent to 7.8 per cent of the population; by 1960 the equivalent figure was 13 per cent. As he concluded, the background context to health care services in 1940s and 1950s was 'one of a changing pattern of disease and an increasing public demand for medical services' (Padley 1961: 2–3).

Thus, despite improved health indicators and an extensive network of curative and preventative services the government's commitment to providing free health care to all at the point of delivery remained constantly under strain in the decades after independence; and the legacy of the colonial period, as exposed by the Cumpston Report in 1950 (Cumpston 1950) continued to present problems. These included a maldistribution of services throughout the island as a result of their ad hoc development. Patient choice exacerbated the overcrowding of popular hospitals, especially the hospitals of the capital, Colombo, where specialist expertise was concentrated. Additionally, hospitals still housed the aged and chronically ill. The hospital sector, whilst it had arguably been a crucial factor in the drive for health care services, absorbed an ever greater share of a limited budget. Preventative health care was increasingly forced to take a back seat; a situation not without its critics within the medical establishment.

The deliverers of health care and the policy makers in the 1950s were fully aware of the need for such medicine buttressed by the ideas of social medicine gaining ground in the West. Dr W.G. Wickremesinghe writing in 1945, before his appointment to the directorship of the medical services, acknowledged that there was a need for professionals to be weaned from their 'Disease Policy' to a 'Health Policy' (Wickremesinghe 1945: 6). Critics of the government six year health plan in 1955 argued that rather than the proposed expenditure on the building of hospitals, resources should be directed to the creation of 'positive health' (Keuneman 1955: 1498). There was much awareness of the need to promote health not just cure the sick. However, the hospitals were the most visible symbol of Sri Lanka's health service and moreover this free health service was ever a 'clear and potent political issue' (Fernando 2004: personal communication). To redress the balance of resources in favour of less visible preventative health care provision was a political minefield that governments of the 1950s and beyond preferred to avoid. In 1970 the then medical superintendent of the General Hospital Colombo, restated this same fundamental question in the press:

> Was it more important to improve sanitation, nutrition, and health education and provide basic facilities for health and patient care of the masses of this

country, or was it more important to go in for sophisticated and expensive programs like heart transplant units, etc, to keep alive the chronically ill?

(*Daily News*, 3 September 1970)

Now that Sri Lanka faces a double disease burden, this issue is ever more acute as public clamour for these 'medical miracles' continues unabated.

## The liberalization boon?

### Choice or inequity: harnessing demand-side strategies for social growth

Sri Lanka's record in the colonial and post-colonial period in improving the health chances of its population was indeed a notable achievement for a low income nation. However in the succeeding decades the sustainability of this success came ever more under threat as economic and political[6] developments and demographic[7] and epidemiological[8] change brought new challenges. Furthermore, the year 1977 marked a major turning point in Sri Lankan governance. The introduction of liberalized economic policies following a change in political regime resulted in a radical reversal in development policy. From being a relatively closed economy with an import substitution growth strategy, it went to one that sought to harness the open economy and adopt export promotion as its 'engine of growth'. This fundamentally changed the context for the making of health policy and demanded a change in the role of the state, yet to be realized even three decades later.

This economic transition has continued for 33 years since 1977, despite a number of political regime changes. It has fuelled social transition[9] as have globalization and the communication revolutions: television, the Internet and the spread of cellular technology. These factors have contributed to changes in lifestyle, eating patterns and stress levels that have had major repercussions on the population's health.[10] Currently ischaemic heart disease, diseases of the respiratory system and neoplasms are the leading causes of mortality in the island. The coinciding of the economic and social transitions with demographic and epidemiological transitions has resulted in a major health crisis now with the rise in the NCD burden in the country, and the corresponding economic burden to be borne by the state and household sectors.

At a policy level, a major reorientation of the health care system is currently under consideration.[11] This is an urgent necessity, as the state seeks to grapple with the financial pressures and dilemmas created by the dual burden of communicable and non-communicable diseases. Sri Lanka has achieved significant success in reducing the impact of CDs, even eradicating poliomyelitis and, more recently, leprosy. However the magnitude of diarrhoea and respiratory morbidity in under five year olds (Department of Census and Statistics 2008: 15), the situation with regard to tuberculosis[12] and the 35,007 dengue cases and 346 deaths reported by the Epidemiology Unit of the Ministry of Health (2009) clearly reflect that the burden of CDs remains sizable.

From colonial times the health system had evolved as a supply-side pro-gramme with the objective of providing free health care to patients, 'close to client'.[13] By 2008 the government sector had 619 hospitals with a bed strength of 65,835 and 411 central dispensaries providing allopathic care (Central Bank of Sri Lanka 2008: 73). The objective of the widespread health care network had been 'close to client care' but current evidence exists of substantial by-passing of the nearest facility, as in the case of childbirth where the bulk of deliveries occur in teaching, provincial or base hospitals and not in rural or district hospi-tals or maternity homes.[14] Likewise the overcrowding of the larger hospitals[15] and the geographical and economic inequities evident in NCD prevention and treatment (Perera and Gunetillake 2006: 8–10) argue for the need for change in health service provision.

International agencies such as the World Health Organization, the World Bank and the Japan International Cooperation Agency are currently strongly advocating NCD care at primary health care level in Sri Lanka. Inequities of provision that go against national objectives of equity and of health for all and such advocacy are now pushing policy makers towards a more demand-oriented approach. Providing choice and ensuring the continuity of treatment 'close to client' can be achieved utilizing existing primary health care facilities but will involve enhancing manpower and infrastructure to provide NCD care. More importantly it will also necessitate changes in drug lists, drug distribution and drug provision regulations that currently limit smaller hospitals to issuing drugs only for short durations. The challenge then is how to formulate, coordinate and regulate a demand-oriented state health system including the parallel private sector in such a way as to maintain equity and social growth to ensure that the legacy of good health achieved by the country, far above that to be aspired to by an economy of such low per capita income, continues in the future.

NCD diagnosis, treatment, interventions and outcomes at present are closely linked to economic and geographical accessibility. NCD clinics are provided by base hospitals, provincial hospitals and teaching hospitals but evidence suggests that access to such care is limited by distance and time. These clinics held during working hours are predominantly utilized by females and the aged.[16] Perera and Gunetillake (2006), using case studies of patients in Colombo, Galle, Anurad-hapura and Moneragala, clearly show how distance and poverty in conjunction lead to inappropriate care patterns whereas poverty in cities still allows access to appropriate proximate care. The gap in state services is covered to an extent by accessing the private sector, but the cost of such care results in burdening of households and often endangers continuous care, essential in the context of NCDs.

The Mission of the Ministry of Healthcare and Nutrition is 'To contribute to the social and economic development of Sri Lanka by achieving the highest attainable health status through promotive, preventive, curative and rehabilita-tive services of high quality made available and accessible to people of Sri Lanka' (Ministry of Healthcare and Nutrition 2009). In pursuit of the ministry objective of 'improving comprehensive health services delivery and health actions' in the context of NCDs, different interventions are currently under discussion. The first proposal is to introduce the WHO-PEN programme to primary health care facilities. The WHO-PEN programme involves ensuring that an essential package of facilities (equipment and drugs) is available and that appropriate protocols are adopted at primary health care institutions to ensure a commitment to regular, low-cost, continuous NCD care. Second, under the auspices of the Japan International Cooperation Agency (JICA) community screening and health education are being piloted in the North Western Province of Sri Lanka. The third possibility is to switch from day to day outpatient care to the concept of 'family practice' within the state sector at primary health care level. Fourth, the introduction of a community nursing service, particularly to take care of the elderly and the chronically ill, is under consideration. Finally, just as the use of family health workers (traditionally known as midwives) was a major contributor to the reduction in maternal and infant deaths (Pathmanathan *et al.* 2003: 135) so the use of field-level NCD educators and change agents to reduce NCD mortality is under discussion.

The challenge of achieving 'good health at low cost' is now more daunting since NCDs are clearly more costly to diagnose and treat than CDs.[17] NCD prevalence is increasing alarmingly in the country, including in the rural sector. Heart disease is the number one mortality factor in the country and the prevalence of pre-diabetes and diabetes has been estimated to be one in five adults (Katulanda *et al.* 2008: 1062). Prevention through health education is clearly cost effective and de Silva (2010: 60) argues for community screening given the major burden imposed on households due to NCDs in the form of indirect costs (mainly lost earnings), psychic costs and the heavy economic burden imposed by the cost of care. Despite the availability of free health care, 'push factors' such as shortages of drugs in the state sector, lack of access to specialist care and delays in gaining interventions such as bypass surgery operate, as well as the 'pull factors' of choice and patient comfort, to propel patients towards the private sector.

The private sector had remained small and had contracted even further in 1964 when private practice by state sector doctors was banned.[18] In 1977 with the liberalization of the economy, private practice by state sector doctors was again allowed. This resulted in a phenomenon dubbed 'channelling': dual affiliation by medical staff to the state sector and the private sector, with the latter taking the form of single practices (often in their homes), group practices and working in health clinics or private hospitals outside state working hours (8.30 a.m. to 4.30 p.m.). This spearheaded the growth of the private sector. This trend continues to date with significant expansion in coverage even to rural and remote areas. The private sector thus has grown rapidly. The number of private hospitals in the country as reported by the Central Bank of Sri Lanka (2008: 73) is 220 with a bed strength of 850. The bulk of patient interactions with the private sector, however, is in the form of outpatient care.

The medical specialist market that involves dual affiliation through 'channelling' is limited to the major towns while the market structure is oligopolistic, with the fees charged by different consultants generally tending to be similar and below the market clearing fee that results in queues and delays in accessing services. Medical officers are involved in private practice throughout the country, generally in close proximity to the state sector institutions they serve. In the case of specialists, given the limited number of such staff, private practice is important in enhancing their service provision, an outcome that is favourable in providing patients with choice and access to specialist services. In the case both of medical officers and of specialists this alternative income avenue also plays an important role in buttressing state sector salaries, important in ensuring employee satisfaction and counteracting overseas migration. Some other categories of health care staff, such as laboratory technicians and physiotherapists, also benefit through dual affiliation. The role of the private health care sector in Sri Lanka is complex: dual affiliation of some health care categories, lack of information on demand and supply in the private sector, and multiple sources of health care provision including indigenous health care providers, result in an unregulated health care market and lacunas in health information and management.

The state clearly has a role to play in the regulation of this private sector. One activity it is currently forced to undertake is the prevention of public sector staff working for the private sector during working hours. More importantly, however, it is also expected to be the guardian of quality in private institutions. The Private Medical Institutions (Registration) Act (No. 21) was finally passed in 2006, more than a decade after it was initially drafted, in a bid to control the private sector. The main activity envisaged in the Act is that health institutions are required to register annually with the Ministry of Health. The physical characteristics of the health institution and the qualifications of private health sector employees are to be inspected during the registration process. Querying financial investment in the health care institution and looking into billing/recording processes also come under the ambit of the Act, as prerequisites for gaining annual registration. Controls relating to the quality and pricing of services are also under discussion as the state seeks to strengthen stewardship and management functions in the private sector in line with the main objective of the Health Development Master Plan of improving health status and reducing inequalities.[19] Given that 52.5 per cent of total health expenditure was in the private sector in 2007 and that 86.7 per cent of this was out of pocket expenditure (WHO 2010), the burden on households is a major concern, necessitating policies for cost containment in the private sector in the future. Parallel to this runs the interest in expanding pre-payment and insurance schemes.

The existence of this strong alternative private sector is both a boon and a challenge to the state sector. It puts pressure on the state to change its role from being primarily that of a provider of health care to one that coordinates, regulates and facilitates health care provision in the country. National health policy should then be directed to optimizing the strengths of the public and private sectors in order to benefit from this synergy and to safeguard the access to health care of the poor in what has clearly become over time a two-tiered health system. The two tiers, it should be noted, are not essentially a reflection of differences in quality of care (the state has well-trained medical specialists, medical officers and nurses and strives to keep pace with the growth in technology in the private sector) but relate to such factors as timeliness of interventions, ease of access, comfort and choice.

An educated population, a widespread state health care network and an active private sector coexist but can the burden of NCDs be reduced as successfully as that of CDs in Sri Lanka through the hitherto successful 'social growth path'? The challenges are many.

First, it should be noted that the double burden encompasses the entire population since poverty does not immunize the poor from NCDs as previously perceived. The Barker hypothesis on the contrary argues that those born underweight (most likely children of poor households) actually have a higher probability of developing coronary heart disease, stroke, diabetes mellitus and hypertension in adulthood if their nutritional status improves over time due to their poor foetal metabolic development in the intrauterine stage. State financing of NCD care then seems crucial. While state health expenditure accounts for close to 50 per cent of total health expenditure in the country and the inpatient burden in particular is being borne significantly by the public sector, the cost of NCD outpatient care, drugs, investigations and interventions is falling on households even in the rural areas.

Second, committing sufficient health financing to expanding NCD provision is a challenge for the state. On the expenditure side, competing demands on the state including defence and rehabilitation, given the recently resolved civil war, are likely to constrain the health budget, though the state is currently ranking health as its second priority expenditure head. Tax revenue which is the primary source of government funding, too, is likely to be limited, given the expected low growth rates in the context of a world recession. Furthermore the poorly designed and implemented tax system in the country has resulted in a tax to GDP ratio of only 14.2 per cent in 2007 (Central Bank of Sri Lanka 2008: 129). In contrast the government expenditure to GDP ratio is 23.5 per cent and the resulting budget deficit constrains current spending and adds to the future expenditure burden in the country through the resulting indebtedness. The country faces major policy dilemmas. Is there a role for an 'essential package' of care defined rather more broadly than is usual in order to cover NCDs as well as CDs? Should rationing if needed occur systematically, based on predetermined criteria rather than on the current ad hoc basis where, for instance, a large number of drugs are provided free but when drug stocks are exhausted, shortages force all patients to purchase drugs privately?

Moreover, though Sri Lanka has a sizeable private outpatient health care sector, the inpatient burden still rests with the state sector. This is due to the very limited role played by private health insurance in the country with only 3 per cent of private health financing being attributed to private health insurance in 2006 (Fernando *et al.* 2009: 17). While prevention and early diagnosis could go a long way in reducing the hospitalization burden, the feasibility of introducing social insurance or methods of providing safety nets to poor patients to access private sector care for interventions such as bypass surgery needs rigorous analysis.

There may also, as in the colonial period, be a role for voluntary charitable donations. Philanthropists are often begged through the media to assist those needing bypass surgery or kidney transplantation either locally or more often abroad. Likewise donations are made to state hospitals: drugs, equipment or even the painting of wards or landscaping of gardens. Such donations are made by individuals, schools, firms and social service organizations. Many hospitals have a hospital committee that seeks to involve the community, particularly private sector organizations, in hospital development. Harnessing such financing that currently happens very much on a person-to-person basis rather than under a planned programme of hospital development or patient needs could enhance service provision, ensure equity of outcomes and improve the responsiveness of the health system.[20]

This problem is likely to be exacerbated as Sri Lanka's population is ageing rapidly (World Bank 2008: 1). This has repercussions both on health conditions and income levels as many people will be in the retired age group, with smaller financial resources, at the very point when their health needs are at a peak. This is not a group that can seek private health insurance as a means of distributing risk since most insurance schemes either do not cover the elderly or have premiums that are heavily biased against them. The state health care system takes care of their needs gratis but travelling for care and accessing appropriate care in a continuous manner in particular is challenging since public transport is often crowded, making it inappropriate for the sick elderly. This is where moving geriatric and NCD care to PHC level (as advocated by WHO) and community-level, home-based care are likely to become crucial to the wellbeing of the elderly.

This section has focused on the challenges of the health system as it faces demographic, epidemiological and socio-economic transition. It has also highlighted the policy options that are currently under consideration as Sri Lanka grapples with its NCD 'epidemic'. Clearly health transition necessitates health system transition. The NCD crisis makes reform imperative. However, whether such reforms allow Sri Lanka to remain a 'model of social growth', a country achieving favourable equity and health outcomes at low cost, will depend on the country's ability to achieve effective health system transition. Whether policymakers are able to swing their thinking regarding health care provision from 'supply side' to 'demand orientation' and be innovative in determining health financing alternatives including the consideration of other options such as the partial subsidization and systematization of rationing in place of free health care will determine the effectiveness of the transition. The problem is to ensure that the challenges of liberalization are met by effective health transition policies that ensure it promotes the health outcomes of the entire nation.

Sri Lanka's role as an exemplar of good health at low cost is clearly under threat in this second decade of the twenty-first century. The double disease burden and demographic transition which now confront it place great pressure on its continuing commitment to providing accessible health care for all. The colonial legacy contributed to an impressive record in the reduction of deaths from CDs and infant and maternal mortality rates commensurate with rich developed nations; and it contributed to a health system founded on equity. Successive governments since independence have resisted the pressure to reform the health system through pathways like user charges and have continued along the supply-side, free health care approach to achieve further successes: eradicating poliomyelitis and leprosy, significantly reducing child diarrhoeal deaths and achieving laudable life expectancy, fertility, maternal and child mortality indicators. That present day policymakers are aware of the dilemmas is evident from the discussions outlined here: but are they, the political leadership and the people, ready to adopt a new paradigm: harnessing demand-side strategies for social growth? Health system transition in this direction seems imperative but such reforms must ensure the safeguarding of equity and the health achievements to date. Undoubtedly, social growth that stemmed from the unlikely source of colonization and that was nurtured even during challenging economic crises and civil war conditions must remain the core of any future reforms.

## Notes

1  Sri Lanka, formerly Ceylon, was a British colony from 1805 until independence in 1948.
2  There is also a thriving independent and government Ayurvedic medicine sector.
3  Interestingly, however, historical chronicles like the Mahawansa and Rajaratnakaraya record the existence of hospitals in ancient Sri Lanka (see Jones 2009: 3).
4  User charges had been in existence from as early as 1903, but the cut-off point was fixed at such a level that Rannan-Eliya and de Mel (1997: 33) prove that in the 1940s over 90 per cent of the population were exempt.
5  It should be noted too that women were admitted to the College on equal terms with men from 1890.
6  Sri Lanka was plagued by a civil war that lasted over 30 years when the Liberation Tigers of Tamil Eelam were fighting for a separate state. While the civil war disrupted health services and adversely affected the availability of health personnel in the conflict areas, the state continued to fund the public service and to provide drugs and equipment. Public health remained a major concern even among the rebels as evidenced by the declaration of 'ceasefires' to coincide with polio immunization from 1995–1999 that allowed for polio eradication in Sri Lanka (WHO 2001). Furthermore, health reports were published for rebel-held areas by the North East Province Provincial Planning Secretariat in 2002 including statistics on diseases such as diarrhoea and respiratory illness. In May 2009 the mass exodus from rebel held areas towards the end of the civil war was a major humanitarian crisis: the government sought to provide health care, nutrition, clothing and shelter to over 265,000 internally displaced persons in the Northern Province which was resolved through the efforts of the state, international aid, NGO cooperation and donations from the general public. As in the case of the Tsunami in 2004, rapid systematic intervention prevented major epidemics among the displaced (WHO-SEARO 2009).
7  Sri Lanka has reached the third phase of demographic transition characterized by a declining birth rate and a relatively stable low death rate. The Central Bank of Sri Lanka *Annual Report* (2009a) records the percentage of the population above age 55 as estimated during its socio-economic surveys to be 7.2 per cent in 1963, 8.9 per cent in 1981/1982 and 14.1 per cent in 2003/2004 with the corresponding values for the population under 14 years reduced from 40.5 per cent to 34.0 per cent to 23.4 per cent.

8  As stated in the National Policy and Strategic Framework for prevention and control of chronic non-communicable diseases (2009) of the Ministry of Health and Nutrition 'Currently, chronic non-communicable diseases are overtaking communicable diseases as the dominant health problem, and are now the leading causes of mortality, morbidity and disability'. The major chronic NCDs that have a significant disease burden are cardiovascular diseases, including coronary heart disease, cerebrovascular diseases and hypertension, diabetes mellitus (DM), chronic respiratory diseases, chronic renal diseases and cancers. Road traffic accidents are also a major health burden in terms of mortality and disability. This document goes on to state that currently ischaemic heart disease including myocardial infarction is the leading cause of mortality in hospitals in Sri Lanka. This report states that no national level disaggregated data exist by gender, ethnicity or sector, but that small research studies have found higher DM rates among urban populations, higher DM rates among females, higher ischaemic heart disease rates among males and about the same rate of hypertension among both sexes.

9  Social transition refers to changes in social structures, institutions, behaviour and interactions that have resulted from international and domestic economic, political, social and cultural dynamics stimulated in this period primarily by the forces of globalization, liberalization and technological developments in transportation, communication and media.

10  *Demographic and Health Survey 2006/2007* reports 7.2 per cent of women in the age group 15–49 as being obese (BMI above 30). Obesity is considered a major risk factor for DM among females and urban dwellers in Sri Lanka (Katulanda *et al.* 2008: 1068).

11  Consultations were held in this regard involving the different Directors of the Ministry of Health, the Provincial Directors of Health Services, the Director General of Health Services and the Secretary to the Ministry of Health in 2009.

12  Tuberculosis continues to be a major public health problem in the country in 2010 with about 9,000 new cases notified every year, of which around 60 per cent are smear-positive pulmonary TB cases (National Programme for Tuberculosis and Chest Diseases 2010). In 2007, cases per 100,000 population based on trends in hospitalization and hospital deaths were 35.2 and deaths 1.4 (Ministry of Healthcare and Nutrition 2007: 31). However the high numbers of TB cases are not linked to HIV/AIDS with the prevalence of HIV/AIDS remaining relatively low at present.

13  A characteristic advocated by the Macroeconomics and Health Commission of the WHO in 2000.

14  In 2007, 33 per cent of births took place in teaching hospitals, 22 per cent in provincial hospitals, 33 per cent in base hospitals; with only 12 per cent occurring in district hospitals, peripheral units, rural hospitals and maternity homes (Ministry of Healthcare and Nutrition 2007: 52), even though these hospitals are staffed by medical officers in addition to nurses and midwives.

15  In 2007, provincial and base hospitals recorded a bed turnover rate of 102.1 and 108.4 (including floor patients) and occupancy rates of 94.8 and 70.0 respectively in contrast to bed turnover rates of 71.0, 71.9 and 77.5 and occupancy rates of 39.4, 40.1 and 40.6 in district hospitals, peripheral units and rural hospitals respectively (Ministry of Healthcare and Nutrition 2007: 53).

16  See de Silva (2007) study entitled 'Financing NCD Treatment: Burden of Out of Pocket Expenditure'.

17  NCDs are more costly than CDs to treat due to being chronic, degenerative diseases involving longer periods of medication and hospitalization. Such diseases often necessitate rehabilitative care as well. The *Review of Costing Studies Conducted in Sri Lanka 1990–2004* (de Silva *et al.* 2007) which collates and summarizes the findings of a large number of costing studies by different authors on different diseases in Sri Lanka, finds NCD care to be far more costly than that for CDs due to the former involving more sophisticated interventions and expensive pharmaceuticals.

18  Specialist private practice was banned in 1972.
19  The main objective of the Health Development Master Plan – improving health status and reducing inequalities – will be achieved by implementing five strategic objectives: empowering the community to maintain and promote their own health; improving comprehensive health service delivery and health actions; strengthening stewardship and management functions; improving the management of human resources for health; and improving health finance, mobilization, allocation and utilization.
20  Responsiveness of the health system refers to how the health system meets the needs of individuals in contrast to that of patients (a concept introduced by WHO in its Health System's Performance Evaluation framework presented in the *World Health Report* (2000). Responsiveness covers aspects such as the quality of basic amenities, prompt attention, dignity and choice.

## References

Central Bank of Sri Lanka (2008) *Annual Report*, Colombo: Central Bank of Sri Lanka.

Central Bank of Sri Lanka (2009a) *Annual Report*, Colombo: Central Bank of Sri Lanka.

Central Bank of Sri Lanka (2009b) *Recent Economic Developments: Highlights of 2009 and Prospects for 2010*, Colombo: Central Bank of Sri Lanka.

Cumpston, J.H.L. (1950) *Sessional Paper III, Report on the Medical and Public Health Organisations of Ceylon*, London: HMSO.

*Daily News* (1970) 'Problems of Our Doctors Listed', 3 September, Lakehouse Library Archive, Colombo.

de Silva, A. (2004) 'Overview of the Health Sector', in S. Kelegama (ed.) *Economic Policies in Sri Lanka (A festschrift in honour of Gamini Corea)*, New Delhi: Sage Publications, 426–444.

de Silva, A. (2007) 'Financing NCD Treatment: Burden of Out of Pocket Expenditure', Report of the Working Group on Financing of the National Commission of Macroeconomics and Health, in *Working Groups on Budgeting and Financing (Study Report 7)*, Colombo: National Commission on Macroeconomics and Health, Ministry of Healthcare and Nutrition.

de Silva, A. (2010) 'Costing of NCD Screening at Primary Health Care Level', Study undertaken for the Japan International Cooperation Agency, Colombo, Mimeo.

de Silva, A., Samarage, S.M. and Somanathan, A. (2007) *Review of Costing Studies Conducted in Sri Lanka 1990–2004 (Study Report 6)*, Colombo: National Commission on Macroeconomics and Health, Ministry of Healthcare and Nutrition.

de Silva, K.M. (1997) 'Sri Lanka: Part I, the Second World War and the Soulbury Commission, 1939–45', in K.M. de Silva (ed.) *British Documents on the End of Empire*, London: HMSO, i–xxxv.

Department of Census and Statistics (2008) *Sri Lanka: Demographic and Health Survey 2006/2007 Preliminary Report*, Colombo: Department of Census and Statistics.

Epidemiology Unit (2009) Ministry of Healthcare and Nutrition, Sri Lanka. Online, available at: www.epid.gov.lk (accessed 10 January 2010).

Fernando, M. (2004) 'Hospitals in Sri Lanka', Personal communication by email, 8 November.

Fernando, T., Rannan-Eliya, R. and Jayasundara, J.M.H. (2009) *Sri Lanka Health Accounts: National Health Expenditures 1990–2006*, IHP Health Expenditure Series, No. 1, Colombo: Institute of Health Policy.

Fleisher, L., Pablo, G., Leive, A., Schieber, G.J., Tandon, A. and Walters, H.R. (2008) 'Introduction to Part 1', in P. Gottret, G.J. Scheiber and H.R. Waters (eds) *Good*

*Practices in Health Financing: Lessons from Reforms in Low- and Middle-Income Countries*, Washington, DC: World Bank, 3–8.

Hewa, S. (1995) *Colonialism, Tropical Disease and Imperial Medicine*, Lanham, MD: University Press of America.

Jones, M. (2004) *Health Policy in Britain's Model Colony: Ceylon, 1900–1948*, Hyderabad: Orient Longman.

Jones, M. (2009) *The Hospital System and Health Care: Sri Lanka, 1815–1960*, Hyderabad: Orient Blackswan.

Kahawita, L.J. (1955) *Annual Medical Report*, Department of Medical Services, Ceylon National Archives, Public Record Office (NA: PRO) Kew: DO 109/29.

Katulanda, P., Constantine, G.R., Mahesh, J.G., Seneviratne, R.D.A., Wijeratne, S., Wijesuriya, M., McCarthy, M.I., Adler, A.I. and Matthews, D.R. (2008) 'Prevalence and Projection of Diabetes and Pre-diabetes in Adults in Sri Lanka-Sri Lanka Diabetes, Cardiovascular Study (SLDCS)', *Diabetic Medicine*, 25: 1062–1069.

Keuneman, P.G.B (1955) *Debates of the Appropriation Bill, Parliamentary Debates*, 15 August, 1498, Sri Lanka National Archives Library, Colombo.

Kynsey, W.R. (1876) *Annual Medical Report*, Department of Medical Services, Ceylon National Archives, Public Record Office (NA:PRO) Kew: CO 57/69), 'Report on the Medical School'.

Ministry of Health (2009) 'The National Policy and Strategic Framework for Prevention and Control of Chronic Non-communicable Diseases', draft document circulated as a mimeo. Online, available at: http://203.94.76.60/NCD/temp/NCD%20Policy%20 English.pdf (accessed 6 February 2010).

Ministry of Healthcare and Nutrition (2007) *Annual Health Bulletin*. Online, available at: http://203.94.76.60/AHB2007/Annual%20Health%20Statistics% 202007.html (accessed 20 January 2010).

Ministry of Healthcare and Nutrition (2009) *National Health Policy: Sri Lanka*. Online, available at: http:/www.health.gov.lk (accessed 14 January 2010).

National Programme for Tuberculosis and Chest Diseases (2010) Website. Online, available at: http://203.94.76.60/TBWeb/index.htm (accessed 12 January 2010).

Ordinance No. 3 (1905) *Ordinance to Incorporate the Council of the Ceylon Medical College*, National Archives, Public Record Office (NA: PRO), Kew: CO 56/16.

Ordinance No. 2 (1905) *Ordinance to Provide for the Registration of Medical Practitioners in Ceylon*, National Archives, Public Record Office (NA: PRO), Kew: CO 56/16.

Padley, R. (1957–1961) *Final Report on Health Statistics Project, Ceylon. WHO Project: Ceylon 45*: 2. World Health Organization, Library Historical Collection: SRL/ DHS/001, Health Statistics, 1961–1977.

Panditaratne, B.L. and Selvanayagam, S. (1973) 'The Demography of Ceylon: An Introductory Survey', in K.M. de Silva (ed.) *History of Ceylon,* Vol. 3, Peradeniya: University of Ceylon, 285–302.

Pathmanathan, I., Liljestrand, J., Martins, J.M., Rajapaksa, L.C., Lissner, C., de Silva, A., Selvaraju, S. and Singh, P.J. (2003) *Investing in Maternal Health: Learning from Malaysia and Sri Lanka*, Washington, DC: World Bank.

Perera, M. and Gunetillake, G. (2006) 'Affordability and Accessibility of Healthcare for Non Communicable Diseases in Sri Lanka: Synopsis of the Sri Lanka Case Study in the Affordability Ladder Programme', *Marga Journal* (Special Issue), April: 1–43.

Rannan-Eliya, R.P. and de Mel, N. (1997) *Resource Mobilization for the Health Sector in Sri Lanka, Data for Decision Making Publication*, Boston, MA: Harvard School of Public Health.

WHO-SEARO (2009) Health Cluster Situation Report. Online, available at: www.searo. who.int/LinkFiles/Sri_Lanka_270709-SitRep.pdf (accessed 12 January 2010).

Wickremesinghe, W.G. (1945) 'A National Health Service for Ceylon', *Journal of the Ceylon Branch of the British Medical Association*, 41(1): 1–12.

Wickremesinghe, W.G. (1950) *Annual Medical Report*, Department of Medical Services, Ceylon, National Archives, Public Record Office, Kew: DO 109/12: 1–2.

World Bank (2008) *Sri Lanka Addressing the Needs of an Aging Population, Report No 43996-LK*, Colombo: World Bank Human Development Unit South Asia Region.

World Health Organization (2000) *World Health Report*, Geneva: WHO.

World Health Organization (2010) National Health Accounts website for Sri Lanka. Online, available at: www.who.int/nha/country/lka.pdf (accessed 10 January 2010).

World Health Organization (2001) 'Health as a Bridge for Peace: Humanitarian Cease-Fires Project'. Online, available at: www.who.int/hac/techguidance/hbp/cease_fires/en/index.html (accessed 10 January 2010).

# 8 Double disease burden in Thailand

## Economic growth and public provisioning

*Paul T. Cohen and Thapin Phatcharanurak*

## Introduction

Since the Second World War the overall health status of Thailand's population has improved considerably. There have been significant reductions in child, infant and maternal mortality and increases in life expectancy, due in large measure to the control of communicable diseases. Over the past few decades there has been a downward trend in rates of morbidity and mortality from communicable diseases (except for the eruption of some new diseases such as HIV/AIDS) and a concurrent upward trend in non-communicable diseases.

That the new health burden of non-communicable diseases and road traffic accidents overlaps with a period of unprecedented economic prosperity raises an important issue concerning the relationship between economic growth and health outcomes. One of the salient features of health transition in Thailand is that major advances in health, especially in communicable disease control, were attained during recession and stagnant economic growth and the critical factor here was public investment in health. Public health is usually associated with state investment. However, in Thailand the standard of public health, over the past 30 years or so, owes much to the growth of civil society and non-government organisations involved in health care – not only through direct investment in health resources but also through political influence on state authorities.

## Decline in communicable diseases and public health

Early public health initiatives in Thailand can be traced back to the American missionary Dan Beach Bradley (1804–1873) and his advocacy of regular cleaning of houses and shallow canals in Bangkok. Government decrees subsequently mandated the cleaning of rivers and canals and culminated in the creation of the Department of Sanitation (*Krom Sukhaphiban*) in 1897 (Davisakd 2007: 315–318). However, these measures were based on miasmic theory (that illness was caused by poisonous vapours from decomposed matter) and it was not until the early twentieth century that germ theory won acceptance in the context of the early modernisation of the Thai state. This was accompanied by a growing elite awareness of the link between national prosperity and a healthy population. Under the nationalistic policies of Field Marshall Phibun Songkhram a National Nutrition Project was initiated to combat the high mortality rate, particularly among children (ibid.: 334–338). It was during Phibun's rule that the Ministry of Public Health was established in 1942.

One of the most successful public health campaigns after the Second World War was the malaria control programme. In 1947 there were 52,034 deaths from malaria alone, with a mortality rate of 297.1 per 100,000 population (Yuwadi 2002: 66). Since 1951, with United States and WHO assistance, malaria control by DDT and later by pyrethroid spraying and other vector-control measures has been expanded throughout the country. By 1977 the malaria death rate had been reduced to 10.9 per 100,000 and to 0.48 per 100,000 in 2006. However, while mortality has steadily declined there have been periodic upsurges in infection rates in the late 1980s and late 1990s and malaria remains a serious problem in some border areas (*Thailand Health Profile 2005–2007*:187).

Vaccine-preventable diseases have also been substantially reduced, especially since the Ministry of Public Health (MoPH) launched its Expanded Programme on Immunisation in the early 1980s to improve coverage of target populations groups such as children and pregnant women. Between 1977 and 2006 the incidence per 100,000 population of measles declined from 20.2 to 5.31, neonatal tetanus from 72.1 to nil, diphtheria from 5.2 to nil, pertussis from 7.2 to 0.11 and poliomyelitis from 2.1 to nil. Only hepatitis B has increased (from 0.09 per 100,000 in 1979 to 5.48 in 2006), possibly due to improved surveillance (ibid.: 176).

Primary health care (PHC) has made an effective contribution to the reduction of communicable diseases. PHC was incorporated into the Fourth Five-Year Development Plan (1977–1981) even before the first international conference on PHC at Alma Ata in 1978. By 2006 Village Health Volunteers numbered 791,383. They have played an important role in vaccination campaigns, communicable disease surveillance, control of malaria and dengue haemorrhagic fever and dissemination of health information.

As a result of these various health interventions life expectancy at birth has increased from a low 52 years in 1960 to 73.7 years in 2006 (ibid.: 161), child mortality has decreased rapidly from 146 in 1960 to 10.4 per 1,000 live births in 2006 (UNICEF 1994: 79–81; *Thailand Health Profile 2005–2007*: 167) and maternal mortality has declined from 374.3 per 100,000 live births in 1962 to 9.8 in 2006 (*Thailand Health Profile 2005–2007*: 164).

## Re-emerging and emerging communicable diseases

However, in recent decades certain endemic communicable diseases have persisted and new communicable diseases have emerged. Some of these diseases – malaria, dengue haemorrhagic fever and HIV/AIDS – reflect broader economic and demographic problems of poverty and human mobility.

## Mobile populations and public health intervention

Human mobility poses particular problems for public health. It often hinders public health interventions due to the difficulties of access and contact and the higher costs involved compared to sedentary populations. In Thailand and neighbouring countries the movement of people is closely linked to poverty and takes a number of forms: cross-border migration of refugees and economic migrants from the poorer countries of Cambodia, Laos and Burma (Myanmar), the circulation of poor Thai farmers within rural areas and rural to urban migration of the poor within Thailand.

Migration has been fuelled by poverty in neighbouring countries of Burma, Laos and Cambodia and the need for low-wage labour in Thailand in fishing, agriculture and industry. The main source of cross-border migration in the west has been ethnic minorities escaping both poverty and political oppression in Burma. In 2004, in the ten western provinces of Thailand that border Burma, there were 400,888 registered migrants (about one-third of the total for Thailand as a whole), a registered refugee camp population of 116,704, and an estimated 500,000 undocumented (illegal) migrants. Multidrug resistant *falciparum* malaria is the major health problem for these populations. While these border provinces have 11 per cent of Thailand's population they report almost 70 per cent of malaria cases (WHO 2009: 1). In the camps morbidity and mortality are relatively low due to good access to diagnosis and treatment (Luxemburger *et al.* 1996: 110). However, the large number of illegal migrants poses a significant problem for national and international health authorities due to the difficulty of locating and monitoring the health of these persons.

Malaria is also still a problem for lowland farmers who have regular contact with forested areas of border regions. Anchalee Singhanetra-Renard has highlighted the health effects of population pressure on land resources in northern Thailand that forces males from land-poor villages into forest work and border activities (swiddening, illegal logging, cattle and other goods smuggling and poaching) and brings them into contact with *Anopheles dirus* – the primary vector of malaria and transmitter of the *Plasmodium falciparum* and which breeds abundantly in the shaded, freshwater pools of the forested hills. Poverty has forced these Thai citizens into fringe or illegal activities that take them 'outside the net of public health or vector control programmes' (Anchalee 1993: 1153). Anchalee concludes that residual insecticide spraying, use of mosquito nets and insect repellent are unsuitable control measures for those continuously on the move and that case detection and therapy (normally excellent in Thailand) are difficult to apply to Thais and non-Thais involved in illegal activities (ibid.: 1153–1154).

Another mosquito transmitted disease (the principal vector being *Culex quinquefasciatus*) is (lymphatic) filariasis which has the potential to develop into disfiguring elephantitis. Nationally the incidence per 100,000 population has been reduced from 8.46 in 1992 to 0.35 in 2006 but, like malaria, filariasis is still a significant health problem in border areas, especially the Thai-Burma border (*Thailand Health Profile 2005–2007*: 188).

Dengue haemorrhagic fever continues to be a serious health hazard, with periodic outbreaks in parts of the country. The disease tends to be highly localised (as the vector mosquito, *Aedes Aegypti*, does not travel far from its breeding place) and is concentrated in urban areas which provide the ideal breeding sites for this mosquito (for example, small water containers). The worst epidemic of the post-war period was in 1958 with a rate of infection of more than 300 per 100,000 population and a mortality rate of 13.9 per cent. There have been a number of other outbreaks since then but over the past 30 years deaths from the disease have declined significantly. The last epidemic occurred as recently as 2008 with 87,494 people infected (138.8 per 100,000 population) but a mortality rate of only 0.12 per cent (101 deaths). Urban slums in Bangkok have increased from 438 slum sites in 1980 to 2,265 in 2000 as a result of rural-to-urban migration (*Thailand Health Profile 1999–2000*: 127). Urban slums are particularly vulnerable to dengue epidemics due to poor access to drinking water and use of ceramic jugs to collect rainwater. Also, symptoms are most severe among the undernourished poor of these slums, especially young children (IRIN 2009: 2).

HIV/AIDS has been a major health problem in Thailand since the late 1980s and is the leading cause of death among the infectious diseases. In 2007 the estimated number of AIDS deaths was 31,000 with the number of people estimated to be living with HIV by the end of 2007 being 610,000 (Avert 2010: 1). HIV infection has also caused the re-emergence of tuberculosis from the mid-1990s following a period of decline (see Figure 8.1).

The main impetus for the HIV/AIDS epidemic was the expansion of the commercial sex industry, both sex tourism and domestic commercial sex. A large proportion of commercial sex workers (CSWs) come from the north. And this region has the highest rate of HIV infection (*Thailand Health Profile 2005–2007*: 194), due to a number of factors: the return of HIV-infected CSWs from Bangkok, a cultural acceptance of male patronage of brothels and increased cash income with which to purchase sexual services, and the frequency of micro-mobility in this region of wage labourers and of lorry drivers, which has facilitated contact between mobile male groups and local CSWs (Thiesmeyer 2001: 3). Furthermore, in the past two decades there has been a significant increase in the trafficking of foreign girls and women (particularly among highland minority groups) for the sex industry in Thailand. Migrant women are especially vulnerable to HIV infection due to their illegal status, language difficulties and little knowledge of HIV/AIDS. They have tended to concentrate at border towns (such as Mae Sai, Chiang Saen and Chiang Khong in northern Thailand), which become junctions for foreign migrants, permanent residents, internal migrants and other mobile groups, and thus high-risk 'hot spots' for HIV infection.

Despite initial apathy and denials the Thai Government launched a massive education and information campaign through radio stations, TV networks and schools and a programme of distribution of condoms in brothels and massage parlours. Consequently, Thailand has been remarkably successful in controlling the epidemic and reversing the spread of HIV/AIDS. By the end of 2007 new

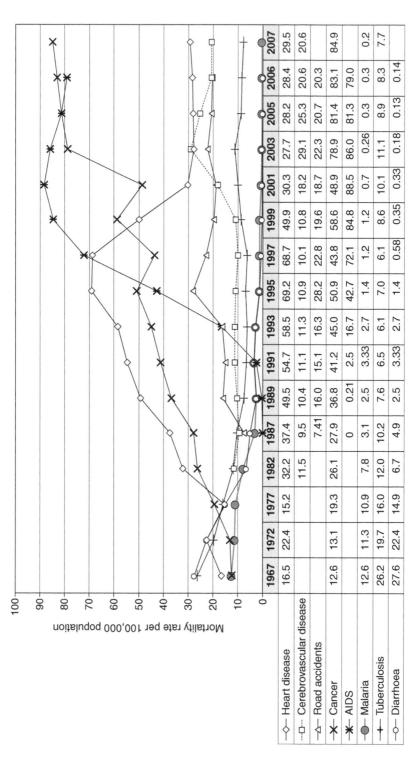

*Figure 8.1* Mortality rates due to major causes of death (sources: (1) *Thailand Health Profile 2005–2007:172, 215*, (2) Bureau of Policy and Strategy 2007).

infections have been reduced from a peak of 143,000 in 1991 to only 13,936 in 2007 (UNGASS 2008: 2).

However, foreign migrants remain a problem both in terms of potential pools of infection and in relation surveillance and treatment. By the end of 2007 there was an estimated two million foreign migrants in Thailand with only about one-third of these registered. Registered workers must have health checks allowing the government to screen for communicable diseases. Those who register have to pay a fee of 1,300 baht (US$40 approx.) to make them eligible for free health care. Migrant health strategy has evolved as a joint effort of government and civil society through a programme called PHAMIT (Prevention of HIV/AIDS among Migrant Workers in Thailand). It is led by the Raks Thai Foundation with seven non-governmental organisation (NGO) partners and one government agency. The programme helps in the training of migrant health volunteers (now numbering about 500 in 30 provinces) to distribute information, education, communication materials and condoms (Thongphit 2009: 1; UNGASS 2008: 47). However, one problem is that many registered migrants are unaware of their rights and may not use health care facilities. Notably the health package for registered migrant workers excludes costly ARV (anti-retroviral drug) treatment. The gap has been filled since 2007 by the NAPHA Extension Programme funded by the Global Fund to Fight AIDS, TB and Malaria. Some illegal migrants have access to ARV treatment through this programme but are often reluctant to visit health centres out of fear of arrest.

The link between HIV/AIDS and cross-border mobility underscores the regional dimension of the disease. The same can be said of new emerging diseases such as SARS and avian (bird) flu. In response to the SARS epidemic of 2003 Thailand instituted effective systems of surveillance, infection control and public information and was able to limit the number of cases of infection to nine with only two deaths. There were 12 reported deaths of humans by May 2005 and, ominously, there were some suspected cases of human-to-human transmission. By the end of July 2009 there was an estimated 100,000 cases of H1N1 flu with 44 deaths.

## Non-communicable diseases

Figure 8.1 reveals significant increases in mortality rates from non-communicable diseases in recent decades.[1] Between 1982 and 1997 the mortality rate for heart disease more than doubled. Since 1997 there has been a decline in the number of deaths due to improvement in people's access to medical treatment and in medical technology. However, hospitalisation for heart disease continued upward from 63.4 per 100,000 population in 1985 to 173.6 in 1997 to 394.6 in 2007 (*Thailand Health Profile 2005–2007*: 207). A comparison of health surveys in 1991/1992 with those of 2003/2004 show significant increases in cholesterol, elevated blood sugar, overweight and obesity in the 35–59 age group – all risk factors for heart disease (ibid.: 117). Bangkok residents had the highest incidence of overweight and obesity (and northerners the lowest) and residents of municipal areas had higher overweight/obesity prevalence than rural residents. Overweight, obesity and lack of exercise have contributed to a sharp rise, since the mid-1980s, in hospital admission rates for diabetes, from 33.3 per 100,000 population in 1985 to 650.4 in 2007 (ibid.: 112, 207).

Another risk factor for heart disease is hypertension. The prevalence of hypertension has increased from 5.4 per cent in 1991 to 22.0 per cent in 2004. The rate of detection has increased. However, there is a low rate of patients receiving medical treatment (ibid.: 208) and the rate of hypertensive patients whose blood pressure is under control is low (Janpen 2003: 237). Furthermore, as hypertension is more prevalent with age, an increase of prevalence of hypertension among aged Thais has occurred both in urban and rural areas (*Thailand Health Profile 2005–2007*: 242). It is likely that, in the light of the increasing number of people aged over 60 years, the prevalence of hypertensive patients will continuously increase and increase the rate of hypertension as a risk factor for heart disease. Hypertension is also the most important cause of cerebrovascular disease (e.g. stroke) and there is an alarming increase in mortality from this disease since 1999 (see Figure 8.1).

Figure 8.1 also indicates is a rising trend in mortality from various forms of cancer and cancer was the leading cause of death in 2007. The incidence of cervical and breast cancer among females increased steadily between 1993 and 2000 (ibid.: 202). Thailand has the highest rate of liver cancer in the world, partly as a consequence of food contamination and inadequately heated food and partly due to liver fluke which is endemic in northeastern and northern Thailand and is caused by eating of uncooked cyprinoid fish. Other cancers are related to toxins from industrial estates and to the 'chemicalisation' of agriculture, with the widespread use of insecticides, fungicides and herbicides.[2] Lung cancer increased sevenfold between 1985 and 1997 and was probably linked to increased tobacco consumption and to air pollution (ibid.: 205).

### Changes in the Thai economy and the economic boom: impact on health

This transition to the predominance of non-communicable diseases is closely linked to changes in the Thai economy, in particular to export-led economic expansion since the mid 1980s, with attendant industrialisation, globalisation and growth of the urban middle class and of urban consumerism.

In the second half of the nineteenth century Thailand became increasingly incorporated into the global economy with the growth of rice exports to the West and to British and Dutch colonies in Asia. The country continued for many years to be economically dependent on rice agriculture. However, in the 1960s the Thai government began to encourage agricultural diversification and the export of non-rice crops. This led to the 'chemicalisation' of Thai agriculture with massive increases in fertiliser and pesticide application.[3]

The government also encouraged import-substituting manufacture and basic industries (e.g. textiles). However, in the late 1970s economic growth slackened in the wake of the global oil crisis and the country entered a period of recession until the mid-1980s. The recession prompted the government to promote export-led growth and the country was soon to experience a 'Golden Age' of economic boom. By 1988 Thailand had become the best performer in the Asian region when GDP growth reached 13.2 per cent (Pasuk and Baker 1995: 151). GDP growth doubled between 1988 and 1992 driven by exports in manufactures and the service industry centred on tourism and fed by foreign investment. During the 1980s the Thai economy was transformed from one that was dependent on agricultural exports to a major exporter of manufactures: between 1980 and 1993 the contribution of agriculture to GDP fell from 27 to 12 per cent and manufacturing's contribution increased from 16 to 26 per cent (ibid.: 153). The early stages of this boom was characterised by the relocation of manufacturing from Japan, Hong Kong and Taiwan to the outskirts of Bangkok (especially from Japan). Later Thai investment flowed out to neighbouring countries in Southeast Asia, including China (Pasuk and Baker 1998: 28, 49–53).

From 1985 to 1995 Thailand's urban population doubled in response to industrial growth and rural–urban migration especially from the poor Northeast. Urbanisation has been accompanied also by the growth of the urban middle class and 'aggressive new urban consumerism' spawned by the economic boom (Pasuk and Baker 1995: 153). Between 1985 and 1995 real income per capita doubled, much of it concentrated in the urban middle class (Pasuk and Baker 1998: 45). Consumerism was characterised by the proliferation in Bangkok and in the large provincial cities of shopping malls, department stores, hypermarkets (owned by Thai, British and French multinational companies), movie cinemas, karaoke booths, video arcades, food courts and fast food franchises, and convenient stores such as 7/11. Motor cars have also become objects of desire for middle-class consumers. Economic stimulus measures and low interest monetary policy has stimulated automobile sales and there is a close correlation between auto sales and road accidents (*Thailand Health Profile 2005–2007*: 220). Consumer capitalism stimulated the growth of the media and of advertising. From 1985 total advertising revenues increased about 25 per cent each year (Pasuk and Baker 1998: 48). TV and advertising in turn helped construct a middle-class lifestyle, including radical changes in patterns of consumption.

Of relevance here is Clarke and Islam's analysis of the 'negative externalities' produced by economic growth for the Bangkok population. They argue that as health levels begin to reach biological limits, it becomes 'increasingly difficult to improve health outcomes, despite increased technology, etc., afforded through economic growth' (2005: 184). Indeed, economic growth may begin to affect health negatively through environmental externalities (e.g. pollution, unhealthy diets and increased smoking and alcohol consumption). Using a 'new welfare economics' approach they set themselves the task of numerically measuring the social and environmental implications of economic growth for health through what they term a HANI index (health-adjusted national income) with adjustments made for inequality, urbanisation, water pollution, air pollution and long-term environmental damage (ibid.: 186). They found that during the economic boom the HANI measure became more distant from the unadjusted measure, reflecting the negative impact of rapid economic growth on the health of Bangkok residents (ibid.: 188).

One of the 'negative externalities' of rapid economic growth has been industrial pollution. Rapid industrialisation that accompanied export-led growth and the economic boom introduced many polluting industries with high health risks for the workforce and nearby residents. Critics have complained that factories are only located in Thailand due to cheap labour and to banish dirty industries from their own countries (Forsyth 1997: 182). Foreign investment during this boom was associated with significant increases in hazardous waste (heavy metals, solvents, oils, and acids and alkalines that are non-biodegradable). Between 1987 and 1989 alone hazardous waste-generating industries (e.g. fabricated metal products, electrical machinery, industrial chemicals, textiles) promoted by the Board of Investment (BoI) increased from 25 to 55 per cent (ibid.: 190). The government responded to these hazards with environmental legislation (the most important being the so-called 'Environment Act' of 1992 which created new government agencies to monitor and enforce environmental safeguards) and by encouraging polluting industries to set up in industrial estates (ibid.: 183, 187). However, Forsyth has argued that during the 1990s the BoI's reluctance to reject foreign investors on environmental grounds and its greater power in relation to government environmental agencies hindered pollution control efforts (ibid.: 193). This situation was changed by the 1997 Constitution and the growing influence thereafter of civil society on environmental policy.

The growing political influence of civil society on industrial pollution control is highlighted by the recent high-profile dispute relating to the Map Ta Phut Industrial Estate in Rayong province (Eastern Seaboard industrial zone). On 29 September 2009 the Administrative Court ordered a halt to work on 76 industrial projects in this estate. The court's injunction was in response to legal action by the Stop Global Warming Association and 42 villagers affected by pollution. The plaintiffs accused the National Environment Board and seven other government agencies of not following Article 67 of the 1997 Constitution which requires projects considered harmful to the environment and people's health to complete health impact assessment reports. These must be screened by an independent body, which has not yet been established (*Bangkok Post*, 12 October 2009). Another NGO, the Eastern People's Network has also been at the forefront of local protests over industrial pollution in Rayong. Serious environmental and health problems have been reported. In 1997 toxic fumes from chemical leaks caused the relocation of a school far from the industrial site (*Bangkok Post*, 1 November 2009). More recent medical research in Rayong province shows the doubling of the incidence rate of cancer in 2001–2003 from that in the year 1997–2000. There has also been a tripling of the rate of new born with physical and chromosome abnormalities during the years 1997–2005. Furthermore, the rate of suicide is 72.17 per 100,000 population which is 11 times the average national rate (*Health of the Thai People* 2008:

61–65). Despite this dire health situation industrialists warned that suspension of the 76 projects would jeopardise 400 billion baht worth of investment (*Bangkok Post*, 19 October 2009), the Finance Minister predicted that the delays could slow the economy by 0.4 per cent and the Industry Minister charged that the environmental and community activists were acting 'like godfathers'! (*Bangkok Post*, 7 October 2009). Towards the end of the year an impasse had been reached between the protagonists, with the only promising solution being the movement of residents near the industrial estate to a new town (*Bangkok Post*, 22 October 2009).

Economic prosperity has also had a negative impact on diet and nutrition. Siriphen (2004) has explored the impact of globalisation, national social and economic development plans and national food and nutrition policy on food consumption and cardiovascular diseases. She argues that Thai social and economic development plans affect directly and indirectly Thai people's dietary behaviour. The growth of per capita income and individual's purchasing power has resulted in more access to food, and the expansion of the food business and media industry affect both the availability of food and individual choice of food. Globalisation, through Free Trade Areas (FTA) and Foreign Direct Investment (FDI), has had a profound influence on the food business. By 2002 bakeries were the leading registered food business. Food franchises in Thailand have also proliferated in recent years and 80 per cent of them comprise heavy fast foods (e.g. from pizza outlets and Sizzler restaurants) while 20 per cent are light fast foods (e.g. Mister Donut). Advertising through the media of ready-to-eat food (such as processed noodles with high carbohydrate and fat levels) fits well with the fast-paced life of the middle and working classes in the urban context and has a deleterious effect on nutrition (ibid.:27). This adds up to a diet that is increasingly rich in fat and sugar and that has magnified the risk factors for cardiovascular disease and diabetes. Eating oily and fatty foods is also a risk factor for hypertension.

## Economic transitions and health

In this section we wish to assess the relative contributions of economic growth and public provisioning over the past 30 years in relation to both communicable and non-communicable diseases in Thailand. In his analysis of the relationship between income per head and health indicators Amartya Sen concludes that 'the impact of economic growth depends on how the *fruits* of economic growth are used' (1999: 44). He contrasts two types of success in the rapid reduction of mortality: 'growth-mediated' and 'support-led' processes. The first works *through* fast economic growth that utilises enhanced economic prosperity to expand social services (including health care). The examples he gives are Taiwan and South Korea. By contrast, the support-led process does not result from fast economic growth but from 'a program of skilful social support of health care, education and other social arrangements'. This process is exemplified by Sri Lanka, pre-reform China, Costa Rica and Kerala (ibid.: 46). We add

Vietnam as another apt example of this type of process. Vietnam was also able to achieve very good health outcomes for its population despite very low income levels, again due to committed state investment in public health and an emphasis on community participation in public health measures. By the early 1990s Vietnam, with an average per capita GDP of only $240, had a life expectancy and infant mortality indicators comparable to Thailand with an average per capita GDP of $1,840 (Purcal and Cohen 1995: 3–4). According to Sen, the 'support-led process' works through priority being given to 'public provisioning', that is, providing social services (particularly health care and basic education) to reduce mortality and enhance the quality of life (Sen 1999: 46). Public provisioning also includes public policies aimed at achieving 'sharing' (ibid.: 49) or 'social participation', a term Marmot uses with reference to Sen's thesis (2002: 43).

Needless to say, the state potentially plays a major role in public provisioning. In Thailand NGOs and civil society have also played a vital and strategic role in the provision of social services (including the promotion of social participation) either directly or indirectly through political influence on the government.

Between 1978 and 1985 the Thai economy was in recession. Indeed, there was an increase in poverty, at least in rural areas as a result of falls in the prices of agricultural products and the stagnation of agricultural production (Dixon 1999: 220). However, despite retarded economic growth there were major advances in health services and the standard of health. A government health report describes this period as achieving 'good health at low cost'. Strategic social investments were crucial to improved health outcomes in a sluggish economy. In the late 1970s the Thai Government committed itself to primary health care. This commitment was due to the combined effect of international pressure and lobbying by prominent officials within the Ministry of Health who, in turn, were influenced by reformist doctors such as Prawase Wasi. Dr Prawase had promoted PHC since the mid 1970s through the Folk Doctor Association and its 'bare-headed doctor' scheme for Buddhist monks, obviously modelled on the Chinese 'barefoot doctors'. The government PHC programme was centred on a system of Village Health Volunteers (VHVs) who were given short-term training in hygiene, immunisation, first aid and the dispensing of basic drugs. These village volunteers aided the government in the expansion of basic immunisation, with coverage increasing from 20–30 per cent in 1982 to 70 per cent in 1986. With a focus on low-cost basic health care the Ministry of Public Health also promoted family planning, maternal and child health nutrition and sanitation programmes. Furthermore, budget allocations minimised investment in large urban hospitals and increased investments at district and sub-district levels. In 1983 the budget for rural health centres and community hospitals combined was, for the first time, higher than that for urban provincial hospitals. Between 1977 and 1987 the number of district hospitals was doubled. There was also a rapid decline in maternal mortality (*Thailand Health Profile 2001–2004*: 407–408). During this period government PHC programmes were supported by NGOs. By

1984 there were 17 NGOs involved in PHC work which was integrated by the Co-ordinating Committee for Primary Health Care of Thai NGOs under the chairmanship of Dr Prawase Wasi.

Between 1985 and 1996 Thailand experienced an unprecedented economic boom, described above. During this decade the MoPH budget increased more than fourfold and the proportion of health budget to total government budget increased threefold in real terms (4.2 per cent in 1989 to 7.7 per cent in 1998) (ibid.: 409). However, a large proportion of the budget was spent on new buildings and sophisticated medical equipment (e.g. CT scanners and MRI machines) and extravagant use of expensive imported drugs (which rose from 27.7 per cent in 1988 to 40.7 per cent in 1997) (ibid.:410). This was accompanied by the expansion of private sector medicine and an internal brain drain from the rural public sector to the urban private sector. From 1987 to 1997 the number of beds in private hospitals increased from 9,974 beds to 29,945 beds and the number of doctors employed by private hospitals increased from 1,094 to 3,244 doctors (ibid.: 410). During this economic boom period there was a significant increase in mortality rates from non-communicable diseases (see Figure 8.1), as a result of the decline in public provisioning in health and the 'negative externalities' associated with rapid industrialisation and the growth of the urban middle class and accompanying lifestyle changes.

The economic boom ended suddenly with the economic crisis of 1997, precipitated by an overvalued currency which slowed down export growth and resulted in a massive current account deficit. Attacks on the local currency caused a huge loss of foreign reserves and rapid currency devaluation. The consequences were bankruptcies, increased unemployment and decreases in income, consumption and in government tax revenue (ibid.: 411). Inequality in income distribution widened and the number of poor increased by one million (Viroj *et al.* 2000: 789).

The crisis led to a significant reduction in the public health budget. Government health expenditure fell at a rate greater than that in the private sector, and the proportion of public expenditures to total health spending declined from 37.8 per cent in 1997 to 32.95 per cent in 2001. The utilisation of private health services (e.g. hospitals) also dropped and the baht devaluation led to high levels of debt and closure of hospital beds by one-third in 2000–2001 (*Thailand Health Profile 2001–2004*: 414). The combined effect of unemployment, increased poverty and reduced government health spending had some negative health effects. The prevalence of underweight schoolchildren increased from 10.5 per cent in 1994 to 12.2 per cent in 1998 and the under-five mortality rate increased from 11.6 per 1,000 live births in 1995 to 16.7 in 1998. At the same time the crisis had some health benefits: there were reductions in road traffic accidents and deaths (due to the decrease in the number of cars), in occupational injuries and tobacco and alcohol consumption (at least until 2003) (ibid.: 413).

The economic crisis of 1997 was a major catalyst for change. It provided the opportunity for people to demand economic and social reform and to return to and advance some of the 'low cost, good health' policies of the 1978–1985 recession. It gave renewed legitimacy to the philosophy of primary health care advocated by reformist doctors and NGOs dating back to the mid 1970s (Cohen 1989: 167–171).

In May 2000 the Cabinet set up a National Health Systems Reform Committee to draft a national health bill with the aim of creating 'a new health paradigm' for public health that was holistic and participatory and promoted equity, efficiency, quality health care, consumer empowerment and self-reliance (*Thailand Health Profile 1999–2000*: 449). The Thai King's post-crisis call for a 'sufficiency economy' (*sethakhit phorpiang*) also gave a royal seal of approval to the philosophy of self-reliance in health care, particularly through the promotion of traditional medicine. The political environment that facilitated health reform was created by the 1997 Constitution. 'The new constitution paved the way for the re-orientation of health and its relation to the general public. It stipulated that health is a human right, which must be protected by the state' (Wiput 2004: 11). Furthermore, the framing of the 'peoples constitution' was itself 'driven by activism from members of civil society' (ibid.: 11). The process of drafting of the National Health Bill was a remarkable example of government social investment in health and in social participation. The drafting followed public hearings in 500 districts and another 20 public hearings on specific health issues (ibid.: 19, 24–25). The national health system reform process culminated in the passing of the National Health Bill in January 2007. Government legislation of 1999 (Act on Operationalisation of Decentralisation), enacted in accordance with the 1997 Constitution, also mandated the decentralisation of public health. The devolution of health services included the setting up of Area Health Boards to take responsibility for the transfer of health facilities to local government organisations (*Thailand Health Profile 2005–2007*: 435). Now local organisations such as municipalities (*tesaban*) and sub-district councils (*ongkan borihan tambon*) have significant responsibilities and budgets for PHC, particularly for malaria and dengue fever control. It is noteworthy that the decentralisation of health embodied in the law was the realisation of a long period of advocacy by NGOs involved in PHC dating back to the 1970s (Cohen 1989: 170).

Universal health care was closely linked to health reform and became a major election promise in the election campaign of the Thai Rak Thai party (led by Thaksin Shinawatra) which won office in January 2001. It became law as part of the National Health Security Act of 2002 (*Thailand Health Profile 2005–2007*: 401). While Thaskin is usually given credit for this popular scheme in fact health system reformists had advocated such a scheme in the 1990s, in particular Dr Sanguan Nittayarumphon who had been influenced by international experiences such as the WHO Public Administration programme. In 1995–1996 a universal health insurance bill was drafted but was not passed into law. After the promulgation of the 1997 Constitution, academics and NGOs drafted the National Health Security Bill (ibid.: 402). By September 2002 74.2 per cent of Thai citizens were covered by the universal health care scheme and altogether 92 per cent had health insurance (including schemes such as the civil servants medical benefits scheme) (ibid.: 408).

We have noted above the participatory nature of the drafting of the National Health Bill. Another outstanding example of the efficacy of social participation in the advancement of better health is that of the HIV/AIDS self-help groups that began in the early 1990s. These groups (formed largely by labourers, peddlers and small traders) emerged in response to discrimination from families, communities and medical institutions that initially focused only on surveillance and control through the promotion of preventive medicine (Tanabe 2008: 165). These self-help groups have formed a new type of 'community of practice' in which people with HIV infection 'acquire knowledge and organise practices for survival ... in a discriminatory environment' (ibid.: 162). In 2006 there were over 900 groups with 20,000 members throughout Thailand as a whole (Lyttleton 2008: 261). Lyttleton argues that in recent years these groups and networks such as TNP+ (Thai People Living with HIV/AIDS) have moved beyond reactive survival strategies in the face social discrimination and medical dominance to become more political, with an 'ability to effect fundamental policy changes' (ibid.: 260). It is not simply that the strength of civil society in Thailand, especially in the 1990s, created the social and political space for these self-help groups to emerge; these groups in recent years have also had 'a formative role to play in civil society' (ibid.: 257). This political influence is exemplified in relation to the distribution of ARVs. Political pressure (in the form of public demonstrations) and legal action against multinational drug companies in 2006 and 2007 by TNP+ and other civil society organisations have led the Thai Department of Intellectual Property to override patents and permit the production of generic medicines through compulsory licensing. In 2005 the Thai Government was also pressured by these groups to include ARVs within a subsidised health scheme. By March 2006 more than 80,000 people infected with HIV were receiving ARV treatment (ibid.: 261, 262).

## Health promotion and non-communicable diseases

One of the major components of post-crisis health reform was the promulgation of the Thai Health Promotion Act in 2001 and the establishment of the Thai Health Promotion Foundation (THPF), a quasi-public agency and autonomous organisation funded by 2 per cent of the excise tax on tobacco and alcohol. The Foundation was a direct response to the growing public concern with the increased mortality from chronic non-communicable diseases and road traffic accidents. The priority programmes of the THPF are the introduction of health promotion, creating awareness about unhealthy behaviour, support campaigns against tobacco and alcohol consumption, and supporting research on health promotion. The THPF's mission is to complement existing MoPH health promotion activities (mostly clinical preventive services) and to network with and support civil society and community-based health organisations (for example, the 144 partner organisation of the Stop Drinking Network and the No Alcohol Campaign) (Phusit *et al.* 2007:17). In 2005 the THPF supported more than 700 projects, with more than one-third of the projects related to tobacco, alcohol and prevention of road traffic injuries (34 per cent), health promotion among specific groups (17 per cent) and community capacity strengthening (16 per cent) (ibid.: 18). The THPF has demonstrated some success in tobacco and alcohol supply control, road safety campaigns and the regulation of alcohol advertisements. With regards to alcohol control one notable achievement has been the passing of the 2008 Alcohol Act that prohibits various forms of alcohol advertising.

However, despite these important health promotion initiatives it is doubtful whether they will have a significant effect on the reduction of chronic non-communicable diseases. In 2005 78 per cent of health expenditure was spent on curative services and rehabilitative care (activities dominated by clinical prevention and personal health services and minimally related to primary prevention), while only 4.8 per cent of total health expenditure was used for public health services and disease prevention, compared to 7.1 per cent in 1994 (ibid.: 13). The policy report by Phusit and others (2007) concludes that the 2 per cent 'sin tax' that funds the Thai Health Foundation 'cannot serve as an adequate financial leverage to halt and reverse the trend of chronic NCD' (ibid.: 15). Revenue collected from the tax was equivalent to US$57.9 million in 2005 – only $1 dollar per capita. The report recommends that the 'sin tax' be *increased* to 5 per cent of the tax on tobacco and alcohol (ibid.: 29). Another obstacle to health promotion and the reduction of non-communicable diseases, highlighted in this report, is that major health funds, such as the Civil Service Medical Benefit Scheme and Social Health Insurance scheme, 'deliberately exclude prevention and health promotion from their benefit packages, on the ground that these two insurance funds are for curative purposes' (ibid.: 27).

## Conclusion

In recent decades Thailand has experienced an epidemiological transition in which non-communicable diseases have replaced communicable diseases as the major causes of morbidity and mortality. This transition has been closely linked to changes in the Thai economy: the commercialisation of agriculture and the recent rapid expansion of Thailand's economy and associated industrialisation, globalisation, the growth of the urban middle class and consumerism. This transition underscores the 'negative externalities' of economic prosperity and invites investigation into the relationship between economic growth, poverty and health with reference to both communicable and non-communicable diseases. The case of Thailand confirms the thesis of Amartya Sen (1999) and others that adequate public provisioning can neutralise the negative health effects of poverty. In Thailand public provisioning is not the exclusive preserve of the state. Rather, in a country with a thriving civil society, NGOs often in alliance with international organisations have played a crucial role in the provision of health services and, in particular, in influencing government health policies and funding. The influence of civil society has been most pronounced since the introduction of the 1997 Constitution, subsequent health reform legislation and public participation in the formulation of national health policy. This includes health promotion in response to the growing problem of non-communicable diseases and road traffic accidents. However, government health expenditure in Thailand is still heavily weighted in favour of curative services and rehabilitative care and some argue there is a need for a substantial increase in 'sin tax' funding for health promotion.

Some communicable diseases also continue to constitute serious health problems, creating a double disease burden for the country. The high levels of morbidity and mortality from vector-borne diseases and HIV/AIDS are related to poverty both within Thailand and in neighbouring countries. However, we have argued that it is not poverty per se that is the problem; rather, it is poverty that pressures people to move both within the country and across national borders and that impedes surveillance and the delivery of health services to mobile and often illegal populations.

## Notes

1 We have included the mortality rate from road accidents in this chart as an important feature of the health transition in Thailand. Deaths from motor-vehicle accidents skyrocketed during the years of rapid economic expansion – from 2,788 deaths in 1985 to 16,727 deaths at the height of the economic boom in 1995 (*Thailand Health Profile 2005–2007*: 216).
2 In addition to causing cancers, pesticide exposure can have a number of serious (acute and chronic) health effects: dermatitis, respiratory diseases, pernicious neurological and behavioural effects, and harmful effects on the reproductive organs and to the immune system (Surasak 2007: 59).
3 Between 1976 and 1990 fertiliser and insecticide application increased about fourfold, fungicides about sixfold and herbicide application increased about 19 times (Dixon 1999: 169).

## References

Anchalee Singhanetra-Renard (1993) 'Malaria and Mobility in Thailand', *Social Science and Medicine* 37(9): 1147–1154.
Avert (2010) 'Southeast Asian HIV & AIDS Statistics'. Online, available at: www.avert.org/aidssoutheastasia.htm (accessed 9 January 2010).
*Bangkok Post* (7 October 2009, Editorial) 'Opportunity not a Setback'.
*Bangkok Post* (12 October 2009) 'The Development Debate: Court-ordered Halt to Activity at Map Ta Phut Underlines the Challenges of Balancing Industrial Development and Prosperity with Quality of Life'.
*Bangkok Post* (19 October 2009) 'In the Hot Seat: Industry Minister Determined to Resolve Map Ta Phut Impasse but Agrees New Models are Needed in the Future'.
*Bangkok Post* (22 October 2009) 'Moving Residents Urged: Senators push Idea for Map Ta Phut Dwellers'.
*Bangkok Post* (1 November 2009) 'The Long March for Environmental Justice'.
Bureau of Policy and Strategy, Office of the Permanent Secretary, Ministry of Public Health (2007) Online, available at: http://bps.ops.moph.go.th/2.3.4-50pdf (accessed 5 January 2010).
Clarke, M. and Islam, S.M.N. (2005) 'The Relationship between National Income and

Health: A New Measure Applied to Bangkok', *Progress in Development Studies* 5(3): 182–198.

Cohen, P.T. (1989) 'The Politics of Primary Health Care in Thailand, with Special Reference to Non-government Organizations' in P. Cohen and J. Purcal (eds) *The Political Economy of Primary Health Care in Southeast Asia*, Canberra: Australian Development Studies Network/ASEAN Training Centre for Primary Health Care Development, 159–176.

Davisakd Puaksom (2007) 'On Germs, Public Hygiene and the Healthy Body: The Making of the Medicalizing State in Thailand', *Journal of Asian Studies* 66(2): 311–344.

Dixon, C. (1999) *The Thai Economy: Uneven Development and Internationalisation*, London and New York: Routledge.

Forsyth, T. (1997) 'Industrial Pollution and Government Policy in Thailand: Rhetoric versus Reality' in P. Hirsch (ed.) *Seeing Forests for Trees: Environment and Environmentalism in Thailand*, Chiang Mai: Silkworm Press, 182–201.

*Health of the Thai People* (in Thai) (2008) Bangkok: Research Institute for Population and Society, Mahidol University, Thailand.

IRIN (UN Office for the Coordination of Humanitarian Affairs) (2009) Online, available at: www.irinnews.org/Report.aspx?ReportId=78586 (accessed 27 December 2009).

Janphen Chuprapawan (2003) *Health of the Thai People Series 2000* (in Thai), Bangkok: Thai Health Institute, Health Systems Research Institute.

Luxemburger, C., Kway Lay Thwai, White, N.J., Webster, H.K., Kyle, D.E., Maelankiri, L., Chongsupajaisiddhi, T. and Nosten, F. (1996) 'The Epidemiology of Malaria in a Karen Population on the Western Border of Thailand', *Transactions of the Royal Society of Tropical Medicine and Hygiene* 90(2): 105–111.

Lyttleton, C. (2008) 'AIDS and Civil Belonging: Disease Management and Political Change in Thailand' in M. Foller and H. Thorn (eds) *The Politics of AIDS: Globalization, the State and Civil Society*, New York: Palgrave Macmillan, 255–273.

Marmot, M. (2002) 'The Influence of Income on Health: Views of an Epidemiologist', *Health Affairs*, March/April: 31–46.

Pasuk Phongpaichit and Baker, C. (1995) *Thailand: Economy and Politics*, Kuala Lumpur: Oxford University Press.

Pasuk Phongpaichit and Baker, C. (1998) *Thailand's Boom and Bust*, Chiang Mai: Silkworm Books.

Phusit Prakongsai, Kanitta Bundhamcharoen, Kanjana Tisayatikom, Viroj Tangcharoensathien (2007) 'Financing Health Promotion: A Case Study on Thailand', Bangkok: International Health Policy Program (IHPP, Thailand), 1 December.

Purcal, J. and Cohen, P.T. (1995) 'The Political Economy of Health and Development in South East Asia' in P. Cohen and J. Purcal (eds) *Health and Development in South East Asia*, Canberra: Australian Development Studies Network, 1–16.

Sen, A. (1999) *Development as Freedom*, New York: Alfred A. Knopf.

Siriphen, S. (2004) 'Political Economy of Food and Cardiovascular Disease', Faculty of Economics, Chulalongkorn University (in Thai). Online, available at: http://hrn.thaihf.org/index.php?module=research (accessed 29 October 2009).

Surasak Buranatrevedh (2007) 'Effects of Pesticides on Health' in P. Kunstadter (ed.) *Pesticides in Southeast Asia: Environmental, Biomedical, and Economic Uses and Effects*, Chiang Mai: Silkworm Books, 59–83.

Tanabe, S. (2008) 'Suffering, Community, and Self-government: HIV/AIDS Self-help Groups in Northern Thailand' in S. Tanabe (ed.) *Imagining Communities in Thailand and Ethnographic Approaches*, Chiang Mai: Mekong Press, 161–188.

*Thailand Health Profile 1999–2000*, Bangkok: Ministry of Public Health (MoPH).

*Thailand Health Profile 2001–2004*, Bangkok: Ministry of Public Health (MoPH).

*Thailand Health Profile 2005–2007*, Bangkok: Ministry of Public Health (MoPH).

Thiesmeyer, L. (2001) 'Mobility, Gender, and Hidden Costs of HIV Risk Households in Northern Thailand', Asia Pacific Impact Research Tool/HIV Impact Assessment 2001, unpublished report.

Thongphit Pinyosinwat (2009) 'PHAMIT: A Program on HIV/AIDS Prevention among Migrant Workers', *Field Actions Science Reports* 3(1): 1–10.

UNGASS (United Nations General Assembly Special Session on HIV/AIDS) (2008) 'Country Progress Report, Thailand'. Online, available at: http://data.unaids.org/pub/Report/2008/thailand_2008_country_progressreport_en.pdf (accessed 8 January 2010).

UNICEF (United Nations Children's Fund) (1994) *Social Indicators of Development*, Baltimore, MD: John Hopkins Press.

Viroj Tangcharoensathien, Piya Harnvoravongchai, Siriwan Pitayarangsarit, Vijj Kasemsup (2000) 'Health Impacts of Rapid Economic Changes in Thailand', *Social Science and Medicine* 51(6): 789–807.

Wiput Phoolcharoen (2004) *Quantum Leap: The Reform of Thailand's Health System*, Bangkok: Health Systems Research Institute.

WHO (World Health Organization), Country Office for Thailand (2009) 'Report of Cases and Deaths in Camps Areas of Work, Border Health (Thailand/Myanmar)'. Online, available at: www.whothailand.org/en/Section3/Section39.htm) (accessed 26 December 2009).

Yuwadi Comphitak (2002) *Medicine and Public Health of Thailand: Progress from the Past* (in Thai), Bangkok: Odeon Store.

# 9 Health transition in Viet Nam

## Resolving past priorities and meeting new challenges

*Michael J. Dibley, Nguyen Hoang Hanh Doan Trang, Tang Kim Hong and Tran Tuan*

**Revolution and wars**

Located in the centre of South East Asia, Viet Nam forms an S-shaped strip on the eastern seaboard of the Indochinese Peninsula, linking to the Asian continent and looking out on the Pacific Ocean. Its land area is about 331,668 square kilometres and the total population in 2010 was 86.9 million (General Statistics Office Vietnam 2010b: 55) making it the third largest country in Southeast Asia. Political and social forces caused radical changes in Viet Nam during the second half of the twentieth century. These changes went far beyond those in the earlier history of the country and have forced dramatic changes in Viet Nam compared to neighbouring countries in Southeast Asia.

These changes started with the French occupation of Viet Nam in the south in 1858. By 1885 France controlled all of the territory as part of French Indochina. Although the emperors of Viet Nam remained on their throne in Hue, all government activities were controlled by French officials. Resistance to the French occupation grew in the early twentieth century, when Vietnamese intellectuals began to establish nationalist and Communist-nationalist, anti-colonial movements. Japan in the Second World War replaced the French Vichy colonial regime and eventually provided an opportunity for the Viet Minh under Ho Chi Minh to take control of northern Viet Nam following the Japanese surrender and to declare the independence of the Democratic Republic of Viet Nam on 2 September 1945.

The French resisted this declaration of independence. In 1946 an armed conflict lasting eight years broke out between the Communist-led Viet Minh and the French and the Vietnamese anti-Communists. With the defeat of the French forces at Dien Bien Phu in May 1954, peace talks were convened in Geneva and an agreement for cessation of hostilities was reached on 29 July 1954 between the Democratic Republic of Viet Nam and France. This agreement provided for a ceasefire, the temporary division of Viet Nam at approximately the 17th parallel into northern (Communist) and southern (Non-communist) governments, and the exchange of those populations desiring to relocate. A planned national election in July 1956 was not accepted by the government in the south which declared its own independence in late 1956.

The United States became involved in Viet Nam in December 1961, starting by sending military advisers at the request of South Vietnamese President, Ngo Dinh Diem, but increasing its military support to the South with US combat forces in 1965 that reached a crest in 1969 with over half a million military personnel involved. Perhaps the peak of this conflict was the Tet offensive in 1968, which, although it weakened the Viet Cong, had a critical demoralizing effect on the Americans and the South Vietnamese Government. Negotiations to end the conflict started in 1969 and the Paris Accords peace agreement was signed on 27 January 1973.

These two Indochina wars and especially the 'American war' caused mass destruction of the natural environment and physical life and pushed Viet Nam, to some extent, '*back to the stone age*' as the Americans said they intended when they launched their bombing raids. The available statistics can only partly describe the war toll that Viet Nam suffered in the period 1955–1975 (see Table 9.1).

Another important change for Viet Nam in this period was the national independence revolution mixed with socialist ideology (lasting for almost 50 years from when the Communist Party was established in Viet Nam in 1930) which removed traditional community organizations and replaced them with a totally new administrative system. Finally, the two Indochina wars forced Viet Nam to use decentralization, local problem-solving and community-based approaches to run government systems, which left the country rich with experience in organizing community campaigns for development goals (McMichael 1976: 51–69;

*Table 9.1* Outcomes of the 1955–1975 war in Viet Nam[1]

*Environment and infrastructure*
- 5 million tons of bombs detonated
- 7.4 million tons of artillery shells discharged
- 150,000 to 300,000 tons of unexploded bombs and landmines across Viet Nam at the end of the war
- 19 million gallons (72 million litres) of herbicides sprayed over 3.6 million acres of farmland and forest (over one-third of the total land mass in South Viet Nam)
- In South Viet Nam: 9,000 of 15,000 rural villages were destroyed or damaged, 12 million population (63%) displaced
- In the North: all five industrial centres were demolished; all 29 provincial capitals were bombed, as well as 2,700 of the 4,000 communes. Virtually every railway and highway was destroyed; 533 (9.5%) of the commune health stations, 94 (27.5%) of district hospitals, 28 (60%) of provincial hospitals and 24 research and specialized hospitals were destroyed or damaged badly.

*Human casualties*
- 3.1 million dead; nearly 2.6 million wounded; 300,000 missing in action (MIAs)
- 50,000 born deformed (allegedly as a result of the chemical defoliant Agent Orange)

Source: Tuan 1995: 6–34; Miron Allukian and Paul 2000: 215–238.

Note 1 Based on Table 2 of the Takemi Research Paper No. 102, Tuan 1995: 6. Further related information on the Viet Nam War can be found in Levy and Sidel 2008: 485.

Tuan 1995: 6–34). These substantial social and political changes have had great influence on how Viet Nam has dealt with health problems following reunification.

## Reunification and reform

Reunification of the country began with the fall of Saigon on 30 April 1975 following a short but intensive military campaign from the north, and the two parts of the country were forged into one state, the Socialist Republic of Viet Nam, on 2 July 1976. The victory in 1975 encouraged the Vietnamese government to launch an ambitious five year plan (1976–1980) where models of the cooperative farm in agriculture, the subsidized state factories in industry, and public health and education networks, in line with the administrative system, were to be expanded to the whole country. Despite the strong political will to implement this massive plan, the lack of resources after several decades of war soon led to an economic crisis. These difficulties became more acute when an American embargo was supported by most Western countries and Chinese aid ceased after Viet Nam ousted Pol Pot's regime in Cambodia in January 1979. As a consequence, Viet Nam faced an overwhelming economic crisis by 1980.

The failure of the 1976–1980 five year plan forced Viet Nam to reassess its performance and direction. The change towards a market-based economy had emerged gradually at the community level soon after the country was united and was seen as an outcome of 'the war, the inefficiencies of the cooperative system, and the inability of agriculture to generate surpluses' (Fforde 1993: 293–325). However, the initial steps away from a centrally planned system had begun to be taken in the early 1980s. These steps included the introduction of the output-contract system, which was formally launched in the agriculture sector in 1981, private classes for students studying for national examinations were informally accepted by the education sector, and the easing of restrictions on private health services and private pharmaceutical sales in Ho Chi Minh City (Dung 1996: 217–230). These tentative changes led to the introduction at the 1986 Sixth Party Congress of a broad range of economic reforms (known as '*Doi Moi*' or renovation), which moved the country from a centrally planned to a market-oriented economy and opened it to foreign investment.

*Doi Moi* started with macroeconomic reforms that returned agriculture to a household-based farming system, removed restrictions on private sector activities in commerce and industry, and decentralized decision-making to managers of state-owned enterprises. All these reforms had an immediate impact on the health sector, but only at the communal level where the cooperative farms were no longer the main source of funds for the commune health system. The health sector remained as a state-wide public system until 1989 when further macro economic reforms were announced. These included a devaluation of the official exchange rate to the parallel market rate, decontrol of prices and an increase in real interest rates to positive levels (Dollar 1993: 207–303). Many of these reforms applied directly to the health sector and there were four major reforms implemented: (1) legalization of private medical practice; (2) the decree on decentralized decision-making for state-owned enterprises extended to the manufacture of pharmaceuticals and condoms, leading to privatization of pharmaceutical production and sales; (3) imposition of user charges for health care, especially in hospitals; and (4) the launching of a national health insurance scheme (Chen and Hiebert 1994: 8). As a result, after 1989, a public–private health care system had been formed in Viet Nam, although continued central government funding for the primary health care services at the commune level has maintained a public health service across the community.

The *Doi Moi* reforms led to a dramatic and rapid improvement in the economy. From 1990 to 1997 the gross domestic product (GDP) increased by 8 per cent annually and since then the annual rate of growth of GDP has remained above 6 per cent (except in 2008), leading to Viet Nam reaching low middle income status by 2009. In 1986 Viet Nam had an agriculture-based economy but with limited agricultural productivity and food shortages, but following the *Doi Moi* reforms agricultural production nearly doubled, making Viet Nam the world's second-largest rice exporter by 2005. This rapid economic change has impacted on the quality of life (see Table 9.2): the poverty rate has halved, the malnutrition rate has dropped from about half the child population under five in the late 1980s to one-third, literacy rates for women have increased, and coverage by preventive health programmes and life expectancy have all increased.

*Table 9.2* Change in socio-economic indicators in Viet Nam, 1985–2009

| Indicators | 1980s | 1993 | 1999 | 2009 |
|---|---|---|---|---|
| GDP per capita (US$) | 157 *(1991)* | 176 | 352 *(1998)* | 1,063 |
| % people under poverty line | N/A | 58 | 37 | 12 |
| Malnutrition rate in under-5 children* (%) Stunting <–2 SD | 60 | 47 | 36 | 29 |
| Percentage of households with access to safe water | N/A | 10.7 | 14.6 | 94 |
| Life expectancy (years) | | | | |
| Male | 63 | N/A | 65 | 70 |
| Female | 68 | N/A | 69 | 74 |
| Under-5 mortality (per 1,000) | | | | |
| Male | – | 42 | 39 | 25 |
| Female | – | 29 | 31 | 23 |
| Literacy rate (%) | | | | |
| Male | 93 | 93 | 94 | 97 |
| Female | 84 | 85 | 88 | 96 |

Sources: Food and Agriculture Organization of the United Nations 1999: 1–24; General Statistics Office Vietnam 2010b: 55; Tuan 2004: 27; UNICEF and National Institute of Nutrition Vietnam 2011: 9; UNICEF Vietnam 2000: 15; World Bank 2011: 60–67; World Health Organization 2011b: 52.

Note
* Data for 1985, 1995 and 1998 from National Institute of Nutrition surveys.

Linked to this rapid expansion of the economy has been the growth of cities in Viet Nam. This is in part driven by the higher productivity in urban areas, which reflect the economies of agglomeration where firms cluster to benefit from economies of scale and better networking (Goldstein and Gronberg 1984: 91–104). The subsequent higher productivity led to more employment opportunities and in-migration from rural areas. Viet Nam is undergoing a double social and economic transition with rapid urbanization which is linked to the move from a centrally planned to a market economy. The three largest urban areas in the county are all experiencing rapid expansion with Hanoi and Ho Chi Minh City growing at about 7 per cent per annum, and Haiphong at about 12 per cent per annum. Overall the rate of urbanization is expected to remain above 3 per cent per annum until 2020 by which time from 35 to 45 per cent of the population are expected to live in urban areas (World Bank and East Asia Infrastructure Department 2010: 1). Urbanization brings important health challenges including non-communicable diseases (cardiovascular diseases, cancers, obesity and diabetes) that are related to unhealthy diets and lack of physical activity. As Viet Nam deals with all its social and economic changes, it is confronted by a 'double burden' of ill health with the newly emerging non-communicable diseases, but a considerable level of communicable diseases and undernutrition related to poverty and environmental risks remains. There are clear indications that this burden of communicable disease and undernutrition has been receding and that this in part has been due to the effective implementation of programmes to control and prevent these problems.

## Responses to communicable diseases

After reunification Viet Nam was confronted with a considerable burden of communicable disease and undernutrition. During the decade from 1975 to 1986 economic stagnation and international isolation meant little progress was made in resolving many of these public health problems. At the time of *Doi Moi* reforms the national burden of disease in Viet Nam was dominated by childhood infections and undernutrition. Diarrhoea and acute respiratory tract infections with underlying undernutrition were the major causes of deaths in children (Chen and Hiebert 1994: 8). Tuberculosis remained common, and cut backs in mosquito control had contributed to a resurgence of malaria. Regional imbalances in the control of infectious diseases and undernutrition meant the diseases of poverty and underdevelopment continued for Viet Nam's poor, despite the socialist transformation of the economy (ibid.: 7).

Even though Viet Nam was extremely poor and had a high burden of infectious diseases and undernutrition, at this time the mortality levels were relatively low compared to other countries of similar economic status (ibid.: 19). Contributing to this mixed health status was the equitable nature of social development in Viet Nam, and even-handed access to the limited health services available. Despite the prolonged colonial and American wars, Viet Nam had attained nearly universal adult literacy (88 per cent) and very high primary school enrolment (ibid.: 3). There was also strong gender equity in these social achievements with equal school attendance for girls and boys, and high female participation in the workforce. This progressive social development may have averted the worst health outcomes but could not completely ameliorate the poverty-related barriers to good health and nutrition. Following the *Doi Moi* reforms the rapidly improving economic situation began to impact on infectious diseases and undernutrition through direct economic benefits to families that improved diet, reduced micro-environmental risks and increased family resources for health, but also through more resources for disease control and prevention programmes provided by the government. To illustrate how Viet Nam has responded to its infectious disease burden, especially after the *Doi Moi* reforms, malaria control is examined in detail below. This brief historical outline of the malaria control in Viet Nam was prepared by the WHO as part of its efforts to document successful malaria control programmes (Schuftan 2000: 1–15).

A malaria control programme was launched in 1958 in the north of Viet Nam following the end of the colonial war with the French. In the early years of this control programme, malaria was reduced by more than 20-fold in the North, although there was much less progress in the South in malaria infested areas. The ongoing war in the South made it all but impossible to implement prevention programmes. Following reunification there was a re-emergence of malaria with a peak in 1991 of over a million cases of malaria and almost 5,000 deaths from 150 outbreaks mainly in central Viet Nam (ibid.: 3–4). Further complicating the situation was the spread of *plasmodium falciparum* (the main type of malaria in Viet Nam) resistance to chloroquine, quinine and sulfadoxine-pyrimethamine. This recrudescence of malaria occurred because of the limited investments in malaria control with a halving of the required budget leading to shortages of anti-malarial drugs and insecticides, combined with large post-war migration of susceptible individuals to high risk endemic malaria areas.

In response to the national malaria crisis in 1991 Viet Nam radically changed its malaria programme strategy from malaria eradication with mass treatment and DDT spraying, to a malaria control programme with distribution of effective anti-malarial drugs through the health system, promotion of impregnated mosquito bed nets and intensive, twice-yearly, residual insecticide spraying and intensive health education and community mobilization involving village heads, Women's Union cadres and commune health staff (ibid.: 3–4). This new programme required a considerable expansion of the resource for malaria control which was achieved as a result of heightened political commitment to malaria control. In 1991, the National Assembly made malaria control a priority national health programme (ranked second amongst government priority health programmes) and greatly increased direct funding from US$540,000 in 1991 to US$6.3 million in 1995. But this political commitment extended beyond the simple declaration of a national health priority and increased allocation of funds.

Following the 1991 epidemic, the malaria programme managers briefed senior authorities directly about the problem and their control strategy and invited them 'to become members of the malaria steering committees from the central to the local level' (ibid.: 7). In 1992, the Prime Minister himself chaired the National Conference on Malaria, the Deputy Prime Minister made repeated visits to observe programme implementation, and the Malaria Programme Central Steering Committee was headed by the Minister of Health. In endemic areas, local malaria programme steering committees were headed by the vice-chairmen of the Provincial and District People's Committees and they committed to programme targets in yearly contracts with the Minister of Health. This engagement in the programme at all levels of government led to genuine understanding of the problems, the rationale for the new approach to control and the practical problems that needed to be overcome for the programme to succeed.

A further key element in the response to malaria was the selection of anti-malarial drugs for the control programme. Artemisinin, derived from a traditional herb found in China and Viet Nam, was found in research in China to be an effective drug for the treatment of *plasmodium falciparum* malaria and free of parasite resistance. The Government in Viet Nam invested in the local production of this new anti-malarial drug and used it to treat malaria especially as other drugs became less effective with developing resistance by the malaria parasite. The resistance of *P. falciparum* to the range of anti-malarial drugs was routinely monitored and treatment guidelines were adjusted to the differing patterns of resistance found in each region of the country. In 1997 a District Level Manual on Malaria Diagnosis and Treatment was developed that was regularly updated to ensure the continued effectiveness of treatment across the country. The full range of anti-malarial drugs was provided free by the government and accounted for approximately 40 per cent of the malaria control budget.

To ensure early treatment and containment of any malaria outbreak a strong epidemiological surveillance system was developed with 400 mobile teams in high endemic districts linked to village health workers who were trained to recognize malaria and collect blood samples for examination. Numerous new microscopic testing points for blood slides were established to ensure early detection of outbreak and the quality of the microscopic diagnosis was maintained through a programme of regular retraining of the microscopists. These measures combined with the ready availability of appropriate anti-malarial drugs and locally adjusted treatment guidelines helped to ensure local outbreaks of malaria did not spread.

An effective strategy of vector control was also introduced in the early 1990s using impregnated bed nets although this component of the control programme was slow to start because of limited donor support. From 1991 to 1996 free bed nets were distributed in high endemic areas and self-purchase was promoted in other areas but all these nets were impregnated at no charge with permethrin twice yearly by staff of commune health stations and mobile district malaria control teams. After 1996 the Government funded free distribution of bed nets in areas of greatest need, but at the same time worked with the Women's Union to promote the purchase of bed nets at half price with UNICEF covering the other half of the cost, and to educate the community about the benefits of using bed nets. By 1999 over 11 million people living in high endemic areas were protected by impregnated bed nets, which was close to the national malaria control target for their use (Schuftan 2000: 4).

This multi-component, malaria control programme was highly successful and from 1992 to 1997 the number of clinically diagnosed malaria cases (without malaria smear confirmation) decreased from 1.2 million to 440,000 per year, the number of deaths decreased from 2,600 to 152 per year and the number of outbreaks decreased from 115 to 10 per year (ibid.: 3). Today, malaria is under control and causes fewer deaths than other infectious disease such as tuberculosis or acute respiratory infections. Across the country the majority of rural and urban areas remain largely malaria free (Ministry of Health Vietnam 2009: 149) but malaria continues to be a threat in about 115 districts in 24 provinces and ongoing surveillance and control are still needed to contain this threat.

Many of the key elements of Viet Nam's success in controlling malaria (and other infectious diseases) are linked to characteristics developed in the prolonged wars following its declaration of independence including the *high level of political commitment* to solving a national problem with concomitant allocation of resources; the effective use the *decentralized health services* with a *vertical programme adjusted to local needs* based on *careful surveillance*; *equitable access* to the key programme elements including drugs and bed nets; *local problem-solving* through the production of a new, efficacious, anti-malarial drug based on local and regional research; and *community-based approaches to mobilize the population* to use of bed nets and to maintain their impregnation with insecticide; and the *engagement of local health cadres to identify cases* and contain new outbreaks of malaria. Will these same characteristics help Viet Nam deal with the emerging epidemic of chronic diseases?

## Emerging non-communicable diseases

Although infectious diseases and undernutrition continue to dominate in the national burden of disease in Viet Nam, their importance has begun to diminish as the history of malaria control illustrates. Progressively, non-communicable diseases (NCDs) are emerging as the dominant health problems, with urban populations leading these changes with their changing diets, increasing consumption of tobacco and alcohol from increased income, and more sedentary lifestyles from mechanized transportation and crowded environments with restricted opportunities for physical activity.

Evidence is appearing to indicate that NCDs are rapidly becoming the major causes of morbidity and mortality in hospitals in Viet Nam. Hospital admissions due to NCDs increased from 39 per cent in 1986 to 68 per cent in 2002 and chronic disease deaths rose from 42 per cent in 1986 to 69 per cent in 2002 (Ministry of Health Vietnam 2003: 177–180). An estimate by WHO showed that, out of 516,000 deaths that occurred in 2002 in Viet Nam, 341,000 (66 per cent) were attributable to NCDs, and the age-standardized mortality rate from NCDs was 664.1 per 100,000 population (Van Minh *et al.* 2009a: 1–8). A population-based study in rural Viet Nam found that 39 per cent of people aged

25–74 years reported at least one chronic disease. More than 10 per cent of them reported having two or more chronic conditions (Minh *et al.* 2008: 629–634).

Morbidity from NCDs has increased since the 1986 *Doi Moi* reforms, and especially after 1996 by which time the economy was starting to accelerate in response to the earlier reforms (see Figure 9.1). Morbidity from NCDs increased significantly from 39.0 per cent of inpatients in public hospitals in 1986 to 66.3 per cent in 2009, while over the same period morbidity from communicable diseases fell from 59.2 per cent to 22.9 per cent (Ministry of Health Vietnam 2007: 171–172; Ministry of Health Vietnam 2009: 183–184). By 2009 statistics from the Ministry of Health showed that morbidity from NCDs was over 2.9 times greater than that of infectious diseases.

Cardiovascular diseases (CVD) are now the leading cause of death in Viet Nam, approximately three times higher than infectious and parasitic diseases, and they accounted for nearly one-fifth of the total burden of disease in 2008. The number of strokes has tripled compared to ten years ago. Coronary vascular diseases have increased sixfold compared to the 1960s (Khan and Khoi 2008: 116–118): in Ba Vi district, a rural district in northern Viet Nam, mortality from stroke was estimated at 73 per 100,000 population, but in Ha Noi and Ho Chi Minh City mortality rates from stroke were much higher, at around 130–131 per 100,000 population (Ministry of Health Vietnam 2006: 48–49).

Results of the National Health Survey 2001–2002 indicated that 15.1 per cent of men and 13.5 per cent of women had high blood pressure. However, only 28

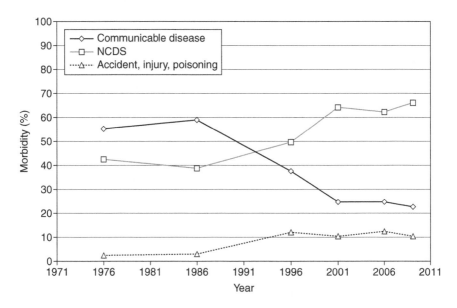

*Figure 9.1* Trends in morbidity patterns of inpatients at public hospitals in Vietnam, 1998–2009 (source: Ministry of Health Vietnam 2007: 171–172; Ministry of Health Vietnam 2009: 183–184).

per cent of men and 42 per cent of women with high blood pressure have been diagnosed with the condition (ibid.: 48–49). The rate of hypertension among adults was 1 per cent in 1960 in northern Viet Nam and increased to 23.1 per cent by 2001 (Khai 2002, cited in Khan and Khoi 2008: 116–118). The prevalence of hypertension also appears to have increased substantially. In 2005, a study in Ba Vi, a rural district in northern Viet Nam, revealed a prevalence of 18.8 per cent for hypertension (Hoang *et al.* 2007: 1–10) whereas in the same population it was only 14.1 per cent in 2002 (Minh *et al.* 2006: 109–115). Similarly, a cross-sectional study conducted in 2005 in two Health and Demographic Surveillance System sites in Viet Nam revealed a prevalence of hypertension (defined as systolic/diastolic blood pressure $\geq 140/90$ mmHg) of 15.1 to 18.3 per cent (Van Minh *et al.* 2009b: 60–67). In Ho Chi Minh City, the cases of hypertension tripled from 16,778 cases in 2001 to 42,848 cases in 2009 (Ho Chi Minh City Health Department 2001–2009).

The National Diabetes Survey, conducted in 2002, showed a national prevalence of 2.7 per cent in adults. This survey also revealed a prevalence of impaired glucose tolerance of 7.3 per cent, indicating the potential for a future sharp increase in diabetes prevalence (Cockram 2006: 361–364). In a HCMC study (Duc Son *et al.* 2004: 371–376) sex, age-adjusted prevalence of diabetes and impaired glucose tolerance were 3.8 per cent and 2.5 per cent, respectively, and three times higher than that observed in Hanoi in 1994 (Quoc *et al.* 1994: 713–722). As a result, Viet Nam is currently ranked in the top ten countries in Asia having the highest number of persons with Type 2 Diabetes and impaired glucose tolerance in the age group 20 to 79 years and it is projected to be at the same rank in 2025. By these methods, in 2007, it was estimated 1.294 million persons had diabetes and 1.175 million impaired glucose tolerance, but this is projected to reach 2.5 million persons and 1.902 million respectively by 2025 (Chan *et al.* 2009: 2,129–2,140).

The levels of overweight and obesity and undernutrition have also been changing rapidly. A recent study reported that the prevalence of adult overweight in Viet Nam has increased sharply from 2 per cent in 1992 to 5.7 per cent in 2002. Significant increases were observed for men and women, in urban and rural areas, and for all age groups (Nguyen *et al.* 2007: 115–121). In 2005, a national survey on overweight and obesity showed that the prevalence of overweight/obesity among the 45–54 age group was around 43 per cent in urban and 17 per cent in rural areas respectively (National Institute of Nutrition Vietnam 2005).

The urban focus of the merging obesity epidemic is most clearly seen in Ho Chi Minh City, the largest city the country with the most rapidly developing economy. The prevalence of overweight and obesity in pre-school children in urban areas of Ho Chi Minh City almost doubled from 2002 to 2005 (21.4 per cent and 36.8 per cent, respectively). The proportion of boys classified as obese in 2005 (22.5 per cent) was three times that in 2002 (6.9 per cent) (Dieu *et al.* 2009: 702–709). Similarly, among adolescents in Ho Chi Minh City, the prevalence of overweight has doubled, and obesity tripled from 2002 to 2004. In 2004 the prevalence of overweight was 11.7 per cent and obesity was 2.1 per cent, while in 2002 overweight was only 5.9 per cent and obesity 0.7 per cent (Hong *et al.* 2007: 194–201). But obesity is not restricted to children and in 2004, a cross-sectional survey of adults in HCMC (Cuong *et al.* 2007: 673–681) revealed that the prevalence of overweight and obesity was high (33.6 per cent in females and 31.6 per cent in males), and progressively increased with age.

The metabolic syndrome, a constellation of signs and symptoms indicating a heightened risk of cardiovascular disease and diabetes that includes elevated blood pressure, serum lipids and abnormal blood glucose, has also been found to be at a relatively high prevalence in adults and even in adolescents in urban Viet Nam. In Ho Chi Minh City a cross-sectional survey in 2004 showed a prevalence of metabolic syndrome in adults of 17.0 per cent in men and 17.6 per cent in women (Trinh *et al.* 2010: 69–78). As well, in Ho Chi Minh City adolescents, the prevalence of metabolic syndrome was reported to be 4.6 per cent in 2007, indicating likely future increases in this condition in adults (Nguyen *et al.* 2010: 141–150).

As the prevalence of overweight and obesity has increased in urban child and adolescent populations, the prevalence of undernutrition has rapidly declined. In Ho Chi Minh City, the prevalence of underweight has decreased in pre-school children aged four to five years, from 10.1 per cent of boys and 10.2 per cent of girls in 2002, to 2.6 per cent of boys and 2.9 per cent of girls in 2005 (Dieu *et al.* 2009: 702–709). Similarly the prevalence in adolescents from Ho Chi Minh City aged 11–16 years halved from 13.1 per cent in 2002 to 6.6 per cent in 2004 (Hong *et al.* 2007: 194–201). National data reveals a higher prevalence of underweight (BMI $< 18.5\,\mathrm{kg/m^2}$) among Vietnamese adults in rural compared to urban areas, but with a steady decline in adult underweight in both areas over time. In 1985 over half the adults in rural areas were underweight (52 per cent) while in urban areas the rate was slightly lower (43 per cent). The level of adult underweight was little changed in 1990 (rural 46 per cent; urban 41 per cent) but had started to decline by 2000 (rural 36 per cent; urban 32 per cent) and had reached substantially lower levels by 2009 (rural 19 per cent, urban 13 per cent) (National Institute of Nutrition 2010). Detailed trend data is not available for Ho Chi Minh City but consistent with the national data the age and sex-standardized prevalence of underweight (BMI $< 18.5\,\mathrm{kg/m^2}$) among Vietnamese adults living in HCMC was 20.4 per cent in 2004 (Cuong *et al.* 2007: 673–681). Despite this national trend for undernutrition in women of reproductive age and under-five children to be falling, the country now faces a double burden of under- and overnutrition.

A group of behavioural risk factors, tobacco use, excess use of alcohol, inadequate intake of fruit and vegetables, and insufficient physical activity, are all predictors of non-communicable diseases. Viet Nam has amongst the highest male smoking rates in the world. In 2002 more than half the adult men (56.1 per cent) reported regular smoking but only 1.8 per cent of women (Ministry of Health Vietnam 2003b). Even after the introduction of tobacco control measures, a survey in 2010 (General Statistics Office Vietnam 2010a: 24–50) found the prevalence of current smoking for males still remained high (47.4 per cent) although slightly lower than in 2002. As in the earlier survey the prevalence of smoking by women remained low at just 1.4 per cent. Most men start smoking when they are young, and 6.8 per cent of boys less than 15 years of age had already taken up smoking; 35.9 per cent began by 17 to 19 years and 44.0 per cent by 20 years or older. A recent survey found that about 65 per cent of smokers report that they smoke in their office and 90 per cent smoke 'sometimes' in their homes (World Health Organization 2011a). Thus the negative impacts of smoking in Viet Nam extend to non-smokers of whom more than two-thirds (68 per cent) reported being exposed to second-hand smoke at home, while amongst non-smoking workers, 49 per cent reported being exposed to second-hand smoke at indoor workplaces (General Statistics Office Vietnam 2010a: 24–50).

In 2004, data from WHO also showed that the prevalence of heavy and hazardous alcohol drinking in Viet Nam was much higher among men (5.7 per cent) than women (0.6 per cent) (World Health Organization 2004: 2). Similarly, the STEPS study in the Mekong delta in 2005 showed that 68 per cent men were current smokers, 87 per cent consumed alcohol and 39 per cent had consumed five drinks or more on any single day in the seven days prior to interview (Pham *et al.* 2009: 291–299).

There are several reports indicating high levels of physical inactivity in adults and adolescents in Viet Nam. In Filabavi district in rural northern Viet Nam in 2005 the prevalence of physical inactivity was high in men (63 per cent) and women (53 per cent) (Ahmed *et al.* 2009: 71). As well, there was 47 per cent of men and 41 per cent of women aged 25–64 years in Ho Chi Minh City in 2005 classified as having a low level of physical activity (Trinh *et al.* 2008: 204–215). Even in adolescents, 24.3 per cent were classified as physically inactive in a study from Ho Chi minh City in 2007 (Trang *et al.* 2009: 1,374–1,383).

Non-intentional injuries are a major cause of death in Viet Nam today. According to the National Health Statistics, the injury mortality rate in 2008 was 43.8 per 100,000 people (Health Environment Management Agency 2010: 22). The rate of injuries has also been increasing in recent times with an average annual increase of 38 per cent in the number of traffic crashes, 52 per cent in the number of injured and 37 per cent in the number of deaths during the 1990s (Vietnam Public Health Research Network 2003: 29–43).

The developing epidemic of NCDs in Viet Nam will increase use of health services and will greatly increase health costs over the coming decades. The estimated cost of NCDs for Viet Nam in 2006 was about US$20 million (accounting for 0.033 per cent of annual GDP). But this estimate will almost double by 2015 if effective interventions are not implemented. The accumulated losses in GDP due to chronic diseases in Viet Nam between 2006 and 2015 could therefore be as much as US$270 million (Van Minh *et al.* 2009a: 1–8).

## Responses to non-communicable diseases

Viet Nam has shown a strong commitment to combating the tobacco epidemic. In 2000, the Government of Viet Nam introduced its National Tobacco Control

Policy (Government Resolution No. 12/2000/NQ-CP), which laid out its policy objectives including: public education; prohibitions on advertising, promotion and sponsorship by tobacco companies; health warnings on cigarette packages; taxes and pricing as disincentives for smoking; development of smoking cessation programmes; and restrictions on smoking in public places. In 2001 it established the inter-ministerial Viet Nam Committee on Smoking and Health. Viet Nam also ratified the WHO Framework Convention on Tobacco Control in December 2004. To strengthen the implementation of tobacco control measures first introduced in 2001, the government issued new regulations in 2007 to further control packaging and labelling of tobacco products; and to regulate public smoking, the retail sale of tobacco products, and tobacco advertising, promotion and sponsorship. More regulations in 2009 provide for sanctions for violations of earlier regulations on the marketing, sale and promotion of tobacco products (Hoang *et al.* 2006: 6–22; Vietnam Steering Committee on Smoking and Health 2011).

These regulations have defined smoke-free public places. Smoking is completely prohibited on public transport and in indoor working areas as well as the following specific public places: schools, kindergartens, health facilities, libraries, cinemas, theatres, community cultural houses and places at high risk of explosion and fire. In other public places (for example airports and railway stations) smoking is permitted, but only in designated smoking areas. Although the regulations allow local authorities to enact smoke-free laws they cannot be more stringent than the national law, thus restricting local tobacco control initiatives. Despite tobacco advertising and promotion being generally prohibited, there are exceptions such as in foreign language print media, and sponsorship and/or financial contributions for events or organizations are allowed but cannot be publicized. Finally, tobacco products are required to have displayed one of two text warnings: 'Smoking may cause lung cancer' or 'Smoking may cause Chronic Obstructive Pulmonary Disease'. The warning must occupy 30 per cent of the displayed package area and be printed in black capital letters on a white background. Although there was a plan to increase the size of the warnings to 50 per cent of the package display area by 2010, the regulations for this requirement are still being formulated. The regulations to control tobacco products represent a promising beginning but vigilance will be required to ensure they expand so that there is, in the future, a substantial impact on the prevalence of smoking. The production of cigarettes in Viet Nam rose steadily until 2005 but has fallen slightly since 2006 after the new tobacco tax was applied. The current tax rate accounts for about 45 per cent of the retail price of a pack of cigarettes although the World Bank recommends that a tobacco tax should account for 66 to 80 per cent of the retail price. From this perspective the tobacco tax rate in Viet Nam is still very low and should be increased.

Almost concurrent with the tobacco control measures has been the development of prevention and control of NCDs. In June 2002, the Prime Minister Nguyễn Tấn Dũng formally approved the National Programme on Prevention and Control of NCDs for the period 2002–2010 (Government resolution number

77/2002/QD-TTg) although it is unclear what specific events triggered this national programme. A national task force was established with a supporting team in the Ministry of Health, and WHO provided technical assistance. This group developed an operational plan for prevention and control and this included the development of a surveillance system, healthy lifestyle education in community demonstration projects, annual national healthy lifestyle campaigns around themes such as detection and management of hypertension or 'Healthy Village Culture', demonstration projects of preventive clinical services for diabetes, hypertension screening and detection and follow-up management, and the establishment of a national NCD network.

The program developed in Viet Nam has been organized to have specific components managed by existing government medical organizations; so the National Institute for Cardiovascular Disease manages the prevention and control of cardiovascular diseases, the National Institute of Oncology (National Cancer Hospital) manages the cancer programmes, the National Institute of Endocrinology, the diabetes programmes and the National Institute of Psychiatry, the mental illness programmes. However, this approach may restrict the integrated approaches needed to tackle NCDs and may lead to too much emphasis on secondary prevention and improved case management, rather than primary prevention.

There is evidence of a substantial financial commitment from the government for NCD control programmes with funding increasing from zero in 2001 to about US$750,000 by 2005 (World Health Organization 2005: 20). Even so, this level of funding is inadequate given the magnitude of the emerging problems and it does not match the level of resources allocated previously to high-priority, infectious disease control programmes.

## Lessons for the future

As mentioned earlier in the chapter, many of the key elements of Viet Nam's success in controlling infectious diseases were linked to characteristics developed in the prolonged wars following its declaration of independence. But these same characteristics may not be as helpful with the emerging epidemic of chronic diseases. The current NCD control programme has attracted a *high level of political commitment*, but the resources required successfully to tackle the problem have not yet been provided.

A very effective strategy for infectious disease control was the use of *decentralized health services* with a *vertical programme* adjusted to local needs based on careful disease surveillance. In contrast, NCDs originate from a complex interaction of rapid social and economic development along with urbanization and cannot be addressed by the health sector alone. Indeed they require multisectoral approaches. Also, NCD control surveillance is less well developed and provides less of the information required for local modification of programmes.

The decentralization of health services may also be promoting less equitable access to services as urban provinces are able to harvest more local resources for programmes from their more rapidly growing economies. Also, national level regulation is required for some control measures, for example, tobacco control, and local problem-solving at the community level may be less important in such cases.

The *community-based approaches to mobilize the population* used in infectious disease control may also be less effective. Often these were involved loud-speakers disseminating messages or promoting programmes in villages and had their origin in warnings during the war about enemy bombing raids. These systems do not work in large urban centres and new approaches will be needed to mobilize communities, perhaps employing new technologies such as mobile phones or the Internet. Furthermore, the behaviours that need to be changed to deal with NCDs often include personal lifestyle behaviours such as smoking, exercise and diet rather than health-seeking behaviours, and these are much harder to change.

It may be possible to engage *local health cadres to conduct screening to detect cases of NCDs*, but this will require a re-tooling of the health system and development of new clinical and preventive skills by these workers. Indeed, the real challenge for Viet Nam will be to develop such new approaches across the board to tackle NCDs and these will amount to fundamental readjustment of the health system if these daunting new public health problems are to be overcome.

## References

Ahmed, S.M., Hadi, A., Razzaque, A., Ashraf, A., Juvekar, S., Ng, N., Kanungsukkasem, U., Soonthornthada, K., Van Minh, H. and Huu Bich, T. (2009) 'Clustering of Chronic Non-Communicable Disease Risk Factors among Selected Asian Populations: Levels and Determinants', *Global Health Action*, 2: 71.

Chan, J.C., Malik, V., Jia, W., Kadowaki, T., Yajnik, C.S., Yoon, K.H. and Hu, F.B. (2009) 'Diabetes in Asia: Epidemiology, Risk Factors, and Pathophysiology', *JAMA*, 301(20): 2129–2140.

Chen, L.C. and Hiebert, L.G. (1994) *From Socialism to Private Markets: Vietnam's Heatlth in Rapid Transition*, Boston, MA: Harvard Center for Population and Development Studies, Harvard School of Public Health.

Cockram, C.S. (2006) 'Diabetes Prevention and Control in Vietnam: A Demonstration Project in Two Provinces', *Practical Diabetes International*, 23(8): 361–364.

Cuong, T.Q., Dibley, M.J., Bowe, S., Hanh, T.T. and Loan, T.T. (2007) 'Obesity in Adults: An Emerging Problem in Urban Areas of Ho Chi Minh City, Vietnam', *European Journal of Clinical Nutritrion*, 61(5): 673–681.

Dieu, H.T., Dibley, M.J., Sibbritt, D.W. and Hanh, T.T. (2009) 'Trends in Overweight and Obesity in Pre-School Children in Urban Areas of Ho Chi Minh City, Vietnam, from 2002 to 2005', *Public Health Nutritrion*, 12(5): 702–709.

Dollar, D. (1993) 'Vietnam: Successes and Failures of Macroeconomic Stabilization', in: B. Ljunggren, ed., *The Challenge of Reform in Indochina*, Boston, MA: Harvard University Press; 207–303.

Duc Son, L.N., Kusama, K., Hung, N.T., Loan, T.T., Chuyen, N.V., Kunii, D., Sakai, T. and Yamamoto, S. (2004) 'Prevalence and Risk Factors for Diabetes in Ho Chi Minh City, Vietnam', *Diabetic Medicine*, 21(4): 371–376.

Dung, P.H. (1996) 'The Political Process and the Private Health Sector's Role in Vietnam', *International Journal of Health Planning and Management*, 11(3): 217–230.

Fforde, A. (1993) 'The Political Economy of "Reform" in Vietnam: Some Reflections', in B. Ljunggren, ed., *The Challenge of Reform in Indochina*, Boston, MA: Harvard Institute for International Development, Harvard University, 293–325.

Food and Agriculture Organization of the United Nations (1999) *Nutrition Country Profiles: Vietnam*, Roma: Food and Agriculture Organization of the United Nations.

General Statistics Office Vietnam (2010a) *Global Adult Tobacco Survey (GATS) Viet Nam 2010*, Hanoi: Vietnam Statistics Press.

General Statistics Office Vietnam (2010b) *Statistical Yearbook of Vietnam 2010*, Hanoi: Vietnam Statistics Press.

Goldstein, G.S. and Gronberg, T.J. (1984) 'Economies of Scope and Economies of Agglomeration', *Journal of Urban Economics*, 16(1): 91–104.

Health Environment Management Agency (2010) *Injury Mortality Statistic in 2008*, Hanoi: Health Environment Management Agency.

Ho Chi Minh City Health Department (2001–2009) *Health Statistics, Ho Chi Minh City*, Ho Chi Minh City Health Department. Online, available at: www.medinet.hochiminhcity.gov.vn/data/news/2011/6/8147/khamchuabenh.htm (accessed 28 November 2011).

Hoang, V.K., Ross, H., Levy, D., Nguyen, T.M. and Vu, T.B. (2006) 'The Effect of Imposing a Higher, Uniform Tobacco Tax in Vietnam', *Health Research Policy and System*, 4: 6–22.

Hoang, V.M., Byass, P., Dao, L.H., Nguyen, T.K. and Wall, S. (2007) 'Risk Factors for Chronic Disease among Rural Vietnamese Adults and the Association of These Factors with Sociodemographic Variables: Findings from the Who Steps Survey in Rural Vietnam, 2005', *Preventing Chronic Disease*, 4(2): 1–10.

Hong, T.K., Dibley, M.J., Sibbritt, D., Binh, P.N., Trang, N.H. and Hanh, T.T. (2007) 'Overweight and Obesity are Rapidly Emerging among Adolescents in Ho Chi Minh City, Vietnam, 2002–2004', *International Journal of Pediatric Obesity*, 2(4): 194–201.

Khan, N.C. and Khoi, H.H. (2008) 'Double Burden of Malnutrition: The Vietnamese Perspective', *Asia Pacific Journal of Clinical Nutrition*, 17 (Suppl. 1): 116–118.

Levy, B.S. and Sidel, S.W. (eds) (2000) *War and Public Health*, Washington, DC: American Public Health Association.

McMichael, J.K. (1976) 'Organising for Health: Selection and Training of Health Personnel', in J.K. McMichael, ed., *Health in the Third World: Studies from Vietnam*, Nottingham: Spokesman Books, 51–69.

Minh, H.V., Byass, P., Chuc, N.T. and Wall, S. (2006) 'Gender Differences in Prevalence and Socioeconomic Determinants of Hypertension: Findings from the Who Steps Survey in a Rural Community of Vietnam', *Journal of Human Hypertension*, 20(2): 109–115.

Minh, H.V., Huong, D.L. and Giang, K.B. (2008) 'Self-Reported Chronic Diseases and Associated Sociodemographic Status and Lifestyle Risk Factors among Rural Vietnamese Adults', *Scandinavian Journal of Public Health*, 36(6): 629–634.

Ministry of Health Vietnam (2003a) *Vietnam Health Statistics Year Book*, Hanoi, Ministry of Health Vietnam.

Ministry of Health Vietnam (2003b) *Vietnam National Health Survey Report, 2001–02*, Hanoi: Medicine Press.

Ministry of Health Vietnam (2006) *Vietnam Health Statistics Year Book*, Hanoi: Ministry of Health Vietnam.

Ministry of Health Vietnam (2007) *Vietnam Health Statistics Year Book*, Hanoi: Ministry of Health Vietnam.

Ministry of Health Vietnam (2009) *Vietnam Health Statistics Year Book*, Hanoi: Ministry of Health Vietnam.

Miron Allukian, J.R. and Paul, L.A. (2000) 'Public Health and the Vietnam War', in: B.S. Levy and S.W. Sidel, eds, *War and Public Health*, Washington, DC: American Public Health Association, 215–238.

National Institute of Nutrition (2010) *General Nutrition Survey of Vietnam 2009–2010*, Hanoi: Ministry of Health Viet Nam.

National Institute of Nutrition Vietnam (2005) *The National General Survey on Overweight and Obesity 2005*, Hanoi: National Institute of Nutrition Vietnam.

Nguyen, M.D., Beresford, S.A. and Drewnowski, A. (2007) 'Trends in Overweight by Socio-Economic Status in Vietnam: 1992 to 2002', *Public Health Nutrition*, 10(2): 115–121.

Nguyen, T.H., Tang, H.K., Kelly, P., van der Ploeg, H.P. and Dibley, M.J. (2010) 'Association between Physical Activity and Metabolic Syndrome: A Cross Sectional Survey in Adolescents in Ho Chi Minh City, Vietnam', *BioMed Central Public Health*, 10: 141–150.

Pham, L.H., Au, T.B., Blizzard, L., Truong, N.B., Schmidt, M.D., Granger, R.H. and Dwyer, T. (2009) 'Prevalence of Risk Factors for Non-Communicable Diseases in the Mekong Delta, Vietnam: Results from a Steps Survey', *BioMed Central Public Health*, 9: 291–299.

Quoc, P.S., Charles, M.A., Cuong, N.H., Lieu, L.H., Tuan, N.A., Thomas, M., Balkau, B. and Simon, D. (1994) 'Blood Glucose Distribution and Prevalence of Diabetes in Hanoi (Vietnam)', *American Journal of Epidemiology*, 139(7): 713–722.

Schuftan, C. (2000) *A Story to Be Shared: The Successful Fight against Malaria in Vietnam*, Geneva: WHO.

Trang, N.H., Hong, T.K., Dibley, M.J. and Sibbritt, D.W. (2009) 'Factors Associated with Physical Inactivity in Adolescents in Ho Chi Minh City, Vietnam', *Medicine and Science in Sports and Exercis*, 41(7): 1374–1383.

Trinh, O.T., Nguyen, N.D., Dibley, M.J., Phongsavan, P. and Bauman, A.E. (2008) 'The Prevalence and Correlates of Physical Inactivity among Adults in Ho Chi Minh City', *BioMed Central Public Health*, 8: 204–215.

Trinh, O.T., Nguyen, N.D., Phongsavon, P., Dibley, M.J. and Bauman, A.E. (2010) 'Metabolic Risk Profiles and Associated Risk Factors among Vietnamese Adults in Ho Chi Minh City', *Metabolic Syndrome Related Disorders*, 8(1): 69–78.

Tuan, T. (1995) *Historical Development of Primary Health Care in Vietnam: Lessons for the Future*, Boston, MA: Harvard School of Public Health.

Tuan, T. (2004) *Community-based Evidence about the Health Care System in Rural Vietnam*, Newcastle, NSW: University of Newcastle School of Medicine Practice and Population Health.

UNICEF, and National Institute of Nutrition Vietnam (2011) *A Review of the Nutrition Situation in Viet Nam 2009–2010*, Hanoi: UNICEF Vietnam.

UNICEF Vietnam (2000) *Vietnam – Children and Women: A Situation Analysis 2000*, Hanoi: UNICEF Vietnam.

Van Minh, H., Lan Huong, D., Bao Giang, K. and Byass, P. (2009a) 'Economic Aspects of Chronic Diseases in Vietnam', *Global Health Action*, 2: 1–8.

Van Minh, H., Soonthornthada, K., Ng, N., Juvekar, S., Razzaque, A., Ashraf, A., Ahmed, S.M., Bich, T.H. and Kanungsukkasem, U. (2009b) 'Blood Pressure in Adult Rural Indepth Population in Asia', *Global Health Action*, 2: 60–67.

Vietnam Public Health Research Network (2003) *Report to Unicef on the Vietnam Multi-Center Injury Survey*, Hanoi: UNICEF.

Vietnam Steering Committee on Smoking and Health (2011) *The National Action Plan for Tobacco Control for 2000–2010*, Hanoi: Ministry of Health Vietnam. Online, available at: www.vinacosh.gov.vn/?mPage=06P20F02 (accessed 28 November 2011).

World Bank (2011) *The World Development Indicators 2011*, Washington, DC: World Bank.

World Bank, and East Asia Infrastructure Department (2010) *Issues and Dynamics: Urban Systems in Developing East Asia*. Washington, DC. Online, available at: http:// siteresources.worldbank.org/INTEAPREGTOPURBDEV/Resources/vietnam-Urbanisation.pdf (accessed 28 November 2011).

World Health Organization (2004) *Country Profile: Global Status Report on Alcohol*, Geneva. Online, available at: www.who.int/substance_abuse/publications/statusreport-alcoholwpro/en/index.html (accessed 28 November 2011).

World Health Organization (2005) *Report on the Regional Evaluation of Non Communicable Diseases Prevention and Control Programme*, Noumea, New Caledonia. Online, available at: www.wpro.who.int/internet/resources.ashx/EDT/NCD.pdf (accessed 28 November 2011).

World Health Organization (2011a) *Vietnam Tobacco Control*, Geneva: WHO. Online, available at: www.wpro.who.int/vietnam/sites/dhp/tobacco_control/ (accessed 28 November 2011).

World Health Organization (2011b) *World Health Statistics 2011*, Geneva. Online, available at: www.who.int/whosis/whostat/EN_WHS2011_Full.pdf (accessed 28 November 2011).

# 10 Singapore

## Health policy and programming in historical perspective and social, political and economic context

*Meng-Kin Lim*

Along with other more populous and economically dynamic countries in the Asia-Pacific region, the tiny island city-state of Singapore (land area: 710 km$^2$; population five million) completed its epidemiologic transition in a very short time. Whereas tuberculosis and pneumonia were the two leading causes of death in the 1950s and 1960s, chronic, non-communicable diseases (NCDs) like cancer, heart disease and stroke are now the leading causes of morbidity and mortality. To appreciate how far Singapore has come, one has only to note that average life expectancy has risen to 81.4 years in 2010, from 62 years in 1957 (the earliest that such a statistic was published), and infant mortality is 2.2 per 1,000 live births, down from an appalling 82 per 1,000 live births in 1950 (Ministry of Health 2010a). The World Health Statistics 2010 ranked Singapore second lowest for infant mortality and ninth highest for life expectancy at birth (World Health Organization 2010: 48).

Its inhabitants enjoy universal access[1] to a high standard of health care at affordable costs. Remarkably, national health expenditure has remained between 3 and 4 per cent of GDP in the past four decades (compared to OECD countries which averaged 9 per cent of GDP (OECD Health Data 2009). The WHO 2000 Report gave Singapore's health care system high marks, ranking it sixth best in the world for overall efficiency (World Health Report 2000). It is fair to say, however, that it was not improved health care per se that was responsible for Singapore's impressive health status improvements; rather, the credit must go to the improved housing, sanitation, nutrition, education and environment that accompanied Singapore's rapid rise as one of Asia's economic miracles: it now boasts a per capita GDP of US$57,200 (purchasing power parity, 2010), surpassing even that of most of the OECD countries (Central Intelligence Agency 2010).

Paradoxically, the dramatic declines in mortality and its new-rich status – good news surely – have combined to generate a fresh set of problems known only too well to developed countries: that rich citizens live longer but have fewer children. In 2009 the total fertility rate was 1.22 (Ministry of Health 2010a). True, the population is relatively young by any standards – in 2009, only 8 per cent were 65 years or older – but assuming the present trajectory holds, 20 per cent of the population will be 65 years or older in 2030 (Ministry of Community Development 1999). The old age dependency ratio, which in 1994 was one elderly dependant to seven working adults, will be one to two in 2030, with serious implications for a whole range of issues: workforce, social security, housing and health, to name a few.

Since health and disease are the result of complex interactions of social determinants in addition to genetic factors, it goes without saying that they are profoundly shaped by the broader context of economic and social development (World Health Organization 2008). This chapter reviews the health policies and prevention and control initiatives of Singapore from a historical perspective and in the context of social, political and economic developments.

## Historical and social context

Singapore was founded in 1819 as a trading outpost of the British Empire. The swampy, mosquito-infested island, which once served as a haven for pirates in the equatorial backwaters of Southeast Asia, drew migrant workers from India, China and the Malay Archipelago – mainly poor and hungry migrants either escaping from the poverty and oppression of their original homelands or simply in search of a better future. It eventually became a thriving centre of commerce in addition to the official headquarters of the British Far East Land Forces.

It would be a fallacy, however, to assume that because Singapore was under British rule for 155 years, it inherited a British-style, egalitarian, national health system. On the contrary, British interest in the health of the locals was initially no different from that displayed by the Belgians, French or Dutch in Africa, Indochina or Indonesia. Western medicine following western expansionism concerned itself mainly with the colonizers. Any spill-over effect invariably involved civil service employees and plantation and mine workers who were predominantly male because they were significant for the wellbeing of the state and economy; women and children, and the poor were neglected. Despite rampant problems of poverty, malnutrition, overcrowding and disease in the nineteenth century, there was no hospital and virtually no medical care for the public in Singapore before 1840. Most local residents went to private traditional practitioners – the Chinese turning to traditional Chinese medicine, the Malays to traditional Malay medicine and the Indians to Ayurvedic medicine.

The first hospital for locals in Singapore (Tan Tock Seng Hospital) was a charity hospital built in 1844 with funds raised by Chinese community leaders. According to historian Mary Turnbull, the laissez-faire government of early Singapore was so distant from the people that an official commission reported in 1875 that "the majority of Chinamen who came to work in these settlements return to their country not knowing clearly whether there is a government in them or not" (Turnbull 1981: 86). She also described post-Second World War Singapore as "a filthy, overcrowded city with barely one-third of the urban population housed satisfactorily" while Philippe Regnier found Singapore society then to be "profoundly non-egalitarian, with 20 per cent of the population in a state of poverty and a virtual absence of social services" (1987: 51).

Even the first (and for the next 100 years, only) western-style medical school was founded in 1905 through the philanthropy of a local Chinese entrepreneur, Tan Jiak Kim, and a petition for its establishment from the local citizens to the Governor, Sir John Anderson. The resulting "Straits and Federal Malay States Government Medical School", with a first batch of 23 students, is the precursor of the National University of Singapore, which now graduates 300 doctors annually.

At Singapore's independence in 1965, public health care was largely tax based and publicly provided, but standards in the decrepit and poorly equipped hospitals were low. In 1960, fewer than 50 doctors in the whole country were in possession of higher qualifications. It was not until the 1970s that medical specialization began in earnest, and not until 1983 that the government responded to the rising aspirations of the people that accompanied their growing affluence with a National Health Plan (Lim 1998: 16–22).

Why did it take almost 20 years after independence before any meaningful reform of the health system was instituted? Because, quite simply, there were other pressing concerns. For Singapore was not granted independence in 1965 on a platter but unceremoniously ejected from Malaysia after a failed, two-year political union with its larger neighbour. Cut off from its hinterland and without any natural resources to speak about (even its water was piped from Malaysia), Singapore faced a most uncertain future.

Two years after independence, in 1967, the Minister of Health, Yong Nyuk Lin, declared matter-of-factly that "health would rank, at most, fifth in order of priority" for funds – "after national security, job creation, housing and educa-tion" (Yong 1967), in that order. It was around this time that the political leader-ship concluded that socialism was not going to bring bread to the table and took an ideological right turn to embrace capitalism, leading to its eventual resigna-tion (or perhaps expulsion) from the Socialist International in 1976. In the end, it trumped the political left (from which it had openly split) in the battle (amidst labour unrest, racial riots and communist insurgency) for the hearts and minds of the hard-working Singaporeans.

Since then Singapore has eschewed, at least rhetorically, egalitarian wel-farism in favour of market mechanisms to allocate finite resources. In practice, this meant using pricing to curb demand but at the same time softening the con-sequences to protect lower income groups. Pragmatism, not ideology, would guide social policies in the decades that followed. As the government and people focused single-mindedly on expanding the size of the economic pie, citizens were encouraged to assume personal responsibility for their own welfare. Real-izing that health-care costs would ineluctably rise as the population aged and technology advanced, the government assiduously avoided policies that would transfer the financial burden to future generations, instead preferring to shift the cost of health care to private pockets (Lim 2004: 83–92).

Singapore's open economy, which thrives on global trade and financial serv-ices, has been consistently given top ranking by the Global Competitiveness

Report of the Geneva-based World Economic Forum. It would not have got there without its strong commitment to open markets, minimal regulation and rule of law. It is not surprising, therefore, that Singapore's health-care sector is highly competitive. Singaporeans have complete freedom of choice between public and private providers. The private sector accounts for 80 per cent of daily outpatient attendances and 20 per cent of hospital admissions. It takes the load off the government as the provider of high-end and more personalized services.

Standards are high, as attested by the steady stream of foreign patients (500,000 in 2009) that flock to Singapore for treatment. All public-sector hospitals and national specialist centres and most private-sector hospitals have been externally accredited by Joint Commission International. The fact that all of Singapore's private-sector hospital groups are listed on the Singapore Exchange reflects the government's favourable disposition towards the commercialization of health-care services. The government has in fact set a target of achieving one million foreign patients, reckoning that it will generate S$3 billion in revenue and create 13,000 new jobs in the process.

Domestically, health care is similarly seen as a consumption activity that should not be offered free at the point of care. The underlying assumption is that if each person were spending his own money instead of the State's, then it would be in his or her interest to manage his or her expenditure, avoid waste and even shop around for value. This principle of "no free lunch" pervades Singapore society, with implications – as we shall see – even for preventive health screening and long term care.

Looking back with the benefit of hindsight, it was indeed very significant that in 1960 the newly elected government of Singapore, barely a year into office, introduced for the first time user fees (50 cents per attendance) at government outpatient clinics. This principle of co-payment, even though the actual recovery was negligible, proved to be a harbinger of things to come. In the government's own words,

> Singapore believes that welfarism is not viable as it breeds dependency on the government. It has adopted a policy of co-payment to encourage people to assume personal responsibility for their own welfare, though the government does provide subsidies in vital areas like housing, health and education.
>
> (Ministry of Education 2011)

Convinced that health care cost is inflationary, and its demand inherently insatiable, the government determined not to let an "entitlement culture" creep in to overburden public finances. It adopted "shared responsibility" as the core principle of its health-care financing policy: government will remain committed to subsidizing health care to make it affordable but Singaporeans able to do so must provide their share. Thus, while the proportion of public spending on health at independence in 1965 was half, by 1990, it had dwindled to one-third. In 2008, Singapore spent about S$10.2 billion or 3.9 per cent of GDP on health care. Out of this the government spent S\$2.7 billion or 1.0 per cent of GDP on health services (Ministry of Health 2010a).

No fewer than five high-level ministerial committees have been convened since 1982 to address long term care issues along with other anticipated needs of the elderly, and the answer has always been the same: there is no magic bullet; financial responsibility for Singapore's elderly lies with the individual, the family and the community (in that order), and only lastly with the state. The landmark 1999 *Report of the Inter-Ministerial Committee on the Ageing Population* reaffirmed the family's responsibility to care for its elderly, with institutional care a measure of last resort. At first glance, such a hands-off approach to the care of the elderly may be misconstrued as rather uncaring and inhumane but on closer examination, it is undergirded by a humane guarantee in 1993 by the government that "no Singaporean will ever be denied needed health care because of lack of funds" (Lim 1998: 20). In other words, both health and institutional care will be available to all, but state funding will remain a measure of last resort.

## Risk factors, morbidity and mortality attributable to chronic, NCDs

The epidemic of NCDs around the world is clearly in evidence in Singapore, where it is the leading cause of morbidity and mortality. According to WHO country data (2004) on the distribution of years of life lost due to three broad categories, NCDs accounted for 73 per cent of years of life lost, while age-standardized mortality rate for all NCDs is 345 per 100,000 population for Singapore. As for the economic burden associated with specific risk factors, a Singapore study estimated that the cost of health care, absenteeism and loss of productivity stemming from smoking-related diseases cost the nation between S\$700 million and S\$800 million in 1997 (Quah *et al.* 2002: 340–344).

Table 10.1 presents the main risk factors underpinning the NCD profile of Singaporeans, drawn from the Ministry of Health's three-yearly household survey conducted in 2007.

## NCD prevention and control policies

As early as 1986 Singapore had launched its National Smoking Control Programme and established a National Smoking Control Coordinating Committee to make non-smoking a social norm and eliminate exposure to passive smoking. The strategy was multipronged including legislation,[2] tobacco taxation, health education and smoking cessation services as well as intersectoral collaboration and community mobilization. Smoking is now prohibited in all public places, tobacco advertising is prohibited and graphic health warning labels on cigarette packs are mandatory.

Singapore's proactive stance is illustrated by banning of cigarette vending machines before they could be introduced and arose from simply looking at the

*Table 10.1* Key risk factors and chronic medical conditions among Singapore residents aged 18–69 years, 2007

*Physical activity*
23.6% exercised regularly during leisure time, up from 20.3% in 2001.

*Cigarette smoking*
13.6% smoked cigarettes daily, about the same proportion as in 2001 (13.8%).

*Alcohol consumption*
1.2% consumed alcohol regularly, up from 0.7% in 2001.

*Obesity*
5.7% are obese (based on self-reported height and weight values; hence likely to be lower than the true prevalence based on actual measurements).*

*High blood cholesterol*
12.5% had been told by a doctor that they had high blood cholesterol.

*Diabetes mellitus*
4.6% reported they had diabetes and were on prescribed medication.

*Hypertension*
12.0% reported they had hypertension and were on prescribed medication.

*Asthma*
6.6% had been told by a doctor they had asthma.

*Arthritis and chronic joint symptoms*
10.1% had been told by a doctor that they had arthritis and also had pain, aching, stiffness or swelling in or around a joint on most days for at least 1 month.

*Mental health*
11.2% and 10.0% were found to have poor mental health when assessed by the WHO-5 and GHQ-12 instruments respectively.

*Dental health*
71.4% brushed their teeth twice a day.

*Self-rated overall health*
66.7% rated their overall health as "very good" or "good", 31.8% "moderate" and 1.4% "bad" or "very bad".

Source: Ministry of Health 2007.

Note
The most recent (not yet published) National Health Survey 2010 findings indicate a 0.65% annual increase in the prevalence of obesity over the past 6 years, from 6.9% in 2004 to 10.8% in 2010 (Health Promotion Board; personal communication).

experiences of other countries. And by introducing legislation early, Singapore prevented the tobacco industry from ever becoming important event sponsors. Increasing retail prices of cigarettes since 1972 have coincided with decreasing per capita consumption. Taxes represent 67 per cent of the average retail price of a pack of cigarettes. When Singapore ratified the WHO Framework Convention on Tobacco Control in December 2003, it was already exceeding the requirements pertaining to tobacco sponsorship, promotion and advertising. The daily-smokers prevalence (aged 18–69 years) in Singapore has declined to one of the lowest in the world – from 20 per cent in 1984 to 12.6 per cent in 2004. However, while the crude prevalence of smoking overall and among males has decreased, it dramatically increased among females from 1992 to 2004, particularly among those aged 18–29 years – a disturbing trend common in many developed countries.

The Government has put its money where its mouth is – financing a broad range of health promotion activities accompanied by supportive legislation. Thus, it launched a National Healthy Lifestyle Programme in 1992 which adopted a multipronged approach to create and foster a supportive environment for Singaporeans to practise healthy behaviour, aided by the media. This includes an annual, month-long campaign, the National Healthy Lifestyle Campaign, with a new focus every year (for example, the Mental Health Education Programme, National Smoking Control Campaign and AIDS) or features (Family Run Run, healthier food in Supermarkets and Restaurants and Telematches) but invariably including mass aerobics; "The Great Singapore Workout" led by the Prime Minister himself, in shorts and all.

In 2001, it took the significant step of establishing a Health Promotion Board with a vision to build a nation of healthy and happy people. The autonomous but state-funded Board targets all segments of the population – the healthy, at-risk and unhealthy – using a variety of strategies and approaches. Its health promotion initiatives focus on primary, secondary and tertiary prevention. It promotes healthy lifestyle practices as well as early detection and management of key chronic diseases. Its programmes include breast screening, cervical screening, childhood injury prevention, community health screening, mental health education, myopia prevention, physical activity, smoking control, nutrition, osteoporosis education and workplace health promotion. Thanks to its efforts, health screening is now fairly common among Singapore residents aged 40 to 69 years (see Table 10.2).

## Infectious disease: down but not out

Despite the striking improvements in living conditions, excellent health care infrastructure, and the virtual disappearance of once-rife infectious diseases like cholera, typhoid and malaria, modern-day Singapore nevertheless faces a real and present threat of infectious diseases. Indeed, Singapore's historic Middleton Hospital, established in 1907 as a quarantine camp for the isolation and treatment of patients with dangerous infectious diseases such as smallpox, plague and cholera, had by 2000 become empty and irrelevant. It was absorbed by the adjacent Tan Tock Seng Hospital (TTSH) and its sprawling grounds earmarked for redevelopment. Diphtheria, typhoid and poliomyelitis have been adequately controlled with Singapore's comprehensive childhood immunization programme, and improved hygiene and public health meant that the hospital was only seeing small numbers of patients associated with the occasional outbreak of chickenpox. Then, in 2003, SARS (Severe Acute Respiratory Syndrome) struck. Because the first two cases were admitted and diagnosed in TTSH, the Ministry

*Table 10.2* Community health screening among adult Singapore residents, 2007

---

*Diabetes blood check*
Among adults aged 40 to 69 years without known diabetes, 72.2% had a blood check for diabetes within the past three years.

*Blood cholesterol*
Among adults without known high blood cholesterol, 78.0% had been screened within the past three years.

*Blood pressure check*
63.9% of those without known hypertension had their blood pressure checked in the past year.

*Breast cancer screening*
83.2% of women aged 50 to 69 years were aware of mammography, up from 46.7% in 2001.
61.3% of women had undergone mammography.
Among women aged 50 to 69 years, 40.9% had a mammogram within the past two years, in line with the recommended screening frequency.

*Cervical cancer screening*
87.4% of women aged 25 to 69 years were aware of Pap Smear tests, up from 69.3% in 2001.
Among women in the 25–69 age group, 74.1% reported that they had ever had a Pap Smear test and 59.2% had the test within the past 3 years, in line with the recommended screening frequency.

*Colorectal cancer screening*
25% of males and 19.8% of females aged 50 to 69 years reported that they ever had a Faecal Occult Blood Test (FOBT).
11.3% of males 13 7.8% of females aged 50 to 69 years reported that they had undergone colonoscopy or sigmoidoscopy at least once.

---

Source: Ministry of Health 2007.

of Health (MOH) decided to centralize the care of all suspected and probable cases of SARS, including pediatric cases, in TTSH. This facilitated the management of SARS patients and reduced the risk of secondary transmission of the disease. Ambulances were diverted and patients at the emergency department with non-SARS conditions who required hospitalization were transferred to other hospitals. It was the SARS crisis that gave impetus to the emergence from the ashes of the now defunct Middleton Hospital of a reorganized and renamed Communicable Disease Centre (CDC) under TTSH, with fresh funding and an urgent mandate as the national referral centre for the diagnosis and management of communicable diseases.

In addition to in-patient and out-patient facilities geared to handling disease outbreaks as well as laboratory facilities to conduct research for better disease management and patient care, Singapore's CDC aims to be a centre of excellence for training and education concerning infectious diseases as well. The latter include not only occasional global outbreaks of pathogens to which Singapore as a regional trade and transportation hub is particularly susceptible but also regionally endemic diseases such as malaria, dengue fever and melioidosis, and emergent ones like HIV, Nipah virus, SARS and H1N1 influenza; the more insidious, less well-publicized infections caused by hospital, drug-resistant micro-organisms are also an important focus.

## Understanding Singapore's health care system

The foundations of the present-day healthcare system were laid in 1983, when the government unveiled its National Health Plan with the objective of building a healthy, fit and productive population through disease prevention and promotion of healthy lifestyles; improving health system cost efficiency; and meeting a rapidly ageing population's growing demand for health care. It laid out an ambitious hospital redevelopment and building plan to bring Singapore medicine into the modern era and then raised the inevitable question: who will pay for all this? The unequivocal answer was that government could not do it alone; everyone must "chip in" and co-pay! The underlying premise – that nothing comes free – was very unorthodox indeed for a government that had ridden to power in 1959 on a democratic socialist platform. The emphasis was individual responsibility for health and self-help health care, with the state as payer of last resort.

## Reforms in health care financing

Any discussion of health policies and programmes cannot be divorced from the incentive structures governing health system financing and delivery. Singapore's unique cost-sharing and risk-spreading "3M" system of health care financing treats the majority of users as co-paying partners while offering special provisions to the minority who cannot afford to pay. Such an approach avoids providing the rich with health care handouts as would be the case under a universal coverage system that ignores income status. It is also designed to counter the moral hazard generally associated with fee-for-service, third-party reimbursement.

How does it work? Medisave was introduced in 1984 as a compulsory health savings account for employees or self-employed persons who are Singaporean citizens or permanent residents. It is tax exempt and interest yielding, and represents 6.5 to 9 per cent (depending on age) of wages earmarked for future hospitalization, day surgery and certain outpatient expenses. As the Medisave account can be used to pay for the hospitalization and other approved medical bills of one's spouse, children or parents there is a small element of risk-pooling within the family; upon the death of the account holder, any unspent balance is passed on to the beneficiaries. In 2008 the combined Medisave accounts of all Singaporeans amounted to S$42 billion – a significant sum considering it is about six times Singapore's annual national health care expenditure. In 2008, eight out of ten Singaporeans admitted to hospitals used Medisave to pay their bills.

Medishield is a voluntary, low-cost insurance scheme designed to protect households from large and unexpected financial losses due to illness; it provides coverage for "catastrophic" illnesses such as heart surgery and liver transplantation for which Medisave is unlikely to be adequate. Premiums can be paid from Medisave. Singaporeans who want more benefits or amenities such as better hospital rooms are free to purchase enhanced "shield" plans offered by private insurers. The government requires these plans, at a minimum, to incorporate the basic Medishield plan while supplementary rider plans provide the desired additional coverage. There are currently 25 such "integrated" shield plans offered by three private insurers catering to the varied health insurance needs of Singaporeans. In 2008, 84 per cent of Singapore's population was covered under MediShield-type plans.

Medifund is the state-funded safety net that takes care of the poor and needy. It was set up in 1993 as a safety net for Singaporeans who cannot afford medical expenses even after government subsidy, Medisave and MediShield. The interest from a large government-sponsored endowment fund (which currently stands at S$1.7 billion) is distributed to both public hospitals and non-profit hospitals run by voluntary welfare organizations, to cover the costs of patients genuinely unable to pay their hospital bills.

## Supplemental health financing schemes and affirmative action

Supplementary schemes are available to alleviate the financial burden of healthcare costs on the elderly. A means-tested public assistance scheme (PAS) provides financial assistance to the destitute, frail or disabled elderly. Although all Singaporeans above the age of 60 are already entitled to a 75 per cent subsidy of the fees charged at government polyclinics (these are one-stop health centres, 18 in all, that provide subsidized outpatient medical care as well as follow-up care for patients discharged from hospitals; they offer a wide range of services including immunization, health screening, health education, laboratory and pharmacy), recipients under PAS are entitled to free medical services. Help from various charitable organizations is also available, and a primary care partnership scheme subsidizes treatment of chronic diseases by private general practitioners and dentists who take part in the government-spearheaded chronic disease management programme (more on this later).

ElderShield, another supplementary, severe-disability insurance scheme to provide insurance coverage to those who require long term care was set up in 2002. Singapore citizens and permanent residents with Medisave accounts are automatically covered under ElderShield at the age of 40, unless they opt out. With premiums payable from Medisave accounts, it provides a fixed payout calculated as sufficient to cover a substantial portion of the patients' out-of-pocket share of subsidized nursing home care or home care, up to a maximum of S$400 per month for six years. The scheme was enhanced in 2007 with the introduction of innovative, supplementary plans from private insurers offering features such as higher monthly payouts, longer periods of coverage and greater options. In 2008 ElderShield covered some 850,000 people out of the 1.2 million (age 40 years and above) who were eligible.

The State also has an ElderCare Fund, to which the government contributes significant amounts annually from its budgetary surpluses. Set up in 2000 and targeted to reach S$2.5 billion in 2010, the fund is intended to cover anticipated increases in subsidies to voluntary welfare organizations that offer care to the elderly. In 2007 Medifund Silver was carved out from Medifund to provide even more targeted support for Singaporean patients aged 65 or over who are unable to pay their bills in public sector hospitals and other Medifund-approved institutions providing intermediate and long term care.

As part of affirmative action, the government periodically pays money (from budget surpluses) into some or all of these savings schemes that belong to low-income families or the elderly. In 2001, for example, the government paid for basic Medishield premiums for two years for all Singaporeans aged 61 to 69, at a total cost of S$110 million. It also set aside S$19 million to help the elderly pay for their ElderShield premiums.

By 2004, S$2.75 billion had been paid into both the Medisave and Medishield top-up schemes for the elderly. In 2008, the government paid up to S$450 per person into the Medisave accounts of all those aged 51 and above – a one-time exercise that cost the government S$220 million. The government also paid S$400 million into the Eldercare Fund in 2008 (bringing its size to S$1.5 billion) and added S$200 million to the Medifund (bringing its size to S$1.6 billion). And in 2009, despite (or perhaps because of) the financial crisis and economic recession, the government topped up Medifund with S$100 million.

A further redistributional element is embedded in the graded system of public hospital wards; these are stratified according to the level of comfort and amenities, thus allowing preferential targeting of subsidies at the lower classes of wards. Patients who opt for C-class (eight-bed) enjoy a wards subsidy of up to 80 per cent, whereas patients who choose A-class (single bed) are not subsidized at all. The MOH estimates that more than 96 per cent of B-class (four-bed) patients and almost 98 per cent of C-class patients should be able to fully pay their bills from their Medisave account.

In January 2009, after discovering that many who could afford the better classes of wards had opted for the heavily subsidized C- and B2-class wards, sometimes crowding out lower-income patients, the government introduced means testing to determine eligibility. It promised that the additional revenue derived from the reduced subsidy for the higher-income groups would go towards subsidizing the lower-income groups; that patients who could not afford the lower classes of wards despite the subsidies would get additional financial assistance through Medifund; and that persons aggrieved by means testing would have their cases reassessed on a case-by-case basis. Because the government has kept to its promise to be flexible at the margins and err on the side of generosity (for example, by being sensitive to the circumstances of retirees and others who are not employed), implementation has not been contentious thus far.

## Reforms in health care provision

There are a total of 11,545 hospital beds in 29 hospitals and specialty centres in Singapore, giving a ratio of 2.6 beds per 1,000 total population. Seven public hospitals (providing multi-disciplinary, acute, inpatient services, specialist out-patient services and 24-hour emergency services) and six national specialty centres (for cancer, heart, eye, skin, neuroscience and dental care respectively) – ranging in size from 185 to 2,064 beds – account for 72 per cent of the beds, while 16 private hospitals (between 20 and 505 beds) account for the rest. In addition, an estimated 12 per cent of daily outpatients are seen by traditional Chinese medicine practitioners in the private sector.

Starting in 1985, and over a 15-year period, the public-sector hospitals and specialist medical institutions systematically underwent a restructuring process, which resulted in them gaining greater autonomy in operational and fiduciary matters. The restructured hospitals and institutions were incorporated, one by one, as independent entities within the meaning of Singapore's Companies Act, each with its independent Board of Directors. Government ownership was, however, retained through a fully government-owned holding company. Matters such as recruitment and remuneration of staff are decentralized, while more sen-sitive issues such as medical fee increases would require the government's approving nod (Lim 2004).

A further move was made in 2000 to reorganize and consolidate the restruc-tured institutions into two "clusters" – Singapore Healthcare Services and National Healthcare Group – each with its own tertiary hospital, supported by specialist medical centres and regional hospitals. Simultaneously, all government polyclinics providing outpatient primary health care came under the manage-ment of one or other of the two clusters. Thus, in one fell swoop, horizontal and vertical integration of all the public sector health care providers – primary, sec-ondary and tertiary – was achieved. The idea behind "clustering" was to generate healthy competition between the two clusters, while allowing each cluster to capitalize on internal synergies and economies of scale. But the situation is not static, the latest evolution being all public sector health care facilities now fall under five broad clusters; Alexandra Health Pte Ltd, Jurong Health Services, National Healthcare Group (NHG), National University Health System and Sin-gapore Health Services (SingHealth) – the last two being Academic Health Clus-ters providing quaternary care while the first three are regional health care clusters, each anchored by a regional hospital working with a variety of primary, intermediate and long term care sector and support services. An Agency for Integrated Care has also been set up by the Ministry of Health to smooth the transition of patients from one care setting to another.

The private sector compares favourably to the public sector in quality of expertise and facilities and is perceived to be better in terms of responsiveness. Prices are not regulated, and in such a free market, willing-buyer–willing-seller, competitive environment, leading physicians and surgeons typically earn consid-erably more than their public sector counterparts. This differential pay gradient has resulted in a steady flow of talent from the public sector about which the government has been quite concerned. But the response has not been to control prices in the private sector, but rather to make careers in the public sector more rewarding and satisfying. More recently, in line with its policy of positioning Singapore as a leading medical hub, the government has signalled that it would like to see the private share of hospital beds in Singapore increase to 30 per cent. It has offered a slew of incentives including the sale of land sites adjacent to existing public sector hospitals.

## Step-down and long term care

Residential long term care facilities that cater to those requiring skilled nursing or rehabilitation services following discharge from acute care hospitals fall into three categories: *community hospitals* which cater to patients who are fit for discharge from acute hospitals but require inpatient convalescent and rehabilitative care; *chronic sick hospitals* which provide skilled nursing and medical care on a long term basis to older persons with advanced, complicated medical conditions; and *nursing homes for the elderly* which provide long term skilled nursing care for older persons who do not have families or caregivers to look after them at home. All these facilities are presently managed either privately or by voluntary welfare organizations and provide important "step-down" health care services to the elderly.

There are now more than 9,200 nursing home beds; about 75 per cent of which are in homes run by voluntary welfare organizations and the rest in privately run homes. Although the government has, as a matter of principle, been discouraging families from sending their elderly to nursing homes except as a last resort, the MOH has recently announced that it intends to increase the number of beds to 14,000 over the next decade, with voluntary organizations and the private sector leading the way.

Under a long-standing incentive policy, the government subsidizes 90 per cent of the capital costs and 50 per cent of the recurring operating costs of facilities run by voluntary organizations. It also provides subsidies (75, 50 or 25 per cent depending on means testing) to needy persons at these facilities. In addition, since 2003 the MOH has extended subsidies to accredited private nursing homes for patients who qualify through means testing. Finally, Medisave can be used for home-based and community-based services that help the elderly to remain in their own homes for as long as possible.

Recognizing that long term care for the elderly will remain fragmented if left to the private and voluntary sectors, the MOH recently grouped them around three of its restructured acute care hospitals according to geographical zones: west, central and east. The geriatric department of the respective hospital would provide professional leadership for the development of step-down care in each zone and to the community hospitals and nursing homes in the form of structured training and quality assurance programmes and shared resources including laboratory services. Selected nursing homes now also serve as "nodal points" that provide a full range of community-based services for the aged.

## Palliative care and end-of-life issues

Despite its attention to other areas of health care, the government has long left palliative care in the hands of charitable and voluntary welfare organizations. A total of 55 per cent of Singaporeans who are terminally ill now die in hospitals, whereas 28 per cent die in their homes. In 2007, hospices cared for 1,200 patients, and an additional 3,200 patients were cared for through five, home-based hospice services. In all, about S\$5 million in state subsidies went to 4,400 patients, an amount the MOH has conceded is small, given the 17,000 deaths here every year. The Singapore Hospice Council estimates that about 70 per cent of people with terminal illnesses are dying without palliative care.

Acknowledging this situation to be unsatisfactory, the MOH has recently announced a range of initiatives to raise the quality of life of the dying, ease their pain and preserve their dignity and support their care (Lim 2008). Plans are afoot to train more doctors (in 2008, there were only 15 doctors working in palliative care in the whole country) and nurses in palliative medicine, creating a national pool of palliative health care professionals and palliative care may even be recognized as a medical subspecialty. The MOH has also announced plans to add 25 hospice places to the 125 currently available at the four existing hospices run by voluntary groups.

The government has also recognized that nursing homes are presently ill-equipped to care for the dying. They frequently send their patients back to the hospital the moment their condition deteriorates. A pilot project studying how to integrate better acute care, long term care and palliative care is underway in six nursing homes, supported by a nearby acute care public hospital with staff trained in palliative care.

A set of guidelines on advance care planning is also being developed for health care professionals so that they can help patients and their families make informed decisions about their treatment plans. A public education effort has also been mounted to get people thinking about end-of-life care long before such choices are imminent.

## Laws on family care and advanced medical directives

Perhaps the most controversial policy implemented so far is the imposition of a legal obligation on children to maintain their parents. With the passage of the Maintenance of Parents Act (1996), Singapore became the world's first country to require adult children to care for their ageing parents.

A less controversial measure is the Advanced Medical Directives (AMD) Act of 1996, aimed at reducing unnecessary suffering of both the terminally ill elderly and their families. The directive states that people medically certified as brain-dead can be relieved of medical life support if they had so willed it when alive and in full possession of their mental faculties. However, fewer than 10,000 people have signed an AMD since the Act came into effect in 1997.

## Chronic disease management programme

One of the more promising, nationwide programmes launched to date is the Chronic Disease Management Programme of 2006. The aim is to shift the focus away from sub-optimal, episodic and reactive care centred on the treatment of symptoms towards a goal of life-long, holistic care that emphasizes prevention and health maintenance. It is a concerted effort to change the way medicine is practised, no less; the programme being predicated on the growing expert consensus that a holistic approach to chronic diseases can achieve better health outcomes than episodic care: for example, by having diabetes patients work closely with their doctors and nurses to maintain good control of their blood sugar, serious and costly complications (such as blindness, kidney failure or foot amputation) can be avoided.

The programme relies on four basic policy approaches: emphasizing primary prevention; creating a supportive environment for the enhancement of health; actively setting goals and assessing results; and promoting effective, well-coordinated activities by the various implementing bodies and stakeholders. It supports the promulgation of disease treatment protocols and provision of training for general practitioners (GPs) and nurse educators in the community to support GPs in educating patients. Trained "wellness coordinators" help the elderly actively manage their conditions and the Medisave scheme now covers payment for outpatient treatment for these conditions.

The programme began in 2006 with four chronic diseases: diabetes mellitus, hypertension, hyperlipidaemia and stroke, for which there are established disease-management protocols. Hospitals would routinely discharge these patients to the care of GPs enrolled in the programme. The GPs would track the patients' progress and take part in hospital-run, continuing medical education programmes to keep them updated on the latest developments in chronic-disease management. The MOH provides the clinical protocols and mounts educational campaigns with the message that GPs are just as good as and less expensive than hospital-based specialists. This message includes assuring the public that the GPs enrolled in the programme are actively upgrading their professional skills. But it will ultimately be up to the GPs to show that the patients with chronic illnesses who require monitoring get better and more responsive services if seen by a regular family physician instead of a hospital-based specialist.

To provide the right financial incentives for shifting the care of such stable, chronic conditions to primary care doctors, the Medisave purse strings were loosened in 2007 to allow patients with the four chronic conditions to use up to S$300 a year from Medisave to copay for their treatment. Following one year of implementation, some 70,500 patients had withdrawn a total of S$15 million to pay for their outpatient treatment. Not only did patients welcome the financial relief of being able to use Medisave money to cover the costs of the consultations, but they also reported travelling shorter distances to see their GPs (than to see hospital specialists) and having an improved relationship with their doctors. Encouraged by this initial success, the government in 2008 added two more conditions – asthma and chronic obstructive pulmonary disease – to the programme. In 2009, schizophrenia and major depression were added to the list.

## Discussion

The relative ease with which health policies are introduced and implemented in Singapore – even when it comes to interventions aimed at lifestyle or behaviour change as in the case of smoking, drug addiction and HIV/AIDS – is attributable to the fact that the paternalistic but democratically elected government has been in power continuously since 1959. It enjoys the huge advantage of being able to pursue, without undue interruption, pragmatic policies, with the longer term "good" in mind.

However, it is not as if unpopular policies are being "rammed down the throats" of hapless Singaporeans. Rather, it is the special government–people relationship developed in the early "sink or swim" years of the fledgling nation's existence that have accustomed the people to placing the common good above self-interest. They had placed their trust in a sagacious government which earned more and more trust as it delivered on more and more of its promises including the "good life". It was therefore not difficult to convince the people that they lived in an imperfect world where free health care in the face of potentially insatiable demand was illusory and potentially ruinous. Neither was it beyond them to grasp that the opposite extreme of fee-for-service, open-ended, insurance-based health care, which only the rich can afford, would be too inequitable.

That there has not been a tradition of state largesse in Singapore is important to understanding why Singaporeans readily accept the hard-nosed health policies of the government. They understand that whether the burden falls on taxes, Medisave, employer benefits or insurance, it is ultimately Singaporeans themselves who must pay – since taxes are paid by taxpayers, insurance premiums are ultimately paid by the people and employee medical benefits form part of wage costs – and that overburdening the state or employers would affect the competitiveness of Singapore's externally oriented economy and, ultimately, their own livelihoods.

Governance in Singapore can be described as "government by expertise". Health care policies are formulated and implemented in a largely top-down process. Often, the MOH forms subcommittees comprising experts to study policy issues, and it does take their inputs seriously. Typically, these committees involve the participation of academics, community groups and the private sector as well.

Thus, a comprehensive review of health care policies ten years after the 1983 National Health Plan produced an important document, the White Paper on Affordable Health Care (Ministry of Health 1993). It laid out Singapore's philosophical approach to health care as follows:

a    nurture a healthy nation by promoting good health;
b    promote personal responsibility and avoid over-reliance on state welfare or medical insurance;

c    provide good and affordable basic medical services to all Singaporeans;
d    rely on competition and market forces to improve service and raise efficiency;
e    intervene directly in the health care sector, when necessary, where the market fails to keep health care costs down.

It was the product of rounds of consultations and deliberations involving various subcommittees. It was coordinated overall by a high-level Ministerial Committee comprising several cabinet-level Ministers and, interestingly, the impetus came from the very top, the Prime Minister himself. In recent years, the government has increasingly adopted the practice of publishing "consultation papers" on its website to obtain feedback before any major health policy change.

The role of the media also deserves mention. Singapore has a high literacy rate of 93 per cent among residents aged 15 years and older. The media in Singapore is openly pro-government. This combination partly explains why the government's marketing of hard-nosed policies has been so effective. Although newspaper editorials criticize government health policies from time to time, they invariably do so in a constructive manner. MOH officials skilled in public relations patiently and politely answer letters of complaint from the public in the newspapers. The media faithfully reports policy speeches, giving politicians and senior health officials ample opportunity to tailor their messages to mass audiences. As well, all the main stream media have regular health columns and even pullouts (one is called "Health Matters") which play an effective role in knowledge dissemination. Newspaper cartoonists even oblige by simplifying the messages into entertaining comic strip form.

## Future challenges

Singapore's greatest, future challenge is its coming "silver-haired tsunami" – the fact that the number of Singaporeans over 65 years will triple between now and 2030, rising from 300,000 to 900,000. The government has, at the time of writing, just announced a range of new measures costing S$500 million over the next five years. New community hospitals will be built to boost capacity to treat chronic diseases such as stroke, heart and kidney failure and other age-related conditions such as dementia, while also enhancing capacity for long term care including rehabilitation, home care and palliative services after patients have been discharged from hospitals. To cope with the surging demand, more than 2,000 nursing home beds will be added over the next five years. Work on five new nursing homes will start within two years including a 300-bed home for patients with psychiatric problems to be ready by 2012. The MOH will also release from its land bank two plots designated for the building of private nursing homes. It will also help two existing homes run by voluntary welfare organizations to relocate to new and larger facilities. Subsidies to intermediate and long term care facilities (including community hospitals, nursing homes and hospices) will be increased to meet growing patient needs. Also announced are a second heart centre and a second cancer centre, two new general hospitals and a third medical university.

Numerous challenges remain, not least of which is the limited evaluation done of the success or otherwise of various control and prevention programmes; for example, the effectiveness of the chronic disease management programmes. There is a need for more consistent health risk behaviour data, especially pertaining to youth. There is also a need to engage stakeholders more meaningfully and mobilize the broader community in order to achieve any measurable impact, for example on obesity rates, over the long term. Additional challenges include high out-pocket costs for medical services and still limited insurance coverage.

Strategies to enhance prevention and control should include empirical investigation of the role of rapid social, economic and cultural change on health risk behaviour including substance use, poor diet, sedentary behaviour, mental health, and health practices and outcomes. Evaluation of policies and programmes should include economic efficiency and cost effectiveness of alternative strategies. There is a need for rigorous studies on several key issues such as patient self-management, comprehensive primary care and provider payment incentives.

Finally, there is considerable scope to strengthen links between research and action, and to bridge the gap between researchers and stakeholders. There should be forums for researchers and policy makers to discuss and prioritize research needs, or for leaders of industry, commerce and civil society to interact with public health policy and research groups on establishing research needs. Research collaborations should focus on providing measurable health improvements for specific populations and should draw on international expertise and experience. Even though government must be part of the solution, it cannot succeed alone.

## Notes

1 The Ministry of Health website contains this assurance: "Our hospitals and healthcare system will never withhold help to a Singaporean because of financial limitations. Yet our philosophy promotes individual responsibility towards healthy living and medical expenses". Online, available at: www.moh.gov.sg/mohcorp/hcsystem.aspx?id=102 (accessed 24 May 2011).
2 The first Singapore laws concerning smoking were passed in the early 1970s and have been periodically revised to incorporate proven international best practices. There are two major legislative instruments: the Prohibition on Smoking in Certain Places Act (1971) and the Control of Advertisement and Sale of Tobacco Act (1991).

## References

Central Intelligence Agency (2010) *The World Fact Book 2010*, Washington, DC: Central Intelligence Agency Office of Public Affairs. Online, available at: www.cia.gov/library/publications/the-world-factbook/geos/sn.html (accessed 24 May 2011).

Lim, M.K. (1998) "Health Care Systems in Transition II Singapore, Part I. An Overview of the Health Care System in Singapore", *Journal of Public Health*, 20(1): 16–22.

Lim, M.K. (2004) "Shifting the Burden of Health Care Finance: A Case Study of Public–Private Partnership in Singapore", *Health Policy*, 69(1): 83–92.

Lim, M.K. (2005) "Transforming Singapore Health Care: Public–Private Partnership", *Annals of the Academy of Medicine of Singapore*, 34(7): 461–467.

Lim, M.K. (2008) "Expanded State Role in the Care of the Dying", *Health Policy Monitor*. Online, available at: www.hpm.org/en/Surveys/University_of_Singapore_-_Singapore/12/Expanded_state_role_in_the_care_of_the_dying.html (accessed 24 May 2011).

Ministry of Community Development (1999) *Burden of Disease Study*, Singapore: Ministry of Health.

Ministry of Education (2011) "Governance Principles". Online, available at: www1.moe.edu.sg/ne/AboutNE/GovPrin.html (accessed 24 May 2011).

Ministry of Health (1993) *Affordable Health Care: A White Paper*, Singapore: SNP U/Publishers.

Ministry of Health (2007) National Health Surveillance Survey. Online available at: www.moh.gov.sg/content/moh_web/home/Publications/Reports/2009/national_health_surveillance_survey_2007.html (accessed 24 May 2011).

Ministry of Health (2010a) "Health Facts Singapore". Online, available at: www.moh.gov.sg/mohcorp/statistics.aspx?id=5524 (accessed 24 May 2011).

Ministry of Health (2010b) "Health System". Online, available at: www.moh.gov.sg/mohcorp/hcsystem.aspx?id=102 (accessed 24 May 2011).

OECD Health Data (2009) Cited in: Pearson, M. "Disparities in Health Expenditure Across OECD Countries: Why Does the United States Spend so Much More Than Other Countries?" Online, available at: www.oecd.org/dataoecd/5/34/43800977.pdf (accessed 24 May 2011).

Quah, E., Tan, K.C., Saw, S.L.C. and Yong, J.S. (2002) "The Social Cost of Smoking in Singapore", *Singapore Medical Journal*, 43(7): 340–344.

Regnier, P. (1987) *Singapore: City-State in South-East Asia*, Honolulu: University of Hawaii Press.

Turnbull, C.M. (1981) *A History of Singapore, 1819–1975*, Singapore: Oxford University Press.

World Health Organization (2000) *The World Health Report 2000 – Health Systems: Improving Performance*, Geneva: WHO.

World Health Organization (2008) *Closing the Gap in a Generation: Health Equity through Action on the Social Determinants of Health Final Report of the Commission on Social Determinants of Health*, Geneva: WHO.

World Health Organization (2010) "World Health Statistics". Online, available at: www.who.int/whosis/2010/en/index.html (accessed 24 May 2011).

World Health Report (2000) *Health Systems: Improving Performance*, Geneva: WHO.

Yong, N.L. (1967) Speech by the Minister of Health at the opening of the WHO Seminar on Health Planning in Urban Development, Singapore, 21 November.

# 11 Learning from the past

## Changing policies concerning the double disease burden in Malaysia

*Wah-Yun Low, Chirk-Jenn Ng, Chiu-Wan Ng, Wan-Yuen Choo and Wen-Ting Tong*

## Introduction

With globalisation, modernisation and urbanisation, the world faces threats from old and emerging infectious diseases and chronic non-communicable diseases (NCDs). Malaysia has not been spared a double disease burden. NCDs contributed to 65 per cent of disability adjusted life years (DALYs) in men and 74 per cent in women while ischaemic heart disease topped the league tables for burden of disease for men and women (see Table 11.1). Risk factors for NCDs (for example, smoking, alcohol, high blood pressure and cholesterol, and overweight and obesity) were also leading causes of the disease burden. On the other hand, infectious diseases were responsible for 9.3 per cent of total DALYs (10.1 per cent in men; 8.1 per cent in women) (see Table 11.1), 85 per cent of which is from mortality. Almost half the burden of infectious diseases is contributed by septicaemia followed by tuberculosis (TB) (13.3 per cent), other infections (13.1 per cent) and HIV/AIDS (11.6 per cent) (Ahmad *et al.* 2004: 48; 60).

Similarly, NCDs headed the causes of death in Malaysia including ischaemic heart disease (20.1 per cent), cerebrovascular disease (10.2 per cent) and chronic obstructive pulmonary disease (3.6 per cent) (with traffic accidents at 6.0 per cent), while communicable/infectious diseases (CDs) such as septicaemia (7.5 per cent) and lower respiratory infections (5.1 per cent) ranked third and fifth respectively.

## Changing socioeconomic and health status in Malaysia

The Federation of Malaya was formed in 1957 when the 11 states of the Malay Peninsula achieved independence from Britain. Malaya became Malaysia in 1963 with the inclusion of Singapore, Sabah and Sarawak. In 1965, Singapore became an independent sovereign nation.

Currently, Malaysia comprises 27.6 million people of various ethnic, cultural and religious backgrounds (Department of Statistics Malaysia 2010: iii). The Malaysian economy has traditionally been based on agriculture (rubber, palm oil and timber) and mining (tin and petroleum) but has now diversified to include

*Table 11.1* The ten leading causes of death and burden of disease by sex in Malaysia, 2000

| Rank | Leading causes of death | | | Leading causes of burden of disease | | |
|---|---|---|---|---|---|---|
| | Disease category | Death | % | Disease category | DALYs | % |
| *Male* | | | | | | |
| 1 | Ischaemic heart disease | 12,142 | 19.2 | Ischaemic heart disease | 164,846 | 10.0 |
| 2 | Cerebrovascular disease | 5,735 | 8.9 | Road traffic accident | 133,789 | 8.2 |
| 3 | Road traffic accident | 5,435 | 8.4 | Cerebrovascular disease | 94,059 | 5.7 |
| 4 | Septicaemia | 4,409 | 6.8 | Septicaemia | 70,232 | 4.3 |
| 5 | Lower respiratory infections | 3,149 | 4.9 | Acute lower respiratory tract infections | 49,649 | 3.0 |
| 6 | Chronic obstructive pulmonary disease | 2,928 | 4.5 | Diabetes mellitus | 47,060 | 2.9 |
| 7 | Cirrhosis | 2,160 | 3.3 | Chronic obstructive pulmonary disease | 45,459 | 2.8 |
| 8 | Nephritis and nephrosis | 1,653 | 2.6 | Hearing loss | 44,566 | 2.7 |
| 9 | Trachea, bronchus and lung cancer | 1,552 | 2.4 | Unipolar major depression | 42,259 | 2.6 |
| 10 | Self-inflicted injury | 1,098 | 1.7 | Cirrhosis | 37,902 | 2.3 |
| | *Total* (111 diseases) | 64,552 | 100 | *Total* (111 diseases) | 1,646,896 | 100 |
| *Female* | | | | | | |
| 1 | Ischaemic heart disease | 9,746 | 21.2 | Ischaemic heart disease | 113,887 | 9.2 |
| 2 | Cerebrovascular disease | 5,555 | 12.1 | Cerebrovascular disease | 86,372 | 7.0 |
| 3 | Septicaemia | 3,926 | 8.5 | Unipolar major depression | 67,211 | 5.4 |
| 4 | Lower respiratory infections | 2,511 | 5.5 | Septicaemia | 57,483 | 4.6 |
| 5 | Nephritis and nephrosis | 1,446 | 3.2 | Diabetes mellitus | 56,390 | 4.6 |
| 6 | Diabetes mellitus | 1,404 | 3.1 | Hearing loss | 38,994 | 3.1 |
| 7 | Road traffic accident | 1,178 | 2.6 | Acute lower respiratory tract infections | 37,890 | 3.1 |
| 8 | Breast cancer | 1,109 | 2.4 | Asthma | 32,815 | 2.6 |
| 9 | Cirrhosis | 1,036 | 2.3 | Road traffic accident | 28,946 | 2.3 |
| 10 | Chronic obstructive pulmonary disease | 1,022 | 2.2 | Osteoarthritis | 26,925 | 2.2 |
| | *Total* (111 diseases) | 45,889 | 100 | *Total* (111 diseases) | 1,240,997 | 100 |

Source: Ahmad *et al.* 2004: 42, 60.

manufacturing (electronic equipment, semi-conductor chips and vehicles), construction and services. The Asian economic crisis in 1997 caused a major setback to economic growth but the country has since recovered. In 2009, the per capita gross domestic product (GDP) was US$7,030, making Malaysia an upper middle-income country according to the World Bank's classification (World Bank 2011).

Economic development has benefitted the majority of Malaysians. National wealth has been invested in social infrastructure, such as schools and health facilities. Primary school fees were abolished in 1962, near universal primary school enrolment was achieved by 1990 and primary education was made compulsory in 2003 (United Nations Country Team Malaysia 2005: 66–86). The health care system with its extensive network of hospitals and clinics provides highly subsidised health services; in 1996, an estimated 50 per cent of the population resided within 10 km of a public hospital and within 3 km of a public health clinic (Institute for Public Health 1997: 73). By 2009, many of the country's social indicators had reached levels approaching those in developed countries: notably, the literacy rate of youths aged 15 to 24 years was 98.6 per cent with no appreciable differences between sexes (World Bank 2011), life expectancy at birth was 77 years and 72 years for females and males, respectively, and the infant mortality rate was 5.7 per 1,000 live births. The maternal mortality rate was 29 per 100,000 live births in 2007.

All these successes have been hard won. At the time of independence poverty was rife. Most people lived in rural areas and lacked access to basic services such as schools, clinics, good sanitation and clean water supplies. Health indicators at that time reflected the impact of such harsh living conditions. In 1957, life expectancy at birth in Malaya was 58 years and 56 years, respectively, for females and males whilst infant mortality rate was 75.5 per 1,000 live births and maternal mortality ratio was 320 per 100,000 live births (Abu Bakar and Jegathesan n.d.: 53).

The nation's social and economic development planning, directed by the Prime Minister's Office, was laid out in a series of five-year development plans, the first of which covered the period 1956 to 1960 (First Malayan Plan). From the beginning, economic planning emphasised improving the living standards of people in the rural areas including expanding rural health services. After the formation of Malaysia, rural health services continued to be a focus under the First Malaysia Plan (1966–1970) but efforts were intensified in the 1960s to control the spread of CDs, the major cause of mortality and morbidity. During this time, national control programmes were established for diseases such as malaria, TB, leprosy, yaws and filariasis (Abu Bakar and Jegathesan n.d.: 118–122). These were successful in containing CDs except perhaps TB. However, over time environmental changes have facilitated the entry of new CDs. For example, increasing urbanisation is said to have contributed to the spread of dengue fever (DF) and dengue hemorrhagic fever (DHF) (Abu Bakar and Shaffee 2002: 23–27). A fatal outbreak of Nipah virus encephalitis in 1998 was associated with fast-expanding pig farms encroaching on the habitat of fruit bats, the natural

*Table 11.2* Historical perspectives on key diseases and policies

| Time | | Communicable disease | | | |
|---|---|---|---|---|---|
| Year | 5-year national development plan | HIV/ AIDS[a] | TB[b] | Malaria | DF and DHF |
| 1956–1960 | 1st MALAYAN PLAN | | | Before 1960 – >200,000 cases | |
| 1961–1965 | 2nd MALAYAN PLAN | | | 1961 –243,870 cases[c] | |
| 1966–1970 | 1st MALAYSIA PLAN | | | 1970 –151,822 cases[c] | |
| 1971–1975 | 2nd MALAYSIA PLAN | | | 1975 –87,432 cases[c] | 1973 incidence rate[k] DF: 5.40/100,000 DHF: 10.1/100,000 |
| 1976–1980 | 3rd MALAYSIA PLAN | | | 1980 –44,226 cases[c] | |
| 1981–1985 | 4th MALAYSIA PLAN | | 1985 –68/100,000 | 1985 –49,528 cases[c] | 1987 – incidence rate[k] DF: 10.40/100,000 DHF: 1.9/100,000 |
| 1986–1990 | 5th MALAYSIA PLAN | 1986–1990 HIV infection: 992 AIDS cases: 23 | | 1986–48,007 cases | 1989 – incidence rate[e] 14.96/100,000 |
| 1991–1995 | 6th MALAYSIA PLAN | 1991–1995 HIV infection: 14,404 AIDS cases: 542 | 1994 – 59.8/100,000 | 1991– 43,545 cases[c] | 1995 – incidence rate[e] 32.79/100,000 |
| 1996–2000 | 7th MALAYSIA PLAN | 1996–2000 HIV infection: 22,994 AIDS cases: 4,158 | 1996 – 58/100,000 | 1996 – 51,921 cases[e] | 2000 – incidence rate[d] 31.6/100,000 |
| 2001–2005 | 8th MALAYSIA PLAN | 2001–2005 HIV infection: 32,219 AIDS cases: 5940 | 1999 – 65.6/100,000 2000 – 65.9/100,000 | 2001–12,780 cases[d] | 2004 – incidence rate[d] 132.5/100,000 |
| 2006–2010 | 9th MALAYSIA PLAN | 2006–2010 HIV infection: 20,803 AIDS cases: 5,689 | 2002 – 59/100,000 | 2006 – 5,294 cases[d] | 2008 – incidence rate[d] 178/100,000 |
| 2011–2015 | 10th MALAYSIA PLAN | | | | |

Sources: (a) Ministry of Health Malaysia and Malaysian AIDS Council 2011. (b) United Nations Country Team Malaysia 2005: 1–229. (c) Tee 2000: 6–9. (d) Ministry of Health Malaysia 2008a: 68. (e) Ministry of Health Malaysia 1995: 91. (f) Ministry of Health Malaysia 1986: volume 5 and 7. (g)

| a-communicable disease | | | | Policies |
|---|---|---|---|---|
| | Hyper-tension | Lung cancer | Cervical cancer | |
| | | | | 1961 – National TB Control Programme (vertical programme) |
| | | | | 1968 – Malaria Eradication Programme |
| | | | | 1969 – Pap Smear Screening Programme introduced |
| | | | | 1975 – Destruction of Disease Bearing Insects Act (DDBIA) |
| | | | | 1986 – Vector Borne Disease Control Programme |
| 86 – NHMS 1[f] (>35 yrs) DM: 6.3% IGT: 4.8% | 1986 – NHMS 1[f] (Definition >160/95) >25 yrs Prevalence: 14.4% | | | 1988 – The Prevention and Control of Disease Act (Act 342) |
| | | | | 1990s – Impregnated bednets for Malaria |
| | | | | 199 – Increased Tobacco taxation until 2003 |
| | | | | 1986 – The First National Health and Morbidity Survey carried out to determine the mortality and morbidity of burden of diseases in Malaysia |
| | | | | 1991 – Healthy Lifestyle Programme: to create awareness on danger of lifestyle diseases, educate on preventive measures and promote healthy lifestyle |
| | | | | 1991 – Healthy Lifestyle Campaign: Prevention and Control of Cardiovascular Disease |
| | | | | 1991 – Cardiovascular Disease Prevention and Control Programme |
| | | | | 1995 – Prevention and control of cancer |
| | | | | 1995 – National TB Control Programme integrated programme) |
| | | | | 1995 – National Healthy Lifestyle Campaign: Prevention and Control of Cancer with the slogan 'Stay Ahead in Cancer' |
| | | | | 1995 – Harm Reduction Programmes for IDUs |
| 96 – NHMS 2[g] (>30 yrs) DM: 8.3% IGT: 4.3% | 1996 – NHMS 2[g] (Definition >140/90) >18 yrs Prevalence: 29.9% >30 yrs Prevalence: 32.9% | | | 1996 – PROSTAR programme |
| | | | | 1996 – National Diabetes Prevention and Control Programme |
| | | | | 1996 – Healthy Lifestyle Campaign: Diabetes |
| | | | | 1996 – National Plan of Action for Nutrition (NPANM I) (1996–2000) |
| | | | | 1996 – Comprehensive National Diabetes Prevention and Control Programme |
| | | | | 1996 – The second National Health and Morbidity Survey (NHMS2) |
| | | | | 1997 – 'Less Sugar, Please' campaign |
| | | | | 1999 – DOTS (directly observed treatment, short course) treatment started |
| | | 2003–2005 Age-standardised incidence rate (ASR)[i] Male: 18.1/100,000 Female: 6.2/100,000 | 2003–2005 Age-standardised incidence rate (ASR)[j] 16.1/100,000 | 2001 – Communication for Behavioural Impact (COMBI) for Dengue Control |
| | | | | 2003 – National Anti-Malarial Drug Response Surveillance Programme |
| | | | | 2003 – Transfer of Training Technology Course in Malaria Control |
| | | | | 2003 – Involvement in WHO Framework on Tobacco Control |
| | | | | 2004 – Control of Tobacco Product Regulation |
| | | | | 2004 – Burden of Disease Study 2004 |
| | | | | 2006 – The 3rd National Health and Morbidity Survey |
| | | | | 2004 – Enactment of the Control of Tobacco Products Regulations in 2004 |
| | | | | 2004 – Anti-tobacco media approach, the 'Tak Nak'(Say No) programme |
| | | | | 2004 – Tobacco Control Act 2004 |
| | | | | 2005 – National Plan of Action for Nutrition of Malaysia (NPANM II) (2006–2015) |
| | | | | 2005 – First Malaysian NCD Risk Factor Survey 2005/2006 |
| 2006 NHMS 3[h] (>30 yrs) DM: 14.9% IFG: 4.7% (18 yrs) DM: 11.6% IFG: 4.2% | 2006 NHMS 3[h] (Definition >140/90) >18 yrs Prevalence: 32.2% >30 yrs Prevalence: 42.6% | 2006 Age-standardised incidence rate (ASR)[i] Male: 19.6/100,000 Female: 7.6/100,000 | 2006 Age-standardised incidence rate (ASR)[j] 12.2/100,000 | 2006 – Malaria Elimination Programme |
| | | | | 2007 – 294 Quit Smoking Clinics set up throughout the country. |
| | | | | 2007 – increase of 25% cigarette excise duty from 12 cents to 15 cents per stick |
| | | | | 2008 – Diabetes and Cardiovascular Diseases Prevention and Control Programme |
| | | | | 2009 – NCD clinic implemented in Putrajaya in April |
| | | | | 2010 – HPV Immunisation in Public School |
| | | | | 2010 – National Strategic Plan for Non-Communicable Diseases (NSP-NCD) |
| | | | | 2011 – Health Awareness Year |

Ministry of Health Malaysia 1996: volume 9. (h) Ministry of Health Malaysia 2008b: xi–xiii. (i) Lim *et al.* 2008: 106; 131. (j) Zainal Ariffin *et al.*, 2006: 70, 80. (k) Chandra Shekhar and Ong 1992/1993a: 126–133. (l) Chandra Shekhar and Ong 1992/1993b: 15–25.

reservoirs of the virus (Chua 2003: 265–275). Thus, despite continued government efforts over the past few decades to control CDs, they remain a cause of suffering for many.

Although economic development has raised living standards, it has brought with it more sedentary but stress-filled lifestyles, smoking and high fat and salt consumption. These significant lifestyle changes coupled with population ageing have led to an upsurge of NCDs such as diabetes mellitus (DM), hypertension and cancers. The 1990s saw the term, 'Healthy Lifestyle', entering the lexicon of health planners and annual national campaigns were initiated in 1991; these focused each year on one particular lifestyle-related disease (for example, prevention of DM in 1996) or a specific lifestyle issue (for example, promotion of mental health in 2000) (Abu Bakar and Jegathesan n.d.: 211). The impact of such campaigns has not been fully evaluated but clearly non-communicable, lifestyle diseases have overtaken CDs as leading causes of mortality and morbidity (Ahmad *et al.* 2004: 1–173). Hence, the latest Malaysia Plan (2011–2015) specifically mentions the Government's intention to continue healthy lifestyle promotion; a testimony to its main policy response to the growing epidemic of NCDs in the country (Economic Planning Unit Malaysia 2010: 2–359).

Malaysia has made great economic and social progress since independence and is on the threshold of achieving developed nation status. However, on the health front the country has not quite emerged from the epidemiologic transition. Both CDs and NCDs still plague the populace although it can be said that the scales are beginning to tip in favour of NCDs. Over the years the Government has devoted substantial national resources to improving health status including programmes targeting specific CDs or NCDs, which have yielded a mixed bag of successes and failures. Its response to various disease threats can best be appreciated by examining public health policies over time vis-à-vis changes in disease patterns (see Table 11.2). The following sections will describe the trends of four CDs – HIV/AIDS, TB, DF and DHF, and malaria – and four groups of NCDs – cardiovascular diseases (CVD), DM and lung and cervical cancers – as well as provide details of policies relevant to the observed trends.

## Communicable diseases

This section will describe the changing epidemiology over the past decades of the four CDs mentioned above. It will also show how the local health authority has responded to their prevention, control and eradication.

### *HIV/AIDS*

HIV/AIDS is a serious concern in Malaysia. Since the first reported case in 1986, the country has witnessed an exponential increase in the number of infected persons. By December 2009, the cumulative number totalled 87,710 with 13,394 AIDS-related deaths (Ministry of Health Malaysia 2010a: 9). The HIV/AIDS epidemic has been described as a concentrated one where the disease is located predominantly within specific high risk populations but is not common in the general population. In 2009, the national HIV prevalence among adults aged 15 to 49 years was only 0.5 per cent (Ministry of Health Malaysia 2010a: 19). However, among injecting drug users (IDUs), female sex workers and transsexual sex workers rates were much higher; at 22.1 per cent, 10.5 per cent and 9.2 per cent, respectively (Malaysian Aids Council 2009: 9). Information concerning the other high risk group, men who have sex with men (MSMs) is limited at the current time.

From 1986, new HIV infections reported annually have increased steadily to a peak of about 7,000 cases in 2002; thereafter they decreased gradually to about 3,000 cases in 2009 (Ministry of Health Malaysia 2010a: 19). The majority of these new cases have been males infected through the use of contaminated drug injection paraphernalia. In 2000, females made up only 10 per cent of all new cases but by 2009, they had doubled to about 20 per cent. Unlike males, the main mode of infection for females was through heterosexual intercourse (Ministry of Health Malaysia 2010a: 20). In short, the initial spread of the disease in Malaysia was among male IDUs. Now, increasingly, females are being infected through sexual routes.

The National Strategic Plan (NSP) to prevent and control HIV/AIDS was developed by the Ministry of Health (MOH) in 1998 (Ministry of Health Malaysia 1998: 1–26). Although the government acknowledged that the bulk of HIV/AIDS was among IDUs, the 1998 NSP lacked concrete measures to control spread within this high risk group (Reid *et al.* 2005: 3–44). Instead, the primary control strategies hinged upon promoting awareness of the healthy lifestyle and behaviour changes needed to avoid infection. An example is the PROSTAR programme initiated by the MOH and targeting youths aged 13 to 25 years. It uses peer education to disseminate messages concerning healthy living and prevention of HIV infection. By mid-2000s, the government came to realise that the epidemic had not abated, especially among IDUs, and this prompted a review of the existing control policies (Ministry of Health Malaysia 2006: 2–20). Failure to halt the spread constituted the only barrier to Malaysia achieving all the Millennium Development Goals (MDGs) set by the United Nations in 2000. Indeed, by 2005, Malaysia had successfully met all the other goals (United Nations Country Team Malaysia 2005: 1–229).

A comprehensive review of the 1998 NSP led to a new strategic plan for 2006 to 2010. This time the government took a more comprehensive approach by focusing on preventing infection, especially among IDUs, as well as treatment, care and support of patients (Ministry of Health Malaysia 2006: 2–20). The new plan was also designed to harness the resources of relevant public agencies and also those of private and non-government organisations (NGOs).

At the core of the 2006–2010 NSP were strategies aimed at IDUs, specifically through the implementation of harm reduction programmes (Ministry of Health Malaysia 2006: 2–20). Malaysia is said to have one of the highest prevalences of injecting drug use in the world (Mathers *et al.* 2008: 1733–1745). In 2002, about 1.33 per cent of adults aged 15 to 64 years were estimated to be injecting drugs.

Thus, government-funded HIV/AIDS prevention programmes for IDUs were sorely needed. Methadone maintenance therapy (MMT) was introduced in 2005 and by 2009 this programme had been made available in 162 government and private facilities across the country including prisons and public hospitals, serving over 10,000 persons (Ministry of Health Malaysia 2010a: 46–47) In 2006, the needle and syringe exchange programme (NSEP) was started, mainly in collaboration with NGOs. By 2009, the NSEP programme had a registered clientele of over 18,000 persons who were provided not only with clean injecting equipment but also with condoms. Currently, MMT and NSEP sites are mainly located in urban areas but there are plans to expand these services to rural areas.

Government policies have also facilitated increased access to effective HIV/AIDS treatment. Anti-retroviral (ARV) drug prices were lowered after the government allowed for the importation of cheaper generic drugs from India in 2004 and for local companies to manufacture generic drugs in the country (Ministry of Health Malaysia 2010a: 56). Currently, many of the first and second line ARV drugs are provided free to HIV/AIDS patients in public hospitals and clinics with the service recently extended to people living with HIV/AIDS in prisons and drug rehabilitation centres (Ministry of Health Malaysia 2010a: 61). Yet, by 2009, only about 10,000 persons living with HIV/AIDS had been started on ARV drugs, a significant number but far short of the estimated 27,000 persons who require them.

The HIV/AIDS programmes since 2005 herald a change in the perception law enforcement agencies and religious bodies have of persons living with HIV/AIDS in conservative Malaysian society; a society where drug use and commercial sex work are perceived as criminal activities. This change in mindset will be essential if the battle against HIV is to be won. Although a good start has been made towards the problem within the IDU community, there remains a lot more to be done for other high risk communities. The feminisation of the Malaysian HIV/AIDS epidemic has begun and it will be crucial that in future all stakeholders in the country contribute decisively to effective public policies.

## TB

TB is an ancient disease associated with poverty and squalor. From the latter half of the twentieth century, socioeconomic improvements generally and better health care delivery specifically, have resulted in a significant reduction in TB incidence especially between the 1970s and 1990s. Notified cases of TB have dropped from 68 per 100,000 population in 1985 to about 58 per 100,000 in 1996 (United Nations Country Team Malaysia 2005: 175).

In 1961, the MOH established the National TB Control Programme which was implemented as a vertical programme with its initial focus on expanding coverage of BCG vaccination among newborns (Sirajoon and Yadav 2008: 124). Other objectives of the programme included early case detection and screening. A directly observed treatment (DOTS) or short course treatment strategy was started in 1999 and continues to be provided free at all public health facilities. In

1999, the national programme was reorganised from a vertical to an integrated programme within other public health delivery programmes (Sirajoon and Yadav 2008: 124).

By the end of 2000, progress in combating TB appeared to have stagnated; indeed, there was an upward trend in the incidence from 58 per 100,000 population in 1996 to 65 per 100,000 in 1999 before it decreased slightly to 59 per 100,000 in 2002 (United Nations Country Team Malaysia 2005: 175).

In addition to the shift from a vertical to an integrated programme, the rise in TB incidence parallelled the increasing numbers of HIV/AIDS cases. The number of patients with twin infections increased steeply from only six in 10,873 TB cases notified in 1990 to 933 cases or 6.5 per cent of the cases reported in 2002 (Aziah 2004: 1). Recognition of the vulnerability of HIV patients to developing active TB led to compulsory screening of all known TB patients for HIV infection. This policy coupled with the availability of health care has helped ensure that the mortality attributable to TB among persons with HIV did not show a comparable increase as the number of HIV and TB co-infections increased (United Nations Country Team Malaysia 2005: 177–178). Another reason for the TB resurgence was the influx of migrant workers. The state of Sabah has one of the highest populations of immigrants, mainly from Indonesia and the Philippines, as well as one of the highest burdens of TB in the country. From 1990 to 2000, immigrants accounted for more than 24 per cent of TB cases detected in the state annually (Dony *et al.* 2004: 8). The government has since instituted compulsory screening for all migrant workers and those found infected with TB will be repatriated to their respective countries after anti-TB treatment has been initiated (Aziah 2004: 1).

Controlling the spread of TB in Malaysia remains a challenge. Despite the early successes, currently TB contributes most to the burden of CDs in terms of mortality and morbidity.

## *Malaria*

Malaysia enjoyed great success in virtually eradicating malaria from densely populated areas, although it remains rampant in some parts of forested areas in Sabah, Sarawak and interior parts of Peninsular Malaysia (Economic Planning Unit Malaysia 2011: 92–93). This success resulted from a series of control measures undertaken during the 1960s (Ministry of Health Malaysia 2000: 87).

Malaria was first documented when ten British civil servants on the island of Penang died from fever during the period 1805–1825. In subsequent years, malaria became the most common cause of death among migrants in Penang. In 1901, with the arrival of a British doctor, Sir Malcolm Watson, the first environmental vector control method in malaria control was introduced in Penang, Klang and Kuala Lumpur. In 1911, the Malaria Advisory Board was formed; this laid the foundation for the implementation of environmental management measures (species sanitation) to curb the spread of malaria in the plantations, estates and urban areas (Ministry of Health Malaysia 2002: 99–100).

From 1960–1964, in line with the WHO Global Malaria Eradication Programme, the Malaysian government carried out a Malaria Eradication Pilot Project. Following its success, the Malaria Eradication Programme in Peninsular Malaysia was launched in 1968 (Rahman 1982: 985). Since then and up to 1980, there was a significant reduction in the number of cases reported; from 243,870 in 1961 to 44,226 in 1980 (Tee 2000: 6). The cases decreased to 7,010 cases (25 per 100,000 population) in 2009. The latest figure shows that most cases are concentrated in Sabah (57.2 per cent) and Sarawak (26.0 per cent), while the remaining cases occur in the interior parts of Peninsular Malaysia, particularly in Pahang and Kelantan (Economic Planning Unit Malaysia 2011: 93). Specific populations have been identified as being at high-risk, notably the *orang asli* (indigenous) population, land scheme workers and army personnel. The influx of migrant workers from malaria-endemic countries, particularly to the palm oil plantations and land schemes, increases transmission (Tee 2000: 7; World Health Organization 2010: 58). The predominant species in Peninsular and Sabah is *P. falciparum* while *P. vivax* is found mainly in Sarawak (Ministry of Health Malaysia 2008a: 70).

In 1986, the malaria control programme was incorporated into the Vector Borne Diseases Control Programme. This new programme aimed to target also other vector borne diseases such as dengue, filariasis, typhus, Japanese encephalitis, yellow fever and plague into the programme. Malaria control activities include focal spraying in localities with outbreaks, active case detection and use of impregnated bed nets to replace DDT residual spraying. The public health care system was reorganised from a three-tier to a two-tier system in the 1970s, thus, making available a widespread network of rural health clinics and better equipped community clinics to a larger population. This enabled early detection and treatment, distribution of prophylaxis, and dissemination of information through educational activities to be implemented throughout the country. However, the control and treatment of malaria was complicated by the emergence of resistance to widely used drugs such as chloroquine. In response the government launched the National Anti-Malarial Drug Response Surveillance Programme in 2003 to monitor drug resistance. During the same period, an international training centre for Transfer of Training Technology Course in Malaria Control was established.

The eradication programme implemented in the states of Sabah and Sarawak in 1961 was initially remarkably successful. However, there was a great upsurge of cases in Sabah from 1975 to 1978. Evidence of resistance of *P. falciparum* to chloroquine emerged as early as 1971 in Sabah and soon after in the northern parts of Peninsular Malaysia and Sarawak (Rahman 1982: 989). In addition, the slowing down of anti-malaria control measures, influx of migrants and inaccessibility of the interior of Sabah, among other factors, proved barriers to eradication. A five-year action plan was implemented in Sabah under the Seventh Malaysia Plan (1996–2000).

Although an increasing number of areas have been declared malaria free, the country has to stay vigilant to sustain these achievements. One of the major challenges is to prevent the reintroduction of malaria in malaria-prone areas. As the incidence of malaria declines in the country, the loss of general immunity within the population is expected to increase. This group will be exposed to risk as domestic travel becomes more common. This is further complicated by drug resistant strains of malaria and declining diagnostic and management skills among clinicians particularly in urban areas. Thus, maintaining pressure on the host–vector–environment transmission dynamics, active surveillance, early warning systems and close monitoring of imported cases are important measures to prevent the reestablishment of the disease. Recognising this, the government continues to support the Malaria Elimination Programme to achieve the MDG-Plus target of complete elimination in Peninsular Malaysia by 2015 and in Sabah and Sarawak by 2020 (Economic Planning Unit Malaysia 2011: 94).

### DF and DHF

Dengue virus infection (DF) is endemic and a major health problem in Malaysia (Poovaneswari 1993: 3–7; Holmes *et al.* 2009: 1–5). The first reported DF in Malaysia was in 1902 and DHF (dengue haemorrhagic fever) in 1962. Ever since, cycles of epidemics have affected the entire country (Poovaneswari 1993: 3). In the last two decades there has been an increasing number of reported dengue cases and from a rate of 14.96 per 100,000 population in 1989 incidence rose to 32.79 per 100,000 in 1995 (Ministry of Health Malaysia 1995: 91), worsening to 132.5 per 100,000 in 2004 (Ministry of Health Malaysia 2008a: 66). This became 178 per 100,000 in 2008 (Ministry of Health Malaysia 2008a: 66). Although DF was more prevalent in children in the early 1970s, there was a major shift towards adults by the 1980s.

In 1973, a significant outbreak of DHF occurred and this prompted the government to implement a series of control measures. Case detection, case treatments, space spraying of insecticides and regular vector surveillance of *Aedes* mosquitoes are common measures to control dengue transmission. The disease became notifiable in 1974. The Destruction of Disease Bearing Insects Act was introduced in 1975 to provide the authority to implement various control measures, and, in 2001, heavier penalties for offenders were imposed (Ang and Singh 2001: 13). Health promotion activities were also intensified. The Dengue Free Schools programme was initiated to educate school children and to recruit them as agents of community participation. The Communication for Behavioural Impact programme was implemented in 2001 for prevention and control of dengue through community participation (Mohd Raili *et al.* 2004: 39) and a nationwide 'Promotion of a Healthy Environment' campaign was launched in 2002 (Abu Bakar and Jegathesan n.d.: 211).

Despite these efforts, DF and DHF are still prevalent. There are many reasons for the dramatic increase in the number of DF/DHF cases in recent years: high rates of population growth, disorganised urbanisation and proliferation of slums, crowding, poor sanitation and waste disposal systems, global warming and rise in global travel, have created epidemiological conditions that favour viral transmission by the mosquito vector, *Aedes aegypti*. But a change in public health policy was probably the major contributing factor. Health reforms in the late 1990s that integrated the vertical organisation structure of the Vector Borne Disease Control Programme into general health services resulted in a major loss of expertise and funding targeted for vector control. The responsibility for vector borne control in major cities and towns was shifted to local governments in 2000. This created a major vacuum in prevention and control arising from lack of expertise, resources and political will within local governments (Kumarasamy 2006: 1).

With the latest figures showing an 11 per cent rise, from 2009 to 2010, in total dengue-related infections, and a 52 per cent increase in dengue-related deaths over the past 20 years, (Director General of Health Malaysia 2010: 1–8), the government has introduced a drastic measure to combat DF and DHF: a field experiment, the first of its kind in Southeast Asia, involving the release of about 6,000 male, genetically modified mosquitoes into an area of uninhabited forest near the town of Bentong in the state of Pahang on 21 December 2010. The *Aedes aegypti* mosquito carries an artificial fragment of DNA designed to curb the insect's fertility by passing on a gene that kills the mosquito at the larval stage of its lifecycle. The project has inevitably sparked criticism from environmentalists and experts who fear that such a measure may cause an imbalance of the ecosystem by creating uncontrollable mutated mosquitoes which in turn may lead to the growth of another insect species and so new diseases (Conner 2011; *Telegraph*, 26 January 2011).

Dengue infections still remain one of the most serious infectious diseases in Malaysia. Many challenges have been identified that need to be overcome. Continued strong leadership, committed action, access to resources, collaborative efforts between institutions, community participation and mobilisation are necessary agents to combat DF and DHF.

## Non-communicable diseases

In Malaysia, the burden of NCDs has grown in the past two decades. This rising trend is particularly noticeable in CVD and its associated risk factors, such as DM (diabetes), hypertension and obesity. However, efforts to prevent and control NCDs did not intensify until recently. This section will focus on the changing epidemiology and policies in four lifestyle-related diseases – CVD, DM, lung and cervical cancer.

### *CVD*

In 1986, the First National Health and Morbidity Survey (NHMS 1) revealed a relatively low prevalence of DM (6.3 per cent) and hypertension (14.4 per cent; Blood Pressure ≥160/95 mmHg) compared to the rest of the world (Ministry of Health Malaysia 1986: vols 5 and 7). However, the prevalence of these conditions has more than doubled in the past 20 years – to 14.9 per cent (DM) and

32.3 per cent (hypertension; BP ≥140/90) based on the Third National Health and Morbidity Survey (Ministry of Health Malaysia 2008b: xiii). The latter survey also shows increases in the prevalence of overweight adults from 16.6 per cent in 1996 to 29.1 per cent in 2006 and obese adults from 4.4 to 14.0 per cent (Ministry of Health Malaysia 2008b: xvii).

CVD topped the league table as a cause of DALYs in Malaysia (Ahmad *et al.* 2004: 1–173). It was responsible for almost one-fifth of the total burden of disease in 2000 and nearly 90 per cent of this burden was due to mortality. Ischaemic heart disease and cerebrovascular disease were the major contributors accounting for 50 and 32 per cent of the cardiovascular burden, respectively.

This epidemic has been attributed to the changing demography and economic and social development over the last few decades. The MOH first recognised the significance of the CVD burden after NHMS 1 in 1986. A Cardiovascular Disease Prevention and Control programme was created in 1991 to reduce risk factors such as hypertension, DM, smoking, hypercholesterolaemia, obesity and physical inactivity (Ministry of Health Malaysia 1995: 110). At the same time, the Healthy Lifestyle Programme was launched to create awareness of lifestyle diseases and promote healthy living (Economic Planning Unit Malaysia 1996: 534).

### *Diabetes*

The policy change in tackling type 2 diabetes is a good example of how the MOH responded to the rising CVD burden. In 2000, DM was responsible for 3.7 per cent of the total burden of disease and ranked sixth in the list of DALYs in the Malaysian Burden of Disease Study. Almost 70 per cent of the burden of DM was contributed by the non-fatal Years Lived with Disability (YLD) component for which DM was ranked second as the leading cause (Ahmad *et al.* 2004: 1–173).

Prior to 1996, policy concerning DM was focused on hospital-based, clinical management and screening for ante-natal mothers. The National Diabetes Prevention and Control Programme was set up in 1996 to promote health and quality of life by preventing and controlling DM, its risk factors and complications (Ministry of Health Malaysia 1995: 114–116). A healthy lifestyle campaign was launched and screening for DM was made available in health clinics and hospitals across the country. In 2000, the National Diabetes Programme was formalised in terms of clinical care provision, establishment of dedicated DM service and teams, and a diabetes resource centre.

Despite these efforts, the prevalences of CVD and DM continue to rise at an alarming rate. A situational analysis of current NCDs prevention and control programmes and activities found that most of these are confined to the health sector and appear disjointed when it comes to intersectoral collaboration (Ministry of Health Malaysia 2010b: 8). There is also a lack of policy on creating a health-promoting, built environment in Malaysia.

Recognising the impact of over-nutrition on the rising prevalence of CVDs and diabetes, the National Nutrition Policy was developed in 2005 to promote healthy eating and active living (Ministry of Health Malaysia 2005: 2–16). In 2010, the National Strategic Plan for Non-Communicable Disease (NSP-NCD) was introduced to tackle the rising trend of CVDs and its risk factors more effectively and efficiently (Ministry of Health Malaysia 2010b: 4–40). The strategic approach is based on the Western Pacific Regional Action Plan for NCDs (World Health Organization 2009: 1–54) and focuses on seven strategies: prevention and promotion; clinical management; increasing patient compliance; action with NGOs, professional bodies and other stakeholders; monitoring, research and surveillance; capacity building; and policy and regulatory interventions.

The key challenge of CVD and risk factor, prevention and control in Malaysia is finding ways to implement and sustain these strategies. This requires leadership, intersectoral partnership and an effective surveillance and evaluation system.

## *Cancer*

Cancer, ranked sixth in the overall burden of disease, is responsible for 6.6 per cent of total DALYs. Almost 96 per cent of the burden of cancer was contributed by the fatal component of burden of disease; in fact, cancer is a major cause of death. Lung, oral and colorectal cancers account for over half of the total burden attributable to cancer in males. In females, it is dominated by breast, colorectal and cervical cancers which together account for 45 per cent of the total burden attributable to cancer (Ahmad *et al.* 2004: 77).

In 2002, there were 26,089 cancer cases diagnosed in Peninsular Malaysia and registered in the National Cancer Registry (males 11,815 and females 14,274). The number decreased to 21,773 in 2006 (males 9,974 and females 11,799). The first report of the National Cancer Registry in 2002 found that the age-standardised incidence rate (ASR) for all cancers was 173.5 per 100,000 (males 168.8 and females 181.9) (Lim *et al.* 2003: 55). In 2006, the ASR declined to 131.1 (males 128.6 and females 135.7) (Zainal Ariffin *et al.* 2006: 8).

In 2002, the top ten most common cancers were lung, nasopharynx, colon, leukaemias, rectum and prostate in men; and in women, breast, cervix colon, ovary, leukaemias and lung cancer (Lim *et al.* 2003: 57). In 2006, the most common cancers were breast, colorectal, lung, cervix, nasopharynx, thyroid gland, liver, stomach, prostate gland and lymphomas (Zainal Ariffin *et al.* 2006: 12); on a gender basis, they were colorectal, lung, nasopharynx, prostate gland, liver, bladder, stomach, lymphoma, leukaemias and brain in males; and breast, colorectal, cervix uteri, ovary, thyroid gland, lung, uterus, stomach, brain and lymphoma in females.

The importance of cancer control was recognised in the National Cancer Control Programme, launched in 1995, to reduce incidence and mortality, and to improve the quality of life of cancer patients through programmes for prevention, early diagnosis, pain relief, palliative care for the terminally ill and legislative initiatives such as control of tobacco use. Emphasis is placed on the optimum utilisation of available resources, appropriate use of technology and active community participation.

In the following sections, lung and cervical cancers will be used to demonstrate how the government has reacted to the rising trend of cancers including strategies to discourage smoking; and, for cervical cancer, screening and, most recently, an immunisation programme.

*Lung cancer*

The 2006 National Cancer Registry shows lung cancer is the second most common cancer among males and third most common overall in Peninsular Malaysia (Zainal Ariffin *et al.* 2006: 12). The ASR was 13.3 per 100,000 population (Zainal Ariffin *et al.* 2006: 9) and mortality rates in 1985, 1990 and 1997 were 2.26, 2.72 and 2.47 per 100,000 population, respectively (Abu Bakar and Jegathesan n.d.: xxxvii).

Tobacco use is the main cause of lung cancer (World Health Organization 2008: 14) which, in Malaysia, accounts for 19 per cent of males and 11.5 per cent of females (World Health Organization 2003: 252–253). National surveys show that cigarette smoking among adults has declined from 24.8 per cent (49.2 per cent in males and 3.5 per cent in females) to 21.5 per cent (46.2 per cent in males and 1.6 per cent in females) (Ministry of Health Malaysia 1996: 16–17; Ministry of Health Malaysia 2008b: x). The MOH initiated an anti-smoking campaign under the National Cancer Control Programme and this included legislating no-smoking areas in government buildings, hospitals and other public places and banning all forms of tobacco advertising. A number of tobacco control activities have been implemented in the past two decades under the Control of Tobacco Products Regulations, 2004, the Tobacco Control Act, 2004 and compliance with the WHO Framework Convention on Tobacco Control in 2003. Other programmes include a more aggressive, anti-tobacco media approach to educate the public about the harm of tobacco such as the *Tak Nak* (Say No) programme in 2004. To November 2007, 294 Quit Smoking clinics had been set up throughout the country. There has also been a steady increase in tobacco taxation; from 1990 to 2003, the import tax increased from RM85/kg to RM216/kg; excise tax, from RM13 to RM48/kg; and sales tax, from 15 to 25 per cent. In 2007, cigarette excise duty was sharply increased by 25 per cent from 12 to 15 cents per stick. Tobacco taxation has proved to be an effective method of reducing cigarette consumption and tobacco-related deaths while increasing revenue for the government (Ross and Al-Sadat 2007: 1,163).

*Cervical cancer*

In 2006, cervical cancer was the third most common cancer among women in Malaysia (Zainal Ariffin *et al.* 2006: 12). A total of 1,074 cases was registered with the National Cancer Registry with an ASR of 12.2 per 100,000 population in

Peninsular Malaysia and with mortality rates for cancers of the cervix and uterus of 0.33, 0.52 and 0.40 per 100,000 population in 1986, 1990 and 1997, respectively (Abu Bakar and Jegathesan n.d.: xxxviii). The cervical cancer incidence rate increased after age 30 and peaked at 60–69 years (Zainal Ariffin *et al.* 2006: 9). Pap smear coverage in the country was less than 2 per cent in 1992, 3.5 per cent in 1995 and 6.2 per cent in 1996 (Nor Hayati 2004). The prevalence rate of Pap smear examination was 43.7 per cent (Ministry of Health Malaysia 2008b: 394) compared to 26 per cent in the National Health and Morbidity Survey 1996. The Government's Pap smear programme was introduced in 1969 for all family planning clients. This programme was again emphasised in the Healthy Lifestyle Campaign in 1995 and now other agencies such as the National Population and Family Development Board, private clinics and hospitals, and university and army hospitals provided Pap smear services for all women aged 20–65 years. In 1995, the National Healthy Lifestyle Campaign – Prevention and Control of Cancer was launched with the slogan 'Stay Ahead in Cancer'. The campaign aimed to educate the public and especially high-risk groups about primary prevention, early detection and healthy lifestyles (Ibrahim 1994: 13)

After Australia developed and administered the Human Papilloma Virus (HPV) vaccine to women aged 12–26 years old, the Malaysian Drug Authority approved the use of the quadrivalent HPV vaccine in October 2006 and the bivalent HPV in 2008. In mid-2010, the bivalent HPV vaccine was given to all 13-year-old girls in government schools. Currently, private organisations, NGOs and the media contribute to creating public awareness of the link between HPV and cervical cancer.

## Conclusion

Demographic and epidemiologic changes have paralleled the country's socio-economic development. In addition, the effects of globalisation, population inter- and intra-migration and sedentary lifestyles due to urbanisation and modernisation have led to an increase in the prevalence of NCDs. While obesity has increased, particularly in urban areas, malnutrition remains a major public health issue in the more remote and rural areas, particularly in East Malaysia. In addition, new and reemerging infectious diseases still pose a major threat and these are partly due to environmental changes arising from climate change and population mobility.

The resurgence of TB and persistent cyclical dengue epidemics are partly attributable to the change in programme administration from a vertical to an integrated approach. Integrated programmes have diluted the focus on specific diseases; and the present generic model has resulted in reduced resources to tackle a particular infectious disease and, hence, less effective prevention and surveillance.

Overall, Malaysian health policies tend to be reactive rather than proactive, with delays in the health authority's response to the changing disease pattern and burden. The HIV epidemic and the exponential increase in cardiovascular diseases were recognised but not dealt with in a timely manner. In addition, most health care programmes and campaigns have not been formally evaluated. Thus, their cost effectiveness and impact remain uncertain.

Lately, the MOH has begun to reassess the development and implementation of health care policies in Malaysia as evidenced by the medium-term National Strategic Plan for NCDs. There is increasing emphasis on multidisciplinary, intersectoral and international collaboration to tackle the rising double disease burden and to build the capacity of the stakeholders (including the community, health professionals and partners, from both the public and private sectors) in terms of research and training.

Both CDs and NCDs will remain a challenge as Malaysia develops from a middle- to high-income country. Lessons must be learned from the past and national CDs and NCDs strategies should be based on accurate demographic and epidemiological data and include participation by key stakeholders. In sum, health policies should be proactive and targeted; and evaluated and revised according to the evolving disease burden.

## References

Abu Bakar, S. and Jegathesan, M. (eds) (n.d.) *Health in Malaysia: Achievements and Challenges*, Kuala Lumpur: Ministry of Health Malaysia.

Abubakar, S. and Shaffee, N. (2002) 'Outlook of Dengue in Malaysia: a Century Later', *Malaysian Journal of Pathology*, 24: 23–27.

Ahmad, F.Y., Amal, N.M., Gaurpreet, K., Mohd, A.O., Vos, T., Rao, V.P.C. and Begg, S. (2004) *Malaysian Burden of Disease and Injury Study*, Kuala Lumpur: Institute for Public Health, Ministry of Health, Malaysia.

Ang, K.T. and Singh, S. (2001) 'Epidemiology and New Initiatives in the Prevention and Control of Dengue in Malaysia', *Dengue Bulletin*, 25: 7–14.

Aziah, A.M. (2004) 'Tuberculosis in Malaysia: Combating the Old Nemesis', *Medical Journal of Malaysia*, 59: 1–3.

Chandra Shekhar, K. and Ong, L.H. (1992/1993a) 'Epidemiology of Dengue/Dengue Hemorrhagic Fever in Malaysia: A Retrospecive Epidemiological Study 1973–1987. Part 1: Dengue Fever', *Asia-Pacific Journal of Public Health*, 6: 126–133.

Chandra Shekhar, K. and Ong, L.H. (1992/1993b) 'Epidemiology of Dengue/Dengue Hemorrhagic Fever in Malaysia: A Retrospecive Epidemiological Study 1973–1987. Part 1: Dengue Hemorrhagic Fever (DHF)', *Asia-Pacific Journal of Public Health*, 6: 15–25.

Chua, K.B. (2003) 'Nipah Virus Outbreak in Malaysia', *Journal of Clinical Virology*, 26: 265–275.

Conner, S. (2011) 'GM Mosquitoes Deployed to Control Asia's Dengue Fever'. Online, available at: www.independent.co.uk/news/science/gm-mosquitoes-deployed-to-control-asias-dengue-fever-2195552.html (accessed 26 April 2011).

Department of Statistics Malaysia (2010) *Population and Housing Census of Malaysia: Preliminary Count Report*, Putrajaya: Department of Statistics, Malaysia.

Director General of Health Malaysia. Week 45/2010 (2010) Re: Press Release, 'Dengue Fever and Chikungunya Situation in Malaysia'.

Dony, J.F., Ahmad, J. and Khen Tiong, Y. (2004) 'Epidemiology of Tuberculosis and Leprosy, Sabah, Malaysia', *Tuberculosis*, 84: 8–18.

Economic Planning Unit Malaysia (1996) *Seventh Malaysia Plan 1996–2010*, Putrajaya: Economic Planning Unit, Prime Minister's Department, Government of Malaysia.

Economic Planning Unit Malaysia (2010) *Tenth Malaysia Plan 2011–2015*, Putrajaya: Economic Planning Unit, Prime Minister's Department, Government of Malaysia.

Economic Planning Unit Malaysia (2011) *Malaysia: The Millenium Development Goals at 2010*, Kuala Lumpur: United Nations Country Team, Malaysia.

Gerard Lim, C.C., Rampal, S. and Halimah, Y. (2008) *Cancer Incidence in Peninsular Malaysia 2003–2005: The 3rd Report of the National Cancer Registry*, Kuala Lumpur: National Cancer Registry, Malaysia.

Holmes, T.P., Perera, D., Muhi, J. and Cardosa, J. (2009) 'Importation and Co-circulation of Multiple Serotypes of Dengue Virus in Sarawak, Malaysia', *Virus Research*, 143: 1–5.

Ibrahim, F.H. (1994) 'Seventh Malaysian Plan for National Cancer Control Program', in Ministry of Health Malaysia (ed.) *Studies of the 6th Malaysian Plan and Preparation of the 7th Malaysian Plan*, Kuala Lumpur: Ministry of Health Malaysia.

Institute for Public Health (1997) *National Health and Morbidity Survey 1996*, Vol. 3, *Recent Illness/Injury, Health Seeking Behaviour and Out-of-pocket Health Care Expenditure*, Kuala Lumpur: Ministry of Health, Malaysia.

Kumarasamy, V. (2006) 'Dengue Fever in Malaysia: Time for Review?' *Medical Journal of Malaysia*, 61: 1–3.

Lim, G.C.C., Halimah, A. and Lim, T.O. (2003) *First Report on the National Cancer Registry Cancer Incidence in Malaysia*, Kuala Lumpur: National Cancer Registry Malaysia.

Lim, G.C.C., Rampal, S. and Halimah, Y. (2008) *Cancer Incidence in Peninsular Malaysia, 2003–2005*, Kuala Lumpur: National Cancer Registry Malaysia.

Malaysian AIDS Council (2009) *Integrated Bio-Behavioral Surveillance: 2009 Report*, Kuala Lumpur: Malaysian Aids Council.

Mathers, B.M., Degenhardt, L., Phillips, B., Wiessing, L., Hickman, M., Strathdee, S. A., Wodak, A., Panda, S., Tyndall, M., Toufik, A. and Mattick, R.P. (2008) 'Global Epidemiology of Injecting Drug Use and HIV among People who Inject Drugs: A Systematic Review', *Lancet*, 372: 1733–1745.

Ministry of Health Malaysia (1986) *The First National Health and Morbidity Survey 1986*, Kuala Lumpur: Institute For Public Health Malaysia.

Ministry of Health Malaysia (1995) *Annual Report 1995*, Kuala Lumpur; Ministry of Health Malaysia.

Ministry of Health Malaysia (1996) *The Second National Health and Morbidity Survey 1996*, Kuala Lumpur: Institute for Public Health Malaysia.

Ministry of Health Malaysia (1998) *National Strategic Plan: Prevention and Control of HIV Infection*, Malaysia. Kuala Lumpur: AIDS/STD Section Disease Control Section.

Ministry of Health Malaysia (2000) *Malaysia Ministry of Health Annual Report 2000*, Kuala Lumpur: Ministry of Health Malaysia.

Ministry of Health Malaysia (2002) *Ministry of Health Malaysia Annual Report 2002*, Kuala Lumpur: Ministry of Health Malaysia.

Ministry of Health Malaysia (2005) *National Nutrition Policy of Malaysia*, Putrajaya: Ministry of Health Malaysia.

Ministry of Health Malaysia (2006) *National Strategic Plan on HIV/AIDS 2006–2010*, Putrajaya: Ministry of Health Malaysia.

Ministry of Health Malaysia (2008a) *Annual Report 2008*, Putrajaya: Ministry of Health Malaysia.

Ministry of Health Malaysia (2008b) *The Third National Health and Morbidity Survey 2006*, Kuala Lumpur: Institute For Public Health Malaysia.

Ministry of Health Malaysia (2010a) *2010 UNGASS Country Progess Report: Malaysia*, Malaysia: AIDS/STD Section Disease Control Section.

Ministry of Health Malaysia (2010b) *National Strategic Plan for Non-Communicable Disease (NSPNCD): Medium Term Strategic Plan to Further Strengthen the Cardiovascular Diseases & Diabetes Prevention & Control Program In Malaysia (2010–2014)*, Putrajaya: NCD Disease Control Division, MOH Malaysia.

Ministry of Health Malaysia and Malaysian AIDS Council (MAC) (2011) *Number of New HIV Infections, AIDS Cases and AIDS Deaths by Gender per Year Reported in Malaysia*. Online, available at: www.ptfmalaysia.org/hiv_aids_in_malaysia.php (accessed 26 April 2011).

Mohd Raili, S., Hosein, E., Mokhtar, Z., Ali, N., Palmer, K. and Marzukhi, M.I. (2004) 'Applying Communication-for-Behavioural-Impact (COMBI) in the Prevention and Control of Dengue in Johor Bahru, Johore, Malaysia', *Dengue Bulletin*, 28(suppl.): 39–43.

Nor Hayati, O. (2004) 'The Wrath of Sexual Malpractice: A Philosophical Outlook on Cervical Cancer in Malaysia', *e-IJM*, 3. Online, available at: www.eimjm.com/Vol. 3-No1/Vol. 3-No1-L1.htm (accessed 26 April 2011).

Poovaneswari, S. (1993) 'Dengue Situation in Malaysia', *Malaysian Journal of Pathology*, 15: 3–7.

Rahman, M. (1982) 'Epidemiology of Malaria in Malaysia', *Reviews of Infectious Diseases*, 4: 985–991.

Reid, G., Kamarulzaman, A. and Sran, S.K. (2005) *Rapid Situation Assessment of Malaysia 2004*, Kuala Lumpur: Centre for Harm Reduction, Macfarlane Burnett Institution, University of Malaya Medical Centre.

Ross, H. and Al-Sadat, N.A.M. (2007) 'Demand Analysis of Tobacco Consumption in Malaysia', *Nicotine and Tobacco Research*, 9: 1,163–1,169.

Sirajoon, N.G. and Yadav, H. (2008) *Health Care in Malaysia*, Kuala Lumpur: University Malays Press.

Tee, A.S. (2000) 'Malaria Control in Malaysia', *Malaria Forum: Information Exchange on Malaria Control in South East Asia*, 5: 6–9.

*Telegraph* (2011) 'Malaysia releases 6,000 GM mosquitoes in attempt to combat dengue fever'. Online, available at: www.telegraph.co.uk/news/worldnews/asia/malaysia/8283598/Malaysia-releases-6000-GM-mosquitoes-in-attempt-to-combat-dengue-fever.html (accessed 26 April 2011).

United Nations Country Team Malaysia (2005) *Malaysia: Achieving the Millenium Development Goals: Successes and Challenges*, Kuala Lumpur: United Nations Development Programme.

World Bank (2011) *World Development Indicators*. Online, available at: http://data.worldbank.org/country (accessed 26 April 2011).

World Health Organization (2003) 'WHO Mortality Database', in *Tobacco Control Country Profile* (2nd edn), Geneva: WHO.

World Health Organization (2008) *WHO Report on the Global Tobacco Epidemic, 2008*, Geneva: WHO.

World Health Organization (2009) *Western Pacific Regional Action Plan for Non-Communicable Diseases*, Geneva: WHO Press.

World Health Organization (2010) *World Malaria Report 2010*, Geneva: WHO Press.

Zainal Ariffin, O., Zainuddin, M.A. and Nor Saleha, I.T. (eds) (2006) *Malaysian Cancer Statistics: Data and Figure Peninsular Malaysia 2006*, Putrajaya: National Cancer Registry.

# 12 Dealing with difficult diseases

## Renovating primary health care to deal with chronic conditions in Indonesia

*Peter Heywood and Terence H. Hull*

## Introduction

This chapter is about the changing pattern of disease in Indonesia over the last 60 years, the changes that are likely in the next 40 years and the challenges that these changes have posed, and continue to pose, for the country's health system.

Any excursion into the health system of a nation presumes a foundation of understanding of social, political, cultural and demographic dimensions that make up the context of both illness and its treatment and control. Indonesia is the largest Muslim nation in the world, and the fourth most populous country, after China, India and the USA. In 2010 the population reached 235 million, spread across thousands of islands straddling the equator. The census counts over 1,000 languages and as many ethnic groups, but the largest groups are the Javanese, Sundanese and Madurese on the central islands of Java (where the capital, Jakarta, is located) and Madura. Following the declaration of Independence from Dutch colonial rule in 1945, and four years of often violent struggle, the nation emerged into the decade of the 1950s as an ambitious democracy with a very weak economy, and a long agenda of social problems, the key ones of which were education and health. In this chapter we review how the struggles to establish a health system to serve the needs of all Indonesians have encountered some very persistent challenges.

The second section presents a discussion of the disease pattern and its context in the period immediately after Independence, a description of the development of the current health system and a summary of the current disease burden. The third section presents projections of the likely disease patterns in the future. The fourth section discusses the demand for health care in the future. The fifth and sixth sections, respectively, summarize the challenges facing the government, and explore the need for a reorientation of the health system.

## Pattern of disease in the years after Independence and development of the health system

At Independence the population of Indonesia was overwhelmingly rural (Frederick and Worden 1993) and poor (World Bank 2006: 7). The demographic pattern was typical of most low income countries at the time – high fertility, high mortality, a high proportion of the population under 15 years of age and low life expectancy. The disease pattern, as well as causes of death, was dominated by communicable diseases, the effects of which were increased by low nutritional status, especially of mothers, infants and young children. The 1972 National Household Health Survey showed infectious diseases to be the dominant causes of death, occupying the first, second and third rank; cardiovascular disease came in at number four; when the survey was repeated in 1980 the rankings were similar except that cardiovascular diseases had moved from fourth place to third (Departemen Kesehatan 1980: 49). Infant mortality rates at the time of Independence were such that one-fifth of infants died before their first birthday (see Figure 12.1). Fertility rates were high – on average a woman had more than five births in a lifetime (see Figure 12.1). This demographic and disease pattern occurred in the context of high levels of poverty (World Bank 2006: 7), limited education opportunities and limited and inadequate public transport infrastructure (World Bank 2007: 27, 73).

This was the demographic and disease pattern that prevailed not only in Indonesia, but also in most low income countries, at the time of the 1978 Alma Ata conference and agreement of WHO member states on the primary health care approach with a particular emphasis on maternal and child health (WHO 1978).

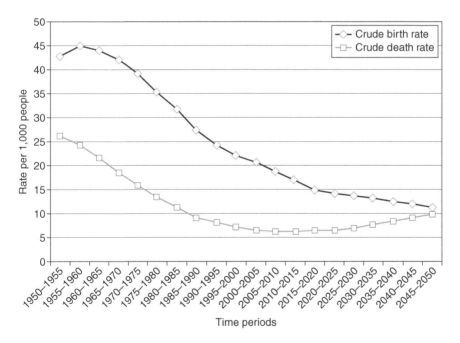

*Figure 12.1* Indonesian demographic transition (source: Population Division of the Department of Economic and Social Affairs of the United Nations Secretariat 2009).

The health system inherited by the Government of Indonesia at Independence was weak, unevenly distributed and much of the population had only limited access to it. At the end of the colonial era the health facilities consisted mainly of public and private hospitals; treatment clinics, most of which were government owned and concentrated on treatment of adults; and maternal and infant health clinics which were mostly government owned (Heywood and Harahap 2009a). The orientation of the system was heavily curative and mostly urban.

This situation – a high burden of disease dominated by infectious diseases and maternal and perinatal conditions and a weak health system – posed an enormous challenge for the new government. The government response was to design and implement a system which sought to bring the facilities and providers closer to the people. Reflecting experience under the Dutch colonial system and a complementary distrust of market forces, the new system had a heavy emphasis on public funding and provision for which the main justification was the need to provide health services for the poor.

The system introduced in the 1950s, based on what was to become known as the Bandung Plan (Leimena 1956: *passim*) and which eventually became the blueprint for the national health system, sought to integrate preventive and curative aspects of health care. The aim was to establish a network of health facilities throughout the country with a health centre at the sub-district level and a hospital at the district level. Initially, new facilities were established by combining those that existed, subsequently new facilities were built. Thus, Indonesia rapidly established a network of health facilities throughout the country – by the mid-1990s there were more than 7,000 health centres, essentially meeting the goal of one for each sub-district, together with over 20,000 health sub-centres. A programme to locate midwives, who were to become key players in the successful efforts to reduce fertility, in villages started in the 1980s.

The health centres were under the direction of a doctor with a standard complement of nurses, midwives, paramedical and administrative staff. To meet this rapid increase in staff needs and ensure their distribution in health centres throughout the country the government, in 1974, introduced obligatory government service for all new graduates in medicine, nursing and midwifery. The staff thus conscripted were made permanent civil servants and assigned to work in various health facilities throughout the country. This approach allowed the government to achieve a much improved distribution of staff and health facilities throughout the country (Heywood and Harahap 2009a).

In addition to these public facilities and providers there is also a limited, but growing, number of private hospitals and other facilities, both of which are usually included in government statistics on the sector. The poorly paid staff of public facilities were permitted private practice after working hours to supplement their income. The private practices of these public servants became, and continue to be, an important source of health care facilities for ambulatory care (Heywood and Harahap 2009b) and, by and large, are not included in government statistics even though these part-time, private solo-providers offer the majority of services available to the public.

The result is that in each district there is a range of facility types (multi-provider and solo-provider), provider types (doctors, nurse[1] and midwives), a range of facility locations (some close, even in the village, others far away at the sub-district headquarters). Some facilities are public, others private, some free, others at which there is a charge. Overall, consumers have a range of provider and facility choices. Many consumers choose the private provider, especially the lower cost nurses and midwives (Heywood and Harahap 2009a).

Significant modifications to the system of compulsory service began in the 1990s as the government realized that it could not afford to continue to employ all new graduates. After a number of additional modifications, compulsory service was finally ended in 2007. A contract system continues for midwives with the aim of placing them in villages. The private sector continues to increase as government hiring is reduced. The flow of new health care providers has increased markedly in recent years as private training institutions have proliferated under a generally lax licensing approach. Most new graduates move straight into private practice without ever serving in a government position, but, as mentioned earlier, this group of providers is largely ignored in government statistics and programmes. The government has only limited information on private providers, even those whose main job is in government clinics. Without an understanding of the numbers and nature of private practices the government has only limited ability to monitor the quality of services they provide.

The effectiveness of the existing health system is further complicated by the radical political, administrative and fiscal decentralization of 2001 under which responsibility for the delivery of services moved to district governments. At the same time, public funding for health services, widely seen as too low during the Suharto era, more than doubled (in real terms) between 2001 and 2006. It was widely expected that these increased funds, together with decentralization and the hope of greater freedom to change budget allocations at the district level, would lead to improvement in the delivery of services as the changed accountability relationships resulted in services more attuned to local needs. Experience at the district level has not fulfilled these expectations as the central government moves to re-centralize many of the functions (Heywood and Harahap 2009c).

Today this is basically a lightly regulated private system for which there is a substantial public subsidy (Heywood and Choi 2010). Assessment of the overall performance of this system is mixed. The delivery of public health functions by the public sector is inadequate. Immunization rates remain low and have shown little if any improvement in the period between 2002–2003 and 2007 (Heywood and Choi 2010; Statistics Indonesia 2008: 180); performance of the tuberculosis control programme is variable and overall performance suboptimal (Ministry of Health 2005: xix). Utilization of ambulatory care services is also low, self-treatment remains the most common response to illness for many and half the patients in the lowest quintile of the income distribution consult private practitioners (Tim Surkesnas 2002: 35; World Bank 2008b: 19). There is great variation between districts in the efficiency with which resources are used (Indonesia NIHRD 2005: 79), and World Bank assessments across districts indicate no relationship between public expenditure on health and immunization coverage or presence of a skilled health provider at birth delivery (World Bank 2008b: 122). The overall quality of care (as measured by knowledge of clinical guidelines) is low (Barber *et al.* 2007: w352).

So, this system is under strain, struggling to maintain its current direction, let alone set a new path in response to more recent pressures. Not only is the overall performance below par, but maintaining the distribution of health facilities and staff achieved during the 1980s will become increasingly difficult now that compulsory service has ended. These factors alone indicate that new service models are needed.

Nevertheless, despite these gloomy assessments, over the last 30 years there have been remarkable changes in the health status and demographic picture in Indonesia. Infant mortality has fallen to 34 deaths per 1,000 live births (2005). The fertility rate has fallen to 2.6 births per 1,000 women of child-bearing age. Contraceptive prevalence is high and life expectancy at birth for males is 68 years and for females 72 years (Statistics Indonesia 2008: 1). Assessing the extent to which these changes are due to the health system per se is complicated by the other massive changes that have occurred at the same time. Over the same period Indonesia has seen rapid economic development with attendant increases in income levels – the proportion of the population living below the poverty line fell from 40 per cent in 1975 to 17 per cent in 2006 (World Bank 2006: 7). For many the jobs that made this move out of poverty possible were in the city. Thus, whereas only 17 per cent lived in urban areas in 1971 (Frederick and Worden 1993), now more than half the population are to be found there (Statistics Indonesia 2008: 3) (see also Figure 12.1). The literacy rate in those aged ten years and over increased from 61 per cent in 1971 to 93 per cent in 2007 with greater increases for females than males. In parallel with the education changes, women are marrying later, and have greatly increased opportunities to participate in the labour force (Statistics Indonesia 2008: 2). Basic infrastructure also improved markedly – e.g. road density almost quadrupled between 1976 and 1996 (Kwon 2006: 4).

No doubt the health system designed and established in the period since Independence has been an important factor underlying these changes. Increased access to basic health services has undoubtedly saved many lives. But it would be a mistake to imagine that the health system was the only factor in this remarkable change over just a 30 year period. Incomes increased, basic education spread, infrastructure improved and most people moved to the city where there was better access to most basic services. And, of course, basic health and family planning services also were introduced and became much more accessible than in the past.

With all these changes has also come a similarly remarkable change in the disease pattern of the Indonesian population. In the 2001 National Household Health Survey (Tim Surkesnas 2002: 16) cardiovascular disease was the leading cause of death, up from number four just 30 years earlier. Infectious diseases, the leading causes of death in 1971, had become number two, significantly behind cardiovascular disease, let alone all noncommunicable diseases (NCDs) combined. At that time, as acknowledged in the 2001 report, there was already a double burden of disease with strong indications that the importance of NCDs would increase even further.

## Future burden of disease

The question now is: what will happen in the future? Can Indonesia expect that the disease pattern will remain much as it is today or are there likely to be further changes? An answer to this question requires projection of the disease pattern into the future. In doing so it is important to take into account the demographic changes and economic development already underway, whether these trends will continue and their effect on the epidemiological picture over the next three decades.

The growth trend in the Indonesian economy is projected to continue (World Bank 2008a: 5) and population will continue to increase for at least another half century, though both projections are subject to wider margins of speculation the farther you look into the future. The population projections assume that both infant mortality and fertility will continue their downward trend (see Figure 12.1); and the proportion of the population living in urban areas is predicted to grow to 80 per cent.

Whilst the disease pattern projections are not available for Indonesia as a whole they have been done for the East Asia and Pacific region. These projections developed by WHO as part of its continuing Burden of Disease (BOD) studies are very likely to be illustrative of where Indonesia will be soon if, indeed, it is not already there. Using their BOD results for 2002 as the starting point, WHO has taken account of increases in population, income, education and technological change in the health system (Mathers and Loncar 2010: 2,012). The population data used for the projections are based on the UN Population Division projections of fertility and net migration and the WHO projected mortality rates. The results are presented in terms of mortality and Disability Adjusted Life Years (DALYs)[2] by region of the world. Indonesia is included in and is a major contributor to the pattern for the East Asia and Pacific region.

A basic summary of the 2002 data together with projections both for deaths and DALYs for 2015 and 2030 are given in Figure 12.2. They show the relative contribution of the various disease categories to the BOD. In summary, in East Asia and the Pacific:

*   In 2002 NCDs accounted for over 70 per cent of all deaths and more than 60 per cent of DALYs, compared with less than 20 per cent of deaths and 25 per cent of DALYs due to communicable diseases. Injuries accounted for 10 per cent of deaths and 14 per cent of DALYs. The general pattern and contribution to the broad disease categories are similar to that already described for the Indonesian National Household Health Survey in 2001 (Tim Surkesnas 2002: 16).

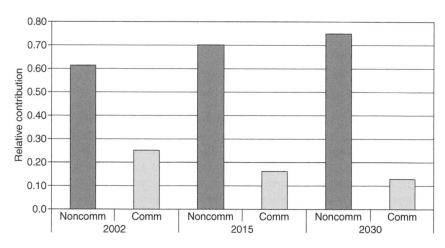

*Figure 12.2* Relative contribution of communicable and noncommunicable disease to disease burden: East Asia and Pacific, 2002, 2015, 2030 (source: adapted from Mathers and Loncar 2010: 2012).

- By 2030 the total number of deaths due to all causes is projected to increase by 44 per cent. Deaths due to NCDs will increase even more, by 66 per cent. Over the same period deaths due to communicable diseases are projected to fall to two-thirds of their current level.
- By 2030 the proportion of all deaths due to NCDs will rise to 83 per cent and the contribution to DALYs from 61 to 75 per cent. The contribution of communicable diseases will fall from 19 to 9 per cent of deaths and to DALYs from 25 to 13 per cent. The main driver of this change is the rapid rise in deaths and DALYs due to NCDs
- By 2030, within the NCDs group the main contributors are projected to be cardiovascular disease (44 per cent), cancers (23 per cent) and respiratory disease (18 per cent), especially chronic obstructive pulmonary disease (COPD), a total of 85 per cent of the noncommunicable group.
- By 2030 deaths due to communicable diseases are actually projected to fall even though the population will grow by about 15 per cent over the same period.

This overall picture at the regional level of a rapid and continuing rise in the importance of NCDs is consistent with evidence on the levels and trends of major risk factors for NCDs in Indonesia. Thus, undernutrition in children under five years has fallen significantly since 1990 (World Bank 2008b: 17), even though it is still higher than desirable levels. This trend is consistent with the sharp fall in the contribution of communicable disease to the overall burden and the continuing fall in infant and child mortality (Statistics Indonesia 2008: 118). Other studies have shown a rise in overweight and obesity in urban children and adolescents, even as underweight persists in some (Julia 2008: 306). The prevalence of smoking, a major risk factor and already at high levels, has risen even further – prevalence among males aged 15–19 years increased from 4 per cent in 1995 to 24 per cent in 2001 (Martini and Sulistyowati 2005: 1). Studies of risk factors in adults indicate increasing levels consistent with the much increased contribution of noncommunicable disease in the future. A 2001 study involving both rural and urban adults of Purworejo District in Central Java (Ng *et al.* 2006: 309) found that more than 40 per cent of rural and urban males and 20 per cent of all women had at least one risk factor for noncommunicable disease. Almost a decade later the levels are likely to be if anything higher. The highest socioeconomic groups in rural areas had levels similar to those in the urban population.

For males:

- more than half smoked, with higher levels in rural groups;
- more than 20 per cent of both groups had raised blood pressure with higher levels in the urban areas; in both areas average pressure increased with age;
- 13 per cent of adult males in urban areas were overweight or obese; in rural areas the prevalence of overweight amongst those in the richest quintile of the income distribution was similar to those in urban areas while other rural men had much lower prevalences;
- 23 per cent of urban men had at least two risk factors.

For women:

- the prevalence of smoking was very low;
- at least 20 per cent in both rural and urban areas had raised blood pressure and levels increased with age;
- almost one-quarter of urban women were overweight or obese.

## Future demand for services?

Even though projections cannot represent the future with certainty, they do present a view of what the future might be like in terms of mortality and morbidity and, as such, provide a basis for anticipating the amount and type of health care the population is likely to demand in the future and for assessing the ability of the health services to respond.

A disease burden projection study in East Java and Central Java (Adeyi *et al.* 2007: 119) provides some indication of what is likely to happen. This study modelled the change in demand for services as a result of population increase (projected to increase by 17 per cent between 2005 and 2020) and rising incomes and estimated the demand for and cost of inpatient and outpatient services in 2020. Treatment rates and cost of treatment were based on information collected in the two provinces in 2005. Depending on assumptions about change in the prevalence of disease, the total number of outpatient visits was projected to increase by between 15 and 48 per cent over the period 2005 to 2030; and the proportion of outpatient visits accounted for by NCDs rose from 54 per cent in 2005 to 71 per cent in 2020. Demand for inpatient bed days increased by between 84 and 124 per cent; and the proportion accounted for by NCDs rose from 67 per cent in 2005 to 79 per cent in 2020. Based on the 2005 rupiah[3] and costs, overall spending for outpatient and inpatient services was predicted to increase from Rp7.5 trillion in 2005 to between Rp14.8 trillion and Rp17.2 trillion; within this amount, the market for NCD treatment was predicted to be at least twice as large in 2020 as in 2005; that is, overall, the demand for health services was projected to rise far more quickly than population alone, and spending on NCDs is projected to double.

The study also estimated the ability of the health system to meet this increased demand for hospital care. In 2005, 38,000 hospital beds (public and private) were available in the two provinces. Estimated demand in 2020 ranged between 53,000 and 64,000, an increase of between 15,000 and 20,000 beds. On 2005 prices and costs, bridging the gap would require a minimum investment of Rp8.7 trillion to Rp15.3 trillion. Meeting the demand for medical personnel to provide the additional services would require an additional 8,000 physicians over the 15-year period, with an estimated training cost of Rp507 billon. The current nurse output was sufficient to meet the increased demand. If these minimal investment costs were to be met from the public budget, up to one-third of future, total public spending on health in these two provinces would be required (assuming public expenditure continued at 2005 levels). At the same time the need for core public health services would continue so the question of how to finance the infrastructure needs becomes crucial. If the future resembles the scenarios presented in the study, maintaining core public health services while providing for health infrastructure will present a serious challenge.

## Where to from here?

This remarkable change in disease patterns and transfiguration in the demand for health care in such a short period of time will pose dramatic challenges for the health system. Originally designed as a publicly funded frontline system to serve a predominantly rural population with a heavy emphasis on infectious disease and maternal and child health, the system is struggling to address the health problems of today, let alone those of tomorrow. In effect, a health system designed for dealing with the "primary burden" of infections, childbearing and accidents is now expected to provide care for a wide range of NCDs. The system is failing to meet this challenge. Effective treatments are not widely available and prevention is not a priority. One immediate implication is that age-standardized mortality rates for NCDs are much higher in Indonesia than they are in high-income countries. The gap represents a burden that falls most heavily on adults, while the rhetoric of the health system is focused almost exclusively on babies, children and mothers (Abegunde *et al.* 2010: 1929).

Improving the performance of the existing system is itself a challenge. But now as Indonesia acknowledges the importance of NCDs, it actually faces two other major challenges: first, how to improve the delivery of services (including public health services) to deal with the remaining problems under the "first burden"; that of communicable disease and maternal and perinatal conditions. At the same time the ongoing economic, social, demographic and epidemiologic changes will challenge the Indonesian health sector's ability to meet the *future* demand for health care to which NCDs will be the major contributor.

Further, this new disease pattern will demand not only a reorientation to NCDs in an increasingly urban setting, it will also require a new type of service. NCDs, often several occurring together, involve different approaches to diagnosis and to treatment (which usually occurs over longer periods of time). Coordination of care, medical records and innovative approaches are all needed (Adeyi *et al.* 2007: 39). On most dimensions, treatment for NCDs is quite different from what is available through the current health system; and contrary to views held by many, NCDs and associated risk factors are not the preserve of the rich; they are equally, if not more, prevalent among the poor (Strong *et al.* 2005: 1581).

In summary, the Indonesian health system is now faced with a task every bit as challenging as the one faced at Independence. Then, the challenge was to establish a health system in a poor country with a large rural population and a high population growth rate in response to a disease pattern dominated by maternal and perinatal conditions and communicable diseases, especially life-threatening, acute episodes of the latter. Driven by these realities, the planners of that day moved from a weak and unevenly distributed system with an urban bias to one which brought basic health care staff and facilities closer to the mostly rural population. Whilst that task is not complete, in the sense that communicable diseases still cause an appreciable portion of the overall disease burden, much has been accomplished. But now, a new and equally critical task faces Indonesia, a country in which poverty rates have fallen, mortality rates are down and replacement levels of fertility are in sight, and where more than half the population now live in urban areas. Indonesia is now a middle income country with greatly improved levels of education and transport infrastructure. The disease pattern is already dominated by NCDs and will be increasingly so in the future. The prevalence of potent NCD risk factors is increasing, bringing with it the need for greater emphasis on prevention, new approaches to treatment, new skills in the providers and a new service delivery model. Like the planners of the earlier period, the planners of today, as well as multilateral and bilateral donors and technical agencies, need to be driven by the current reality and what we know will happen in the medium term to the types of diseases and disability to be faced. It is vital that the drivers are the realities of today rather than, as happens too often, the ideas of the past (Fuster and Voute 2005: 1512). The ability to respond to this new challenge in the new context will have a fundamental bearing on the way Indonesia develops in the next 30 years.

## A new health system?

The dual challenge of completing the first agenda and responding to the current and future demand for services for NCDs requires a reorientation of the current Indonesian health system.

But the problem of reorienting is proving to be intractable. The MoH (Ministry of Health) has been implementing the Bandung Plan for more than 40 years and changing policy direction is difficult. Civil servants who have known no other system and do not have the skills to imagine anything different, want to keep going with the emphasis on MDGs (Millenium Development Goals).[4] They receive support from the international donors who, by and large, feel the same. After all, it is the donors and agencies who drive the MDG agenda. So the rhetorical emphasis is, as it was 50 years ago, on moving services to the rural population, even though much of the rural population is now in the cities and even more want to be there. Moreover, the MoH continues to increase the number of doctors, nurses and midwives employed as permanent civil servants, in essence reinforcing the old approach.

The MoH moves in one direction and the population moves in the other. And decentralization means that coordination between the various levels of government, each responding to a different political situation, is hard to achieve.

Perhaps the best example of the difficulty of changing direction is human resources for health at the district level. Over the last two years the central government has been converting district level contract staff to permanent civil servants. At the same time the province whose role was significantly curtailed under decentralization and is now keen to get back into the game has also been appointing doctors, nurse, midwives under provincial contracts. Further, the districts have been appointing staff on local contracts even though there are central regulations that prohibit this practice. In the public rhetoric many of these personnel changes have been justified in the name of reducing maternal mortality. The problem is that even as the various levels of government make these appointments, often with the emphasis on village midwives, the midwives are moving from the villages to health centres and urban areas where private practice opportunities are greater. Increased numbers of public sector doctors, nurses and midwives also mean increased numbers of part-time private practitioners as they offer health care services outside official hours. Frequently, these new permanent civil servants draw patients away from the public sector to their own practice. The total volume of services provided to patients remains approximately the same but there is a shift to the private sector for treatment even as the public sector wages bill increases.

In the name of the MDGs politicians at all levels are adding new providers to the public payroll. There is little coordination between the various levels and at no point is there discussion of the needs of the health sector as a whole, now or in the future. No one is looking at the broader picture or beyond the next election.

To move beyond this short term, unbalanced approach, what is needed at the national level is a real attempt to envision and then implement the health system that Indonesia will need for the next 20 to 30 years and to use the substantial public subsidy given to this lightly regulated private system in creative ways. This will require attention to at least seven broad points.

First, what are the best service models for the various parts of a very diverse country? Answering this question will require at least entertaining the notion that the health centre, the iconic institution around which the current service delivery model was built, may have reached its use-by date. At the very least, different approaches in different geographic regions are needed.

Second, recognizing that the quality of services in the current system is low is a vital first step to improving it. This will be an important point in devising a new service model, especially one in which there are incentives for good quality rather than a race to the bottom as occurs at the moment.

Third, financing the health system in a way that promotes equity and quality, with an emphasis on the special characteristics of NCDs, is vital. There is little point in large-scale public financing of a low-quality health system. It would be better to work on quality first and then on how it should be financed.

Fourth, any new approach to the health sector and quality of services will need to pay explicit attention to the mix and level of skills required of the service providers. The fact is that many current providers have very inadequate skills relating to NCDs. It is a massive task to revamp the skills set of the current workforce and to ensure that those being trained now and in the future are better prepared for a disease pattern dominated by NCDs.

Fifth, the experience in high income countries with their own NCD epidemics clearly points to the need to place much greater emphasis on prevention. Ironically, this important emphasis of the health system devised more than 50 years ago has been lost and must be rediscovered.

Sixth, even if prevention campaigns are successful, meeting the increased demand for the quantity and type of services required means a massive investment in more hospitals; a demand that the public purse will not be able to meet by itself. Private investment in hospitals is critical to meeting this demand and to allowing public funds to concentrate on ensuring that public health functions are improved and equity of access ensured.

Finally, all of this demands leadership by the Ministry of Health, a leadership that embraces the whole sector – public and private – in a way that values, promotes and evaluates innovation for it is change that is required; a change that allows different approaches and then assesses them. Because the appropriate role of government differs by administrative level, it also demands a leadership that reassesses the role of district, provincial and central governments with emphasis on mitigation of market failures as well as improved equity and quality. The need is to build a health system appropriate to the Indonesian health problems of today and, more importantly, tomorrow.

## Notes

1 Although private practice by nurses is illegal, it is widely acknowledged that they do practise privately. By some estimates they are the most numerous group of private providers (Heywood and Harahap 2009a).
2 Disability-Adjusted Life Year (DALY) is a single measure to quantify the burden of diseases, injuries and risk factors. DALYs for a disease or health condition are calculated as the sum of the Years of Life Lost (YLL) due to premature mortality in the population and the Years Lost due to Disability (YLD) for incident cases of the health condition.

3 One US dollar is approximately equal to rupiah 10,000.
4 The Millennium Development Goals (MDGs), eight international development goals, were adopted at the United Nations Millennium Summit in 2000. They include targets to reduce the child mortality rate by two-thirds and the maternal mortality rate by three-quarters between 1990 and 2015.

## References

Abegunde, D.O., Mathers, C.D., Adam, T., Ortegon, M. and Strong, K. (2010) "The Burden and Costs of Chronic Diseases in Low-Income and Middle-Income Countries". *Lancet*, 370: 1929–1938.

Adeyi, O., Smith, O. and Robles, S. (2007) *Public Policy and the Challenge of Chronic Noncommunicable Diseases.* Washington, DC: World Bank.

Barber, S.L., Gertler, P.J. and Harimurti, P. (2007) "Differences in Access to High-Quality Outpatient Care in Indonesia". *Health Affairs*, 26: w352–w366. Online, available at: http://content.healthaffairs.org/cgi/reprint/26/3/w352 (accessed 7 March 2010).

Departemen Kesehatan (1980) *Survai Kesehatan Rumah Tangga 1980: Laporan. Badan Penelitian dan Pengembangan Kesehatan.* Jakarta: Departemen Kesehatan.

Frederick, W.H. and Worden, R.H. (1993) *Indonesia: A Country Study.* Washington, DC: GPO for the Library of Congress. Online, available at: http://countrystudies.us/indonesia/ (accessed 7 March 2010).

Furster, V. and Voute, J. (2005) "MDGs: Chronic Diseases are not on the Agenda". *Lancet*, 366: 1512–1514.

Heywood, P. and Choi, Y. (2010) "Health System Performance at the District Level in Indonesia after Decentralization". *BMC International Health and Human Rights*, 10: 3. Online, available at: www.biomedcentral.com/1472–698X/10/3 (accessed 12 May 2010).

Heywood, P. and Harahap, N.P. (2009a) "Health Facilities at the District Level in Indonesia". *Australia and New Zealand Health Policy*, 6: 13. Online, available at: www.anzhealthpolicy.com/content/6/1/13 (accessed 12 May 2010).

Heywood, P. and Harahap, N.P. (2009b) "Human Resources for Health at the District Level in Indonesia: The Smoke and Mirrors of Decentralization". *Human Resources for Health*, 7: 6. Online, available at: www.human-resources-health.com/content/7/1/6 (accessed 12 May 2010).

Heywood, P. and Harahap, N.P. (2009c) "Public Funding at the District Level in Indonesia: Sources, Flows and Contradictions". *Health Research Policy and Systems*, 7: 5. Online, available at: www.health-policy-systems.com/content/7/1/5 (accessed 12 May 2010).

Indonesia NIHRD (2005) *Indonesia: Sub-National Health System Performance Assessment.* Jakarta: National Institute of Health Research and Development, Ministry of Health, Indonesia.

Julia, M. (2008) "Tracking for Underweight, Overweight and Obesity from Childhood to Adolescence: A 5-Year Follow-Up Study in Urban Indonesian Children". *Hormone Research*, 69: 301–306.

Kwon, E. (2006) *Infrastructure, Growth, and Poverty Reduction in Indonesia: A Cross-sectional Analysis.* Manila: Asian Development Bank.

Leimena, J. (1956) *Public Health in Indonesia: Problems and Planning.* Jakarta: N.V. v/h G.C.T. Van Dorp and Co.

Martini, S. and Sulistyowati, M. (2005) *The Determinants of Smoking Behavior among Teenagers in East Java Province, Indonesia.* Washington, DC: World Bank.

Mathers, C.D. and Loncar, D. (2010) "Projections of Global Mortality and Burden of Disease from 2002 to 2030". *PLoS Medicine*, 3: 2010–2030.

Ministry of Health (2005) *Tuberculosis Prevalence Survey in Indonesia 2004. Jakarta: National Institute of Health Research and Development.* Jakarta: Ministry of Health, Indonesia.

Ng, N., Stenlund, H., Bonita, R., Hakimi, M., Wall, S. and Weinehall, L. (2006) "Preventable Risk Factors for Noncommunicable Diseases in Rural Indonesia: Prevalence Study using WHO STEPS Approach". *Bulletin of the World Health Organization*, 84: 305–313.

Population Division of the Department of Economic and Social Affairs of the United Nations Secretariat (2009) *World Population Prospects: The 2008 Revision.* Online, available at: http://esa.un.org/unpp (accessed 20 February 2010)

Statistics Indonesia (2008) *Indonesia Demographic and Health Survey 2007.* Jakarta: Statistics Indonesia.

Strong, K., Mathers, C., Leeder, S. and Beaglehole, R. (2005) "Preventing Chronic Diseases: How Many Lives Can We Save?" *Lancet*, 366: 1578–1582.

Tim Surkesnas (2002) *Survei Kesehatan Nasional. Laporan Studi Mortalitas 2001. Pola penyakit penyebab kematian di Indonesia. Badan Penelitian dan Pengembangan Kesehatan.* Jakarta: Departemen Kesehatan.

WHO (1978) Declaration of Alma-Ata. International Conference on Primary Health Care, Alma-Ata, USSR, 6–12 September. Geneva: World Health Organization.

World Bank (2006) *Making the New Indonesia Work for the Poor: 2006 Indonesia Poverty Assessment Report.* Washington, DC: World Bank.

World Bank (2007) *Spending for Development: Making the Most of Indonesia's New Opportunities. Indonesia Public Expenditure Review 2007.* Washington, DC: World Bank.

World Bank (2008a) *Indonesia: Country Partnership Strategy 2009–2012*, Washington, DC: World Bank.

World Bank (2008b) *Investing in Indonesia's Health: Challenges and Opportunities for Future Public Spending.* Washington, DC: World Bank.

# 13 Evolution, revolution and devolution

## A cross-sectional analysis of the emergence of the double disease burden in the Philippines

*Giselle M. Manalo, Angelito Umali, Jaime Galvez Tan, Gabriel Carreon, Angelo Manalo and Alberto Romualdez*

### Introduction

Long before Magellan landed on Philippine shores on 16 March 1521, the Philippines' first inhabitants were a nomadic people, the *Aeta* tribe. They were followed by Nusantao seafarers and finally western Malayo-Polynesian groups (Solheim II 1981: 16–20; Solheim II 1984–1985: 77–85; Bellwood *et al.* 2006: 1–5; Solheim II 2006: 1–5). Later came immigrant traders from Fujian and Guangdong provinces in Southern China who settled before the Spanish conquest. In fact, many indigenous leaders (*datus* and *rajahs*) in the Philippines were of mixed Filipino and Chinese ancestry. Given this cultural mix and a deeply entrenched colonial regime of nearly four centuries (De Bevoise 1997: 113–124), the Filipino people are defined by their history and diverse geographical, social, cultural, economic and political characteristics. These pose unique challenges for public health.

Considered a middle income country with one of the highest population growth rates averaging 2 per cent in the region (AIM-USAIDS 2008: 4; National Statistics Office 2009: 23), the Philippines has sadly declined from its post-Second World War position of growing wealth and power, second only to Japan. Today's sluggish economy notably lags behind the evolving Tiger economies in the region. An intractable resistance to reforms by deeply entrenched interests, a politics of patronage, systemic inefficiencies and myopic reform measures dogged by persistent corruption are some of the reasons for this economic decline. These are all rooted in the complex interplay of Philippine history, culture and policy.

However, in very recent years, the Philippine economy has enjoyed positive gains. In 2007, the economy was at its strongest with a gross domestic product (GDP) real growth rate of 7.34 per cent, the highest in over three decades. Ten per cent of GDP came from remittances to family members from overseas

Filipino workers (US Library of Congress 2006: 11). Yet the gap between rich and poor has widened markedly with official statistics indicating nearly five million families living in poverty. The 2006 Human Development Report revealed over 30 million poor Filipinos were living on less than a dollar (US) daily (AIM-USAIDS 2008: 5; CIA 2008: 1). More alarming is the increase of food-poor Filipinos to over 12 million (National Statistics Office 2008: 1–25). The population poverty incidence was 32.9 per cent in 2006 and it was higher in rural areas; with southern Mindanao having the highest incidence (Human Development Network 2005: 108–112). In 2007, the national unemployment rate was 7.35 per cent (Galvez Tan 2003: 1–3; AIM-USAIDS 2008: 5; National Statistics Office 2009: 52–54; United Nations Development Programme 2009: 168).

The population stands at 92 million and is estimated to reach 102 million by 2015. By 2029, it will have doubled (AIM-USAIDS 2008: 9; National Statistics Office 2009: 23–25). The 2008 US Census Bureau International Database reported Filipino average life expectancy at birth to be 71 years while the National Statistics Office reported the 2010 life expectancy projection for males as 67.61 years and females as 73.14 years.

Although adult literacy levels for both genders have consistently been in the ninetieth percentile, there is a gap that favours women regarding completion of basic education, vocational training and higher education. High drop out rates among male students have been observed in primary and secondary schools. Fewer men pursue further education and vocational training (Department of Education 2008: 1; National Statistics Office 2009: 31–36; US Library of Congress 2006: 9).

With over 7,107 islands comprising the Philippine archipelago and a total land area of 300,000 km², the country boasts abundant natural resources and a rich eco-marine life that once earned her the title, "Pearl of the Orient Seas". While there are three major islands – Luzon, Visayas and Mindanao – the country's archipelagic character is divisive and this is powerfully magnified by regional differences; there are 18 administrative regions, 81 provinces, 136 cities, 1,495 municipalities/towns and 42,008 villages or *barangays* (National Statistics Coordination Board 2008: 1–2; National Statistics Office 2009: 79–83; US Library of Congress 2006: 7–8).

Situated along the earthquake/tropical cyclone belt and the Pacific "Ring of Fire", the Philippines is frequently vulnerable to natural disasters such as volcanic eruptions, typhoons, earthquakes, massive floods and landslides. The Philippine Atmospheric, Geophysical and Astronomical Services Administration reports that the country experiences approximately 20 earthquakes annually and on average 19 to 21 tropical cyclones, of which two are super typhoons, per year (United Nations Development Programme 2001: 1–2; World Health Organization 2007: 1). The health implications of these disasters are massive and in 2009, typhoons Ketsana and Parma destroyed homes, hospitals, medical centres and public infrastructure, crippling the country's disaster response network. Acute communicable diseases were the leading causes of mortality and prompt management of chronic diseases was delayed (United Nations Development

Programme 2001: 1–2; Emergency Disasters Database 2007: 1–3; World Health Organization 2009: 5–12).

### The influence of the colonial past

Spain's over 300 year rule succeeded in bringing Filipinos under the influence of the Roman Catholic church. The Philippines is one of two predominantly Christian countries in Asia. Using religion as a powerful tool to perpetuate fear and obedience among the masses, the Spanish regime laid the foundation of a feudal health care system that was going to have far-reaching influences on how Filipinos currently perceive, behave and relate to each other particularly in matters of governance.

At the turn of the twentieth century, Spain ceded the Philippines to the United States under the Treaty of Paris (US Library of Congress 2006: 1–4). From 1902 to 1946, the United States controlled the Philippines, retaining the feudal system that Spain had implemented. Although a restricted Commonwealth government was established in 1935, it was short lived as history once again intervened. The Second World War ushered in the Japanese occupation of 1942–1944.

The Philippine government and its political structures are based on the US model. It is defined as a republican form of democracy with executive, bicameral legislative and judicial branches (US Library of Congress 2006: 4, 19–21). In 2003, the Philippines was designated by the United States a major non-North Atlantic Treaty Organization ally; it was the fourth largest recipient of US military aid and overseas development assistance (US Library of Congress 2006: 23–24).

While developmental efforts have been attempted by various administrations, health inequities have continued to worsen due to increasing poverty, maldistribution of financial resources, a health personnel haemorrhage, weak governance, mushrooming graft and ingrained socio-cultural perceptions that affect health care delivery. In the southernmost islands of Mindanao where the poorest of the poor are concentrated, health outcomes are alarming. Filipinos in these areas have shorter life expectancies and succumb to communicable diseases. Complicating the situation is a long-standing, secessionist movement which has contributed to unstable conditions and deterred this region's economic development (Human Development Network 2005: 8–11, 16–18, 65–67, 98).

This chapter will discuss the evolution of the double disease burden via a health system approach, highlighting issues that led to the current health scenario. It will identify critical disease priorities over the past decades and chronicle the transition to chronic non-communicable diseases (NCDs). It will expand on key developmental issues such as decentralization, lifestyle/dietary changes and health personnel migration, analysing the challenges posed by these issues and their health implications. Finally, measures to address existing gaps and strengthen current programmes will be suggested.

## Deconstructing the Philippine public health care delivery system and the emergence of the double disease burden

The Philippines continues to suffer from a heavy communicable disease burden; latest data reveal pneumonia, diarrhoeal diseases, bronchitis, influenza, tuberculosis, malaria, chicken pox and dengue are eight of the ten leading causes of morbidity (National Statistics Office 2008: 1–6; 2009: 47–51) While HIV prevalence remains very low at less than 0.1 per cent, risky behaviours amongst vulnerable groups and the persistent presence of tuberculosis (coupled with increases in multiple drug-resistant tuberculosis (MDR-TB)) may lead to a dual HIV/TB epidemic (Philippine National AIDS Council and UNAIDS 2008: 5–8; Portero and Rubio 2006: e539).

Mosquito-borne diseases like malaria, dengue and filariasis are an ever-present threat in endemic areas. Malaria and lymphatic filariasis can be found in regions with the highest incidence of poverty of which the most affected are indigenous people (Galvez Tan 2003: 1–5; World Health Organization 2009: 9–12).

Chronic NCDs comprise the leading causes of death in the country: heart diseases, cerebrovascular diseases, cancer, lower respiratory diseases, diabetes, kidney diseases with tuberculosis, pneumonia, assault/injury and conditions during the perinatal period rounding off the list (National Statistics Office 2009: 47–51).

Average life expectancy at birth has slowly increased to 71 years, but this is about 15 years fewer than that of the developed world. Current health indicators reveal staggering numbers – 80,000 Filipino babies die each year from preventable diseases while 3,000 mothers die unnecessarily (Romualdez 2008:1). Closer examination shows remarkably wide rural/urban disparities with rural health outcomes equivalent to the least developed countries while urban health outcomes are comparable to those of developed countries (Romualdez 2008: 1–2; National Statistics Office 2009: 47–51). Though government health expenditures have increased to 3 per cent of gross national product (GNP), this is below the WHO-recommended allocation of 5 per cent for developing countries (Bautista 2001: 7; AIM-USAIDS 2008: 5). With half of total health expenditures sourced from out-of-pocket payments, the Philippine health system is largely private sector and profit oriented, benefiting the "haves" rather than the "have-nots".

## How did the Philippine health picture get to this point?

### *Evolution of the health system*

Public health in the Spanish period saw the creation of some basic institutions and services. Hospitals provided general medical services, treated communicable diseases and cared for orphaned children and the mentally ill.

Other developments included a public health laboratory, the first medical school, forensic medicine facilities and the construction of piped waterworks for the prevention of waterborne communicable diseases. Noteworthy was the creation of the Board of Vaccinators to prevent smallpox (Valenzuela-Tiglao 1998: 3–5).

During the American occupation, achievements in school education and public health stood out. But both systems were used by the Americans to serve their own economic and political interests. Public health programmes were carried out to encourage productivity, develop an industrial workforce and to allay opposition to the American colonizers. The provision of these services helped win the Filipino people's trust.

Efforts in the early years of the American occupation centred on the control of epidemics (smallpox, cholera and plague) and other communicable diseases (diarrhoea, leprosy and malaria), and *beri-beri*; a Board of Health and health units were established and general sanitation improved. The Philippine Assembly period (1907–1916) saw the establishment of a functional public health system able to monitor common communicable diseases; and provide vaccination, sanitation and nutrition programmes as well as the creation of civic organizations, notably the Philippine Tuberculosis Society, that eventually paved the way for comprehensive work on tuberculosis (Valenzuela-Tiglao 1998: 6–12).

During the Jones Law period (1916–1936), the United States experienced political and economic instability due to the Great Depression and this had repercussions locally. The health status of Filipinos declined. Mortality and morbidity rates rose largely due to communicable diseases (tuberculosis, leprosy, cholera, typhoid, malaria and smallpox) and *beri-beri*. It was not until the late 1930s when Commonwealth status was granted that the public health system eventually recovered. The Rockefeller Foundation extended considerable support by providing skills training for Filipino health professionals and by funding the establishment of the School of Hygiene and Public Health.

Public health continued to prosper during the Commonwealth period (1936–1942) and under a Filipino president. While socioeconomic and political issues remained significant, public health received proper attention evidenced by an increase in budgetary appropriations, construction of more hospitals for tuberculosis and leprosy patients and the establishment of sanitation facilities throughout the country. The Department of Public Health and Welfare was created and it introduced a Maternal and Child Health programme. Health education in schools gained momentum. The Bureau of Census and Statistics could now provide a better assessment of Filipinos' health status. Local health facilities and human resources were properly allocated (Valenzuela-Tiglao 1998: 13–21).

The promising public health advance during the American period suffered a setback under the Japanese Occupation of 1942–1944. Public health and sanitation activities were all paralysed and communicable disease epidemics broke out. There was widespread malnutrition and destruction of public health facilities, and skeletal health services could only deal with emergency cases. After liberation, the United States Public Health Service equipped with developmental funds from the US Congress gave massive support to the Commonwealth government's rehabilitation efforts. Programmes to control communicable disease and advance general sanitation were re-established; public health facilities were reconstructed. As the country's public health system slowly recovered from the ravages of war, the Philippines gained her independence in 1946 (Valenzuela-Tiglao 1998: 22–23).

Under a regime of postwar international cooperation, several agencies lent assistance to the country. The United States launched its Philippine Rehabilitation Program which later led to a mutual assistance and cooperation agreement between the US Economic Cooperation Agency (currently USAID) and the Philippines to provide continuous support for development of health services in all areas in the country, particularly underserved rural areas. Likewise, United Nations agencies initiated various developmental projects. Later the WHO Western Pacific Regional Office was established in Manila (Valenzuela-Tiglao 1998: 24–25).

As communicable diseases dominated the health scene in the mid to late 1940s, rehabilitation efforts focused on the re-establishment of the following: a centralized health laboratory, a National Chest Centre, a tuberculosis case registry, mass BCG vaccinations and research on larvicidal usage to control malaria. The Institute of Nutrition (currently the Food and Nutrition Research Institute) was given the task of addressing the exceedingly high prevalence of malnutrition.

In the 1950s, the first group of exchange visitors programmes with the United States commenced. The goal then was for Filipino health workers to receive advanced training and bring back the skills to improve quality of health services (Ronquillo 2005: 16–18). Thus, began the migration of Filipino health professionals that would later lead to a massive exodus of health care workers to the US, Middle East and other parts of the globe, creating a gaping health personnel black hole in the country.

In the 1960s, a structural reorganization of the Department of Health into regional, provincial and municipal health offices was introduced in order to reach underserved rural areas. Among public health measures prioritized were dental health, malaria education, schistosomiasis control, family planning, disease intelligence and food and drug administration (Valenzuela-Tiglao 1998: 27–30).

### Revolutionizing change

As it gradually became apparent that the majority of Filipinos living in rural and remote communities had no access to health care services, a revolutionary public health strategy was implemented – the Rural Health Unit (RHU) Programme. The RHU became crucial to the delivery of essential health services to improve the country's overall health status.

The RHU Programme trained rural health midwives to work alongside volunteer community health workers. They became the frontline health care providers at the community level. The Philippine Rural Reconstruction Movement introduced a fourfold approach to rural development by integrating livelihood, education, health and governance. The Rizal Development Project created the framework for the rural health care delivery system, and World Bank Population Loans provided support for capacity building among primary health care workers. The enactment of the Philippine Medicare Act, it was hoped, would bring essential medical services to more Filipinos and provide a viable means of payment for their medical care.

Public health grew stronger with these developments but the proclamation of martial law by President Ferdinand Marcos in 1972 affected access and delivery of these programmes particularly in Mindanao where the volatile armed conflict between military and *Moros* escalated (Human Development Network 2005: 66–69).

Major breakthroughs during this period included use of improved antibiotics and the adoption of primary health care nationwide through an integrated health care delivery system that functioned alongside an independent private sector network. (Romualdez 2009a: 1) Community-based health programmes continued with the launching of oral rehydration therapy for diarrhoeal disease control. Primary, secondary and tertiary health care strategies were developed. Public health research made inroads with the creation of the Nutrition Council of the Philippines, the Philippine Council for Health Research and the Research Institute for Tropical Medicine. These institutions became central to public health operations during the early 1980s, as globalization swept across the world breaking barriers on how information was communicated and shared, and impacting on how societies interacted with one another. Increasing travel and overseas work opportunities exposed Filipinos to new health threats the most striking of which was HIV/AIDS.

Amidst such rapid developments came a very significant change that catapulted Philippine politics on to the global stage – the "People Power" Edsa Revolution of 1986. It was an emphatic declaration by a country clamouring for social justice, meaningful democracy and people empowerment. While the Edsa revolution restored democratic government, the effects on the health sector were mixed. Effective implementation of public health programmes was still largely dependent on the priorities and interests of individuals leading the Department of Health and its associated agencies.

Under the new government, a number of health policies and programmes revitalized the public health system. The Milk Code promoted breast feeding and ensured proper use of breast milk substitutes when necessary. The Generics Act aimed to ensure an adequate supply of affordable and safe generic drugs to give consumers the right of informed choice. The Magna Carta for Public Health Workers advocated improvement of social and economic well-being of health workers, developed their skills to enhance effective delivery of health programmes and encouraged health workers to remain in government service; and the Safe Motherhood Programme sought to improve maternal health outcomes (Valenzuela-Tiglao 1998: 38–40).

Department of Health initiatives reinvigorated health promotion, changing the public's perception of health by instituting clever and innovative, media-friendly programmes. Amongst these were the National Immunization Day, the Mother-Baby Friendly Hospital Initiative, the Promotion of Traditional Medicines, the Centre of Wellness Hospitals, the Doctors to the Barrios programme and an anti-smoking campaign (Valenzuela-Tiglao 1998: 42–46).

The National Health Insurance Law was enacted in the early 1990s to give Filipinos partial coverage of their hospital care (Romualdez 2009a: 1).

### Devolution of health services

The late 1980s and early 1990s ushered in an era of technological advancement. The advent of the Internet not only revolutionized telecommunications it also transfigured work, lifestyle, attitudes and behaviour. Working Filipinos and students belonging to the middle and upper income groups were adopting a more westernized lifestyle. Long sedentary work hours were accompanied by unhealthy dietary patterns, increased stress levels, diminished physical activity and increased alcohol consumption and smoking. The world had become smaller and the pace of life much faster as more Filipinos flocked to urbanized areas for studies, employment and a better quality of life.

In the Philippine Senate there was strong support for decentralization of health administration. Theoretically it would improve community participation, fostering a sense of local ownership and strengthening services. Devolution involved the transfer of authority, decision-making power and responsibility from the national government to the intermediate and local governments (Magno 2001: 34–36; Dumogho 2006: 1–3).

In 1991, the Local Government Code granted unparalleled authority to local government units (LGUs) at provincial, city and municipal levels to engage in health care delivery (Bautista 2001: 30; Dumogho 2006: 2–6; Magno 2001: 34–48; Grundy *et al.* 2003: 220–222; Romualdez 2009a: 1).

However the preparation for this transfer of health care delivery was extremely inadequate. Most mayors and governors (also called local chief executives at the city/municipal and provincial level respectively) were not equal to the task. There was heavy reliance on equally unprepared physicians who discovered they lacked the necessary skills, knowledge and attitudes required of them by their new responsibilities (Magno 2001: 38–43; Manalo 2004: 1–3). While well-resourced upper class and better governed LGUs in the National Capital Region managed to cope with the magnitude of administrative and financial responsibilities, the majority was left to provide services with very meagre resources and limited technical know-how. This led to widespread frustration and demoralized community health personnel working on limited funding from their local governments as the latter's priorities were not necessarily health oriented. The quality of tertiary hospital care and preventive rural health services progressively deteriorated. Structural referrals, monitoring and evaluation network systems between city/municipal, provincial and regional levels became disjointed and eventually disintegrated (Magno 2001: 34–47; Obermann *et al.* 2008: 343–349).

Despite good intentions, the devolution of health services in the Philippines led to undesirable effects that further fragmented the public health care delivery system, reinforced distressing inequities, worsened health outcomes, revealed incompetent local governance and ill-prepared health care workers against a background of a long-standing health personnel haemorrhage (Department of Health 1999: 7–15; Manalo 2004: 1–3; Galvez Tan 2003: 1–2; 2005: 1; 2009: 3; Carreon 2007: 6–8; Romualdez 2008: 13–14; Romualdez 2009a: 1–2).

Since its implementation nearly two decades ago and through three post-Edsa administrations, the Department of Health has responded resolutely to these problems and implemented reforms tailored for a devolved public health system. The Health Sector Reform Agenda targets more effective coverage of national and local public health programmes, increases access to health services, especially by the poor, and reduces the financial burden on individual families (Department of Health 1997: 4; 1999: 15–17). Other strategic frameworks were the National Objectives for Health and the *Four*mula One for Health – a modification of the Health Sector Reform of 1999 targeting health financing, human resources for health, health service delivery, health regulations, health sector governance and health information systems (Department of Health 2005: 1; Romualdez 2009a: 1). Recognizing the real threat of the double disease burden, programmes have been developed geared towards both communicable disease and NCDs (Department of Health 2009: 13–14).

## Key issues in the emergence of the double disease burden

As developed countries eradicated major communicable diseases in the 1950s and 1960s, the Philippines battled against pneumonia, malaria, dengue, schistosomiasis, diarrhoeal diseases and tuberculosis. A slight decline in mortality and morbidity rates resulted from comprehensive primary health care programmes and improved access to antibiotics. Morbidity and mortality rates for heart disease, stroke and cancer (NCDs) remained low (Ngelangel and Wang 2002: S52; Galvez Tan 2009: 1).

The epidemiological shift became apparent in the early 1980s when NCDs insidiously crept up national statistical charts (see Figure 13.1). Demographic surveys in the mid-1990s revealed a shift from 7:3 (communicable to NCD) to 3:7 ratio.

On closer scrutiny, the epidemiologic transition may have occurred alongside the change in government in 1986. During the Aquino and the subsequent Ramos administrations, as wealth began to decentralize, the implementation of the Comprehensive Agrarian Reform Programme had ushered in economic growth in the more developed urban and provincial areas. However, the land reform was unsuccessful in the poorer provinces of Bicol, Samar and the Autonomous Region of Muslim Mindanao. This factor may have widened the gap between rich and poor. Furthermore, wealth decentralization leading to lifestyle changes may have contributed to the shift in the disease burden to NCDs (Galvez Tan, 2009: 3–5; Department of Health and National Epidemiology Centre 2004: 52–56, 82–83).

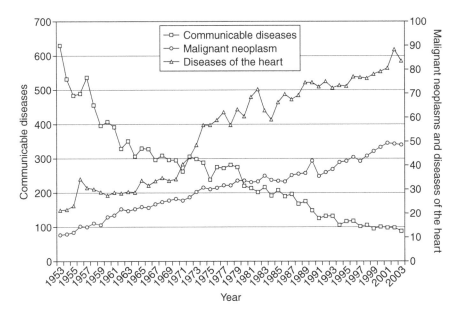

*Figure 13.1* Mortality trend: communicable diseases, malignant neoplasms and diseases of the heart per 100,000 population, the Philippines, 1953–2003 (source: Philippine Health Statistics 2004: 203).

As the political situation stabilized, foreign economic investments poured in. Rapid urbanization and internal migration of Filipinos occurred as employment opportunities somewhat improved. These events brought a radical change in lifestyle, work habits and diet among Filipinos. Shopping malls and fast-food restaurants proliferated across metropolitan and provincial areas nationwide. Consequently, Filipinos ate out more frequently adapting to a westernized diet of high caloric and high fat content (Pedro *et al.* 2006: 206, 210–220; Department of Science and Technology – Food and Nutrition Research Institute 2008: 12–14; National Economic and Development Authority 2008: 7).

The average food intake shows more fish, meat, poultry and eggs; more sugars, syrups and less complex carbohydrates. Filipinos have been found to eat less fruits and vegetables as these natural foods became more expensive due to trade liberalization (Pedro *et al.* 2006: 210–216). The National Nutrition Survey (2003) reported 8.5 per cent of adult Filipinos have high blood cholesterol compared to 4 per cent five years ago.

The ease of marketability of fast foods has accelerated with numerous street food stalls, convenience stores popping up at every corner, "drive thru" hamburger franchises and take-away/delivery services proliferating. Advances in information technology (Internet and tri-media) have made it all very attractive and within easy reach. Dining out at these fast-food chains has become a family's special treat.

Instant noodles, soup packets and pre-packed ready-to-eat meals with lesser nutritional values, higher fat and sodium content are considered time savers. As urbanized lives became frenetic and stressful, working Filipinos found less time to buy and cook fresh produce. Over the years, adult Filipinos have gradually become more overweight, from 16 per cent in 1993 to 26 per cent in 2008, increasing at an average rate of 0.67 percentage points per year (Department of Science and Technology – Food and Nurtition Research Institute 2008: 16–17). High fat, sugar, salt and high calorie diets with a sedentary lifestyle in addition to smoking and alcohol consumption predispose a person to heart diseases, hypertension, stroke, diabetes, cancer and kidney diseases.

However, the flip side of the coin is that the poorest of the poor who live mostly in rural and more remote provinces barely have anything to eat. Such is the double burden of malnutrition in the Philippines – over- and undernutrition. Most overweight Filipinos belong to the 40 to 59 age group; while malnutrition affects the most vulnerable groups – pregnant women, infants, children and indigenous groups with low socioeconomic status. Childhood obesity is still low but numbers are slowly increasing (Department of Science and Techology – Food and Nutrition Research Institute 2008: 22; National Economic and Development Authority 2008: 15–16).

Another significant factor contributing to this epidemiological transition is the ten million overseas Filipino workers (OFWs) (Dayrit and Dolea 2005: 14; Galvez Tan 2005: 3–4; Ronquillo 2005: 16; AIM-USAIDS 2008: 5; Romualdez 2009b: 2). Considered to be a major contributor to the country's economic development and relatively stable economy in light of the global financial crisis, OFWs are remitting US$17 billion a year (National Statistics Office 2009: 65–67). This accounts for the 60 per cent of the population receiving monthly remittances of between US$100 and $1,000. This extra source of income provides Filipinos with an improvement in living standards but not necessarily healthier lifestyles.

Leading cancer types in the country are lung, breast, cervix, liver, colon and rectum, prostate, stomach, oral cavity, ovary and leukaemia. Cancer prevention awareness is quite poor and patients usually see a doctor when it is too late (Ngelangel and Wang 2002: S52–S53). Early detection and prompt action increase survival rates which currently are relatively low.

Meanwhile tuberculosis (TB) continues to be a leading cause of mortality and morbidity. The Philippines is still one of the 22 high burden disease countries despite meeting 2005 TB global targets, 100 per cent DOTS (Directly Observed Treatment Short Course chemotherapy) coverage and stronger public–private partnerships. HIV testing in tuberculosis patients is still an area of need. It may be argued that the low prevalence of HIV/AIDS does not warrant regular testing but so far no evidence-based explanation exists to explain the low prevalence. Questions still remain whether this is an accurate assessment of the HIV/AIDS picture in the Philippines, given the millions of Filipinos overseas, continued presence of sexually transmitted diseases and powerful sociocultural attitudes, perceptions and behaviours concerning sex and HIV/AIDS.

Recent complications to the TB burden are multiple drug-resistant tuberculosis (MDR-TB) and extremely drug resistant tuberculosis (XDR-TB). This is a concern as second line drugs for MDR-TB are more expensive and treatment time is longer. However, there is no treatment available for XDR-TB. Perceived challenges for MDR-TB treatment are accurate and prompt diagnosis, difficulties with patient compliance, treatment centre access for remote/rural areas, procurement of quality assured medicines, continuous drug supply, side effects from anti MDR-TB drugs, funding shortages, HIV co-infection, limited numbers of health care workers and adequate monitoring and follow-up. The Philippine government has allocated funds for TB control including MDR-TB treatment. However, most of the current funding for MDR-TB comes from international agencies (Tupasi *et al.* 2000: 1126–1132; Tupasi 2006: 549). Alternative sources of funding have to be found for these programmes to be sustained.

As prevention is crucial, identifying the causes of MDR-TB, whether patient based or health system based, is imperative. Once identified, all stakeholders must act quickly before the rates of MDR-TB or XDR-TB escalate. It is incumbent on the Department of Health to ensure that procurement of anti-TB drugs are regularly monitored for quality assurance to prevent substandard drugs from being distributed to health centres, thus compounding the MDR-TB problem. Likewise, generic drugs sold in markets or procured by the government should undergo rigorous bio-A testing and their results made transparent to the public (Kanavos *et al.* 2002: 24).

Because TB patients are susceptible to HIV, monitoring of HIV is essential. In 2007, an estimated 7,490 Filipinos were considered living with HIV. At risk populations are female sex workers (FSWs), men who have sex with men, injecting drug users and male clients of FSWs. Knowledge of AIDS and sexually transmitted diseases varied. Attitudes among sex workers combine fatalism and indifference (De Bevoise 1997: 128–130).

De Bevoise (1997) noted that FSWs believed personal hygiene, inspection of clients and self-medication would prevent STDs and HIV/AIDS; and fewer than 40 per cent intended to request their clients to wear a condom. Inadequacies are apparent with the HIV surveillance system and cases may be under-reported due to stigma and other sociocultural reasons. Nevertheless, complacency is out of the question. Increasing incidence of unsafe sex, low condom usage and a high TB burden make HIV/AIDS a disease priority. A potential dual epidemic must be averted at all cost (De Bevoise 1997: 130; Bosch 2003: 1; Philippine National AIDS Council 2005: 55–60).

## Responses to the double disease burden and key health system issues

### Government

The Department of Health has instituted reforms, as already noted. These programmes and policy frameworks have set the course towards safe, affordable and quality health care for all Filipinos. Attempts at stronger intersectoral collaborations between government agencies have been instituted so that health could be made a valuable component in the development goals of the country. Civil society groups springing from the business sector, non-government organizations (NGOs), independent and religious organizations and the academic sector have been involved in public health programmes to bridge the gaps in the public health care delivery system. How effective have these strategies and partnerships been?

Although the Philippine economy may have fallen behind the rest of her Asia-Pacific neighbours, over six decades overall health indices have incrementally improved. Reductions in mortality rates may have slowed down in the last decade, but average life expectancies have risen; basic health services have become accessible; sanitation facilities have achieved relevant coverage; and arguably the country seems to be producing more than enough health personnel for health care delivery. But many of these health workers leave the Philippines and work overseas (Department of Health 2009: 17–18; Galvez Tan 2005: 1–3; Ronquillo 2005: 16–17).

The most notable pioneering interventions in the public health sector are the establishment of a National Health Insurance Programme intended to achieve progressively universal social health insurance cover, the Generics Act meant to make quality low-cost medicines readily accessible and the "Sentrong Sigla" Movement designed to turn primary health care facilities into centres of wellness through the achievement of a number of quality operational standards. The Health Sector Reform Agenda became the first strategic framework to address the fragmentation of a devolved health care delivery system by instituting five complementary reforms concerning health financing, public health programmes, hospital systems, health regulations and local health systems implemented as a single package. The development of the National Objectives for Health (1994–2004 and 2005–2010), on the other hand, provided the first technical road map by which programmatic targets, indicators and strategies were set for the achievement of the country's health goals. The launch of *Four*mula One for Health in 2005 became the newest vehicle for instituting health sector reforms redesigned to be implemented with speed, precision and better coordination (Department of Health 2005: 1).

Programmes aimed at reducing the burden of communicable diseases include the TB-DOTS, CARI (Control of Acute Respiratory Infections), CDD (Control of Diarrhoeal Diseases), the Expanded Programme on Immunization for vaccine-preventable diseases and various control programmes for rabies, leprosy, HIV/AIDS, malaria, filariasis, dengue and schistosomiasis. The country's response to the global issue of re-emerging infections such as SARS (severe acute respiratory syndrome), avian influenza and "mad cow" disease was commendable. While neighbouring countries reported significant levels of morbidity and mortalities, the Philippines responded quite well by isolating and controlling its spread (Department of Health 2009: 177–178).

Instituting programmes to address the rapid rise of chronic NCDs in the country became a major challenge for the DOH amidst ongoing struggles to control infectious diseases. A Healthy Lifestyle programme was implemented to promote balanced diets and physical activity. Control programmes for cardiovascular diseases, diabetes, chronic respiratory diseases, cancer, kidney diseases, mental health disorders, accidents and injuries were also established. Database and registry systems were set up to keep track of noted degenerative and lifestyle-related diseases (Department of Health 2009: 181–204). While progress with tobacco control and anti-smoking advocacy has been slow over the years due to sociopolitical opposition involving rich landowners, tobacco companies and obstructive trade practices, significant strides had been made to limit advertisements on billboards. Today cigarette packs have clear warning labels, though graphic pictures might be added. Reduction in sporting and cultural sponsorships and tri-media exposure were huge steps. Hopefully, a total ban on advertisements and sponsorships will happen in the immediate future (Galvez Tan 2009: 13–14).

### *Private sector*

Civic organizations, NGOs and other stakeholders have taken up the cudgels for health. The League of Corporate Foundations comprising large and influential corporations practising Corporate Social Responsibility (CSR) has been regularly cooperating with the Health Department in the implementation of various health programmes and initiatives. The Zuellig Foundation, a non-profit organization, runs a health management programme for health sector development focusing on improving local governance for health in order to provide efficient and quality health services (Zuellig Foundation Inc. 2007: 1). Technical and financial support have also come from international aid agencies like the United Nations, International Committee of the Red Cross, USAID, AUSAID, Japan International Cooperation Agency, World Vision, Oxfam, Save the Children, Plan International and Deutsche Gesellschaft fur Technische Zusammenarbeit.

Several medical, nursing, health science and allied health schools have restructured their respective curricula to become more responsive to public health issues. A few schools have two to four year community based academic programmes with specific requirements that students from regional areas return after graduation to serve their home communities (Manalo 2000: 5–6; Romualdez 2009b: 1). Public health institutions have been conducting monitoring and evaluation studies to aid development of public health programmes. The Asian Institute of Management, in a joint collaborative partnership with the Local Government Academy – Department of Interior and Local Government, the Ford Foundation and various development agencies pioneered the *Galing-Pook* (a place or community) initiative to identify outstanding local governance practices which then can be replicated (AIM Policy Center 2007: 103–109; Galvez Tan 2009: 10).

Given these numerous strategies, the country's health picture appears promising. However, closer examination may suggest otherwise. The wealthier and better performing regions can mask the dire health outcomes of poorly performing regions such as the Autonomous Region of Muslim Mindanao, the Zamboanga peninsula, the Bicol region, Eastern Visayas and Mimaropa (National Statistics Office 2008: 1–25).

Although the Depatment of Health instituted various reform agendas, only a few LGUs apart from the designated pilot areas have effectively implemented them. This could very well explain the low performance impact of the health sector reforms throughout the country (Galvez Tan 2009: 7–12).

If devolution caused confusion about roles and responsibilities among LGUs, the national level was not exempt. The Department of Health was also unprepared for the change. Ironically, it felt it had lost power as it was no longer involved with programme implementation despite responsibilities that included setting regulatory standards, encouraging health promotion and human resources development.

With the devolved structure, donor agencies tended to bypass the national government and go straight to the provinces. However, the Department of Health believed that such funding had to go through national agencies first, and funding was only to be released after local governments complied with technical standards for programme implementation set by the department. Since health programme management had already been devolved to the local governments, the DOH may have felt ineffective in its new role simply providing technical assistance (Galvez-Tan 2009: 10–14).

The private health sector remains inaccessible to the poor and the public health sector that serves them can be inefficient with overcrowded tertiary hospitals and under-utilized primary and secondary hospitals (Dorotan and Mogyorosy 2004: 28–29).

The current health information system is relatively inefficient and requires restructuring to benefit provincial and municipal levels; for example, the National Demographic and Health Survey. It can be better utilized for development planning.

The national health insurance programme (PhilHealth) which was supposed to reduce inequity in health care financing unfortunately facilitates it. Institutions that serve wealthy clients receive the highest share of reimbursements. Employed PhilHealth members receive the highest benefits compared to sponsored low income PhilHealth members (Romualdez 2009a: 2).

A total of 60 per cent of Filipinos die without getting medical attention from a professional health worker. Most health care professionals prefer to work in urban areas; while the few village health workers and midwives are the frontline health care providers in rural health units. Unfortunately, many schools that produce health care professionals, especially nurses, train their students for export. These graduates are out of touch with the actual needs of the health care system and prioritize professional advancement over community service. In the late 1990s, as developed countries faced nursing shortages, active international recruitments took place offering very attractive conditions that the Philippines could never match (Ronquillo 2005: 17). At the turn of the twenty-first century, because of poor working conditions in government hospitals, limited opportunities at private hospitals and the lure of lucrative nursing jobs abroad, a substantial number of doctors switched to the nursing profession. On average tens of thousands of Filipino nurses leave the Philippines to work overseas annually (Galvez Tan 2005: 2–4). This personnel haemorrhage entails catastrophic consequences for the country.

## Looking to the future

### *Integrated approach to communicable disease control and non-communicable diseases*

A primary health care approach is necessary so that integrated, long term programmes can address the double burden holistically and rationally at all levels of care (Carreon 1982: 152–155; WHO 2008: 12–14). Short term, single disease-focused interventions do not work and lack a sense of direction. It is important to conduct background qualitative research to devise culturally appropriate and effective preventive and promotive programmes. Understanding health beliefs and health seeking behaviours among Filipinos is crucial to the success of a health care system (Auer *et al.* 2000: 653–655; Tan 2008: 1).

A study of health care practice in a rural community revealed that health beliefs were influenced by both traditional perceptions and modern medical views (Palaganas 2003: 106–127). In ethnic minority communities in northern Luzon, traditional and modern systems of health care co-exist. By working together, they enhance service delivery by establishing transparency and trust among members of the community. They could be models for the rest of the country (Yang-ed *et al.* 2009: 66–83).

### *Multisectoral collaboration and public health mainstreaming*

All sectors of Philippine society, even those not traditionally involved in health, need to be engaged. Departments of Trade, Education, Transportation, the Environment and Urban Planning, to name a few, all have massive impacts on health. Very little attention is given to coordinating strategies to gain maximal outcomes. Public and private coordination needs to be strengthened. Support for regulating bodies should be strong so they can do their job efficiently and without fear. Undesirable and unethical practices at different levels of health care delivery should be stopped. Genuine commitment to participatory approaches, transparency and accountability will be required.

### *Health personnel development*

That 70 per cent of all health workers are in the private health sector serving only one-third of the population who can afford to pay for their health care, while the remaining 30 per cent of the workforce take care of majority of the Filipinos too poor to afford private services is clearly an ineffective system. The loss of personnel overseas has exacerbated the problem. Social accountability must be pursued by medical, nursing, public health, dental, allied health, pharmacy and midwifery academic institutions. As most of the teaching and training has been directed towards working overseas, it is high time action is taken to review curricula, integrate primary health care approaches to make them more community relevant and produce culturally competent, multi-skilled graduates who will best serve the country's health needs. Concerted action by the Commission on Higher Education, the Professional Regulations Commission and all health professional groups will be necessary (Manalo 1996: 1–3; 2004: 1–5; Carreon 2007: 1–8; Romualdez 2009a,b: 1–2).

Alternative sources of health manpower may be considered. There has to be a stronger push for training, accrediting and integrating traditional healers (*herbolarios*) and midwives into health care delivery as they are the first line of choice for the majority of poor Filipinos and ethnic minority groups (Caragay 1982: 159–163; Yang-ed *et al.* 2009: 64–84). Public health undergraduate and postgraduate education has to engage a wider group of students from non-health backgrounds and, possibly, work with programmes in Social Sciences and Development, Law, Health Economics and Education.

A proposed National Health Service Act for all health professions, development of inter-professional, rural polyclinics, capacity building for and skills training of local health workers through high-level negotiations with foreign countries importing Filipino nurses and, possibly, finding a use for Filipino alumni overseas are only a few of the more feasible strategies that may be employed to solve the problem (Manalo 2000: 1–6; Bautista 2001: 25–30; Dayrit and Dolea 2005: 11–15; Galvez Tan 2005: 1–6; Ronquillo 2005: 16–19; Carreon 2009: 5).

### *Community, municipal, regional and national governance*

Elected local and national officials have to be educated in matters of health and development policy, and advocacy and implementation, so they can carry out their responsibilities free of the politics of patronage. Legislation focusing on health and development is urgently needed. Local government expenditure on health needs to increase. A health financing scheme that clearly benefits the poor and marginalized, and ends advantages for the "haves" has to be constructed.

There is a need for visionary, ethical, action-oriented leaders with transparent administrations committed to public health and education who can "negotiate and steer", not "command and control" (WHO 2008: 8–14). Solutions require innovation, lateral thinking and a bottom-up approach. Collaborations between LGUs can be strengthened by sharing best practice models and successful community strategies so these measures can be replicated and positive health outcomes sustained regardless of a change in government.

In the end, the efficiency with which any programmatic intervention can deliver its outcomes will depend largely on how well health systems are managed. Unless everyone – government leaders, policy and law makers, the private sector, health care workers, academia and community members – acquires relevant knowledge and skills, develops cultural competency beyond a token level and has the conviction to act expediently and respond effectively to the double disease burden, all past achievements in public health will crumble to dust and make dreams of a healthier future virtually impossible to realize.

## Acknowledgements

This chapter is the product of generous assistance from so many people and institutions that it is not possible to mention everyone: Secretary of Health Francisco T. Duque, Undersecretary of Health Mario Villaverde, Kenneth Ronquillo and DOH staff; at the National Epidemiology Center, Agnes Benegas and Eric Tayag; at the Health Policy Development and Planning Bureau, Frances Rose Elgo; National Statistics Office staff; at the Department of Interior and Local Government, Local Government Academy, Jean de Pano; Provincial Government of Southern Leyte; City Government of Olongapo; United Nations Population Fund; at the Zuellig Foundation, Kenneth Hartigan Go and Tony Faraon; Plan Philippines; and at the University of the Philippines, Ramon Arcadio, Nina Gloriani, Lucy Rabuco, Portia Marcelo, Delen dela Paz and Ruben Caragay.

## References

AIM-USAIDS (2008) *USAID Country Health Statistical Report Philippines*, Country Health Reports, Washington DC: Analysis Information Management Communication Activity and United States Agency for International Development.

AIM Policy Center (2007) *Pinoy Cities on the Rise: Philippine Cities Competitiveness Ranking Project*, Manila, Asian Institute of Management Policy Centre. Online, available at: www.policy.aim.edu/downloads/Publications/pccrp_2005.pdf (accessed 26 November 2009).

Auer, C., Sarol, J., Tanner, M. and Weiss, M. (2000) "Health Seeking and Perceived Cause of Tuberculosis among Patients in Manila, Philippines". *Tropical Medicine and International Health*, 5(9): 648–656.

Bautista, V. (2001) *Challenges to Sustain Primary Health Care in the Philippines*, Quezon: University of the Philippines.

Bellwood, P., Fox, J. and Tryon, D. (2006) *The Austronesians Historical and Comparative Perspectives*, Canberra, ANU E Press.

Bosch, X. (2003) "HIV Mystery in the Philippines". *Lancet Infectious Diseases*, 3(6): 320.

Caragay, R. (1982) "Training Indigenous Health Workers: A Philippine Experience". *World Health Forum*, 3(2): 159–163.

Carreon, G.G. (1982) "The Role of the Hospital in Primary Health Care". *World Health Forum*, 3(2): 152–155.

Carreon, G.G. (2007) "A Trio of Challenges: A Path to Constructive Social Activism". *University of the Philippines Newsletter Manila*, 293: 1–8.

Carreon, G.G. (2009) Interview on Double Disease Burden in the Philippines. Interviewed by G. Manalo, Sydney, Australia.

CIA (2008) *The World Factbook*, Washington, DC: Central Intelligence Agency. Online, available at: www.cia.gov/library/publications/the-world-factbook/geos/rp.html (accessed 12 November 2009).

Dayrit, M. and Dolea, C. (2005) "Human Resources for Health from a Global Perspective" in E. Garilao, M. Tolosa and A. Go (eds), *Health Intel Annual: Influencing Paradigms of Health & Governance*, Makati: Zuellig Foundation, 1–29.

De Bevoise, K. (1997) "A History of Sexually Transmitted Diseases and HIV/AIDS in the Philippines", in M. Lewis, S. Bamber and M. Waugh (eds), *Sex, Disease and Society: A Comparative History of Sexually Transmitted Diseases and HIV/AIDS in Asia and the Pacific*, Westport, CT: Greenwood Press, 113–138.

Department of Health (1997) *Health Sector Reform Agenda*, Manila: Department of Health.

Department of Health (1999) *Health Sector Reform Agenda 1999–2004*, Manila: Department of Health and United States Agency for International Development. Online, available at: www2.doh.gov.ph/hsra/hsra/copyright-pg.pdf (accessed 29 October 2009).

Department of Health (2005) "*Four*mula One for Health." Online, available at: www.doh.gov.ph (accessed 29 October 2009).

Department of Education (2008) *Basic Education Statistics Fact Sheet*, Manila: Department of Education.

Department of Health (2009) *National Objectives for Health 2005–2010*, Manila: Department of Health.

Department of Health and National Epidemiology Centre (2004) *The 2004 Philippine Health Statistics*, Manila: National Statistics Office.

Department of Science and Technology – Food and Nutrition Research Institute (2008) *7th National Nutrition Survey*, Manila: Department of Science and Technology.

Dorotan, E. and Mogyorosy, Z. (2004) "Let us Make our Local Health Systems Work", in C. Bodart and K. Obermann (eds), *Applied Research for the Health Sector Reform*, Manila: Department of Health and German Agency for Technical Cooperation, 1–127.

Dumogho, E. (2006) "Relevant Provisions of the Local Government Code of 1991". Presented at Comparative Study Tour on Local Government Administration and Management, Development Academy of the Philippines. Online, available at: www.pcij.org/blog/wp-docs/Dumogho_LGC_Relevant_Provisions.pdf (accessed 20 January 2010).

Emergency Disasters Database (2007) "Philippines Natural Disasters". Online, available at: www.em-dat.net/disasters/Visualisation/profiles/countryprofile.php (accessed 12 October 2009).

Galvez Tan, J. (2003) "The Elimination of Lymphatic Filariasis: A Strategy for Poverty Alleviation and Sustainable Development – Perspectives from the Philippines", *Filaria Journal*, 2(12): 1–5.

Galvez Tan, J. (2005) "The National Nursing Crisis: 7 Strategic Solutions." Online, available at: www.pcij.org/stories/2005/nursing-crisis-galvez-tan.pdf (accessed 29 October 2009).

Galvez Tan, J. (2009) Interview on Double Burden of Disease in the Philippines by G. Manalo and A. Umali, Manila, Philippines.

Grundy, J., Healy, V., Gorgolon, L. and Sandig, E. (2003) "Overview of Devolution in the Philippines", *Rural and Remote Health*, 3(2): 220–229.

Human Development Network (2005) *Peace, Human Security and Human Development in the Philippines*, Philippine Human Development Report, 2nd edn, Manila: Human Development Network, United Nations Development Programme and New Zealand Agency for International Development. Online, available at: http://hdn.org.ph/2005-philippine-human-development-report-peace-human-security-and-human-development/#download (accessed 6 December 2009).

Kanavos, P., Lim, J. and Pascual, C. (2002) *Philippines Health Policy Note: On Improving the Poor's Access to Affordable Drugs*, Manila: World Bank Human Development Unit.

Magno, C. (2001) *"The Devolution of Agricultural and Health Services" 2001 Report*, Manila: Social Watch Philippines. Online, available at: www.aer.ph/index. php?option=com_content&task=view&id=293&Itemid=65 (accessed 28 November 2009).

Manalo, A. (1996) "Rural Polyclinics: A Concept for Health Delivery to Provincial Areas Utilizing Private Physician Graduates of a Community Oriented Medical School". Unpublished paper presented at the Network of Community Oriented Medical Institutions for Health Sciences Annual Conference, Egypt.

Manalo, A. (2000) "Thoughts on Accreditation and Standardization of Philippine Medical schools". Unpublished paper presented at the Association of Philippine Medical Colleges Annual Convention, University of the Philippines College of Medicine, Manila.

Manalo, A. (2004) "The Doctors of Tomorrow: A Proposal for a Pilot Training Program to Provide Holistic 5 Star Doctors for the Philippine Countryside". Unpublished paper presented at a Strategy Meeting, University of the Philippines College of Medicine and Philippine General Hospital, Manila.

National Economic and Development Authority (2008) "Nutrition in the Philippines: A Continuing Challenge". *DevPulse*, 12(16): 1–2.

National Economic and Development Authority and United Nations Country Team (2007) *Philippines Midterm Progress Report on the Millenium Development Goals*, Manila: National Economic Development Authority.

National Statistical Coordination Board (2008) *NSCB Philippine Standard Geographic Code Summary*. Online, available at: www.nscb.gov.ph/activestats/psgc/NSCB_ PSGC_SUMMARY_2008Dec31.pdf (accessed 14 November 2009) and www.nscb. gov.ph/activestats/psgc/NSCB_PSGC_SUMMARY_2010Jun30.pdf (accessed 12 July 2010).

National Statistics Office (2008) *2008 National Demographic and Health Survey*, Manila: National Statistics Office.

National Statistics Office (2009) *The Philippines in Figures 2009*, Manila: National Statistics Office.

Ngelangel, C. and Wang, E. (2002) "Cancer and the Philippine Cancer Control Program". *Japan Journal of Clinical Oncology*, 32(suppl. 1): S52–S61.

Obermann, K., Jowett, M.R., Taleon, J.D. and Mercado, M.C. (2008) "Lessons for Health Care Reform from the Less Developed World: The Case of the Philippines". *European Journal of Health Economics*, 9(4): 343–349.

Palaganas, E. (2003) *Health Care Practice in the Community*, Manila: Educational Publishing House.

Pedro, M.R.A., Benavides, R.C. and Barba, C.V.C. (2006) *Dietary Changes and their Health Implications in the Philippines*, Los Banos: Institute of Human Nutrition and Food, University of the Philippines.

Philippine Health Statistics (2004) *Mortality Trend: Communicable Diseases, Malignant Neoplasms and Diseases of the Heart Philippines 1954–2004*, Manila: National Statistics Office.

Philippine National AIDS Council (2005) *Fourth AIDS Medium Term Plan 2005–2010*, Manila: Philippine National AIDS Council Secretariat.

Philippine National AIDS Council and United Nations Programme on HIV/AIDS (2008)

*UNGASS-Country Report of the Philippines January 2006 to December 2007*, Manila: Philippine National AIDS Council Secretariat.

Portero, J.L. and Rubio, M. (2006) "Multidrug-Resistant TB in the Philippines: Totem and Taboo". *Public Library of Science Medicine*, 3(12): e539.

Romualdez, A. (2008) "Universal Health Care for Filipinos". Presented at University of the Philippines Centennial Lecture, University of the Philippines, Manila.

Romualdez, A. (2009a) "Needed Changes in the Health Sector". *Malaya Opinion*, Manila: Malaya Press.

Romualdez, A. (2009b) "Reforming Health Workforce". *Malaya Opinion*, Manila: Malaya Press.

Ronquillo, K. (2005) "The Philippine Human Resource for Health Master Plan", in E. Garilao, M. Tolosa and A. Go (eds), *Health Intel Annual: Influencing Paradigms of Health and Governance*, Makati: Zuellig Foundation, 1–29.

Solheim II, W.G. (1981) "Philippine Pre-history", in G. Casal, R.T. Jose, Jr., E.S. Casino, G. Ellis and W.G. Solheim II (eds), *The People and Art of the Philippines*, Los Angeles: Museum of Cultural History, University of California: 16–83.

Solheim II, W.G. (1984–1985) "The Nusantao Hypothesis: The Origin and Spread of Austronesian Speakers". *Asian Perspectives*, 26(1): 77–88.

Solheim II, W.G. (2006) "Origins of the Filipinos and Their Languages". Ninth Philippine Linguistics Congress, Quezon, Department of Linguistics, University of the Philippines.

Tan, M.L. (2008) "Culture and Health". *Philippine Daily Inquirer*, Manila, PDI Press. Online, available at: http://opinion.inquirer.net/inquireropinion/columns/view/20081114-172102/Culture_and_health (accessed 26 November 2009).

Tupasi, T. (2006) "Multidrug-Resistant TB in the Philippines: Authors' Reply". *Public Library of Science Medicine*, 3(12): e549.

Tupasi, T., Radhakrishna, S., Co, V.M., Villa, M.L., Quelapio, M.I., Mangubat, N.V., Sarol, J.N., Rivera, A.B., Pascual, J.L., Reyes, A.C., Sarmiento, A., Solon, M., Solon, F.S., Burton, L. and Mantala, M.J. (2000) "Bacillary Disease and Health Seeking Behavior among Filipinos with Symptoms of Tuberculosis: Implications for Control". *International Journal of Tuberculosis and Lung Diseases*, 4(12): 1126–1132.

United Nations Development Programme (2001) "The Philippines Disaster Management Programmes". Online, available at: www.undp.org/cpr/disred/documents/publications/corporatereport/asia/philippines.pdf (accessed 24 October 2009).

United Nations Development Programme (2009) "Table G: Human development and index trends, Table I: Human and income poverty", in United Nations Development Programme (UNDP) (ed.), *Overcoming Barriers: Human Mobility and Development: Human Development Report 2009*, New York: Palgrave Macmillan. Online, available at: http://hdr.undp.org/en/media/HDR_2009_EN_Complete.pdf (accessed 14 December 2009), http://hdrstats.undp.org/en/indicators/74.html (accessed 14 December 2009) and http://hdrstats.undp.org/en/countries/country_fact_sheets/cty_fs_PHL.html (accessed 14 December 2009).

US Library of Congress (2006) *Country Profile Philippines*, Washington, DC: Federal Research Division. Online, available at: http://lcweb2.loc.gov/frd/cs/profiles/Philippines.pdf (accessed 17 December 2009).

Valenzuela-Tiglao, T. (1998) *A Century of Public Health in the Philippines*, Manila: University of the Philippines, Manila, Information, Publication and Public Affairs Office.

World Health Organization (2007) "Philippines Natural Disasters". Online, available at: www.wpro.who.int/internet/files/eha/tookit_health_cluster/EM-DAT%20%20Philippines%20Natural%20Disaster%20Profile.pdf (accessed 8 November 2009).

World Health Organization (2008) *The World Health Report 2008: Primary Health Care Now More Than Ever*, Geneva: WHO Press.

World Health Organization (2009) *Public Health Risk Assessment and Interventions: Tropical Storm Ketsana and Typhoon Parma: The Philippines*, Geneva: WHO Press.

Yang-ed, E.J., Samaniego, E.S. and Minger, J.G. (2009) "Health Practices and Beliefs among some Ethnic Groups in Benguet". *University of the Cordilleras Research Journal*, 1(3): 64–84.

Zuellig Foundation Inc. (2007) "Reaching the Community, Sound and Progressive Health Policy for the Filipino People, Makati". Online, available at: www.zuelligfoundation. org/v2/?s=zffhistory (accessed 10 December 2009).

# 14 The double disease burden in Papua New Guinea

*Vicki Luker*

Papua New Guinea does not fit the more usual profile of the 'double disease burden'. The phrase applies to developing countries that shoulder a growing load of 'new' chronic noncommunicable diseases (NCDs) in addition to the burden of 'old' infectious diseases (Marshall 2004: 556; WHO 2007: 14; WHO 2010a: 2). To use the World Bank's classification of countries into high, upper-middle, lower-middle and low income (though income is not the only criterion of development), this double burden is particularly pronounced in the 'lower-middle income' aggregation. Here about two-thirds of deaths are caused by NCDs but about one-quarter are still caused by infectious diseases, together with nutritional and perinatal conditions (WHO 2011a: 10). Today most of humanity lives in countries that fall within this income classification, which includes the first and second most populous nations in the world, China and India, plus fourth-placed Indonesia. It also includes Papua New Guinea (PNG).[1]

Yet in PNG, infectious disease predominates as a cause of sickness and death. Only in a small number of nations, mostly in sub-Saharan Africa, is this now the case (WHO 2011a: 9–10). Among the Pacific Islands states and territories, PNG's proportion of the national disease burden attributable to NCDs is also by far the smallest (SPC 2011). Indeed, the Pacific Islands region is experiencing an 'NCD crisis' (PIFS 2011: annex 2). PNG's weighting of the 'double disease burden' points to underlying conditions and processes somewhat different from those prevailing in most other countries.

The rise of NCDs is often understood in terms of the 'epidemiological transition'. According to Omran's classic formulation, populations move from 'traditional' demographic and health regimes characterized by high fertility, high infant mortality, low life expectancy, and death from epidemics and famine, to 'modern' regimes of low fertility, low infant mortality, long life expectancy, and sickness and death from chronic, degenerative diseases (Omran 1971: 509–538). According to Omran, transition in the West was driven by 'industrialisation', but the actual causes of 'epidemiological transition' vary in different circumstances and are much debated (Caldwell 2001: 159–160; Riley 2001: 6–31). In the twentieth and twenty-first centuries they seem broadly implicated in those catch-all processes of 'development' and 'modernisation', and a certain inevitability about 'epidemiological transition' is usually assumed. Yet PNG's modern history of health change departs in striking ways from this script and one should resist confident assertions about the future.

The challenges posed by NCDs to development have only recently been propounded with any force. Because NCDs tend to afflict adults, cause protracted ill-health and kill sufferers too soon (generally sooner in poorer countries), they diminish available human resources and strain families. Because the medical treatment of NCDs is long term and often resource intensive, NCDs make heavy demands on health services – which, in countries under the double burden, are also trying to reduce infectious disease. And partly because NCDs have historically been associated with rich people and rich countries – and in developing societies were noticed first among elites (Trowell and Burkitt 1981: xiv; WHO 2010a: 2) – recognition of their wide and widening spread among poorer people in the developing world was delayed. Global development agenda have generally concentrated on infectious disease. Thus the Millennium Development Goals (MDGs), launched in 2000 as an international framework for development, target the human immune deficiency virus (HIV), tuberculosis and malaria; the omission of NCDs has since been described as 'irrational' (WHO 2011a: 37).[2] Even in sub-Saharan Africa, to which the MDGs were fundamentally geared and where these three infectious diseases are so destructive, the hitherto poorly recognized extent of NCDs has been spotlighted and their imminent preponderance predicted (WHO 2011a: 9).

As this chapter will show, some of the archetypically modern NCDs have increased in PNG too. These are diseases routinely characterized as 'modern', 'western' or as diseases of 'lifestyle', and discussion here will focus on coronary heart disease, stroke, cancer, chronic respiratory disease, and diabetes. Although the list of 'modern' NCDs is longer, these five are usually emphasized in talk about the rise of NCDs in developing countries (WHO 2005: 36). Their intermediate risk factors are raised blood pressure, raised blood glucose, abnormal blood lipids, and obesity. Common modifiable risk factors are an unhealthy diet (too rich in fats and sugars and too poor in micronutrients and fibre), insufficient physical exercise, and the smoking of tobacco. Excessive alcohol consumption is stressed as a modifiable factor too (WHO 2005: 49; WHO 2011a: 19–20). Non-modifiable risk factors are age and heredity. Globalization, urbanization, and population ageing are often highlighted as underlying determinants (WHO 2005: 48).

Yet these modern NCDs are not widely based in PNG and there is a danger of overestimating them. Conditions may be even less favourable for their prevalence in PNG than in sub-Saharan Africa, to which PNG in some health contexts is compared. There is also a danger of misconstruing the 'modern'. Contrary to any preconceptions that infectious diseases are 'traditional', the greater burden of 'modern' disease in PNG is not in the form of the 'modern' NCDs (which are only a portion of the country's NCDs more broadly defined) but in the diversifying range of infectious diseases. These constitute a pressing and complicated impediment to development.

PNG's double disease burden does, however, encapsulate a perceived policy dilemma: whether to provide health services that meet demands for the better treatment of modern NCDs or to prioritise the needs for universal basic health. In practice, the two are difficult to reconcile in PNG's circumstances. Although the current national health plan, like its predecessors, vigorously commits to the latter, the former commands some de facto political advantages, discussed below. In conclusion this chapter reflects on the potential to respond in some measure through primary health to both chronic and acute conditions (terms not exactly synonymous with noncommunicable and communicable disease), while acknowledging the inherent limitations of medicine in producing improvements to the health of populations – in PNG or anywhere. But first, the scene must be set.

## PNG: the setting

PNG gained independence from its colonial administrator, Australia, in 1975. Comprising the eastern half of the great island of New Guinea, PNG dwarfs the other 21 state and territory members of the Pacific community in both land area (462,840 km$^2$) and population (*c.*6,774,955 in mid 2010) (SPC 2010). Most Papua New Guineans (87 per cent) live in small, dispersed villages and rely heavily on subsistence and cash-cropping (PNG 2003: 7). By international but not Pacific Island standards, PNG's urban populations are tiny. In 2000, the four largest cities were the capital, Port Moresby (with 254,158 people, now perhaps 350,000 or more), the port of Lae (78,692, now maybe 125,000 or more), Arawa in Bougainville (31,462), and Madang (28,547).[3] Infrastructure, including roads, is meagre. Government services often function poorly and have receded from many communities. Despite the recent, rapid uptake of mobile phones, many people still have little access to modern means of communication. Although revenues from extractive industries have enriched a few and PNG is embarking on a new phase of massive resource development (some describe PNG as 'a mountain of gold, on a sea of oil, surrounded by gas' (Chandler 2011a)) nevertheless poverty in many rural areas and among the urban disadvantaged is grave (Bourke and Allen 2008; Storey 2010: 5–8). No other Pacific Islands nation has a wider gap between rich and poor (Abbott and Pollard 2004: 32). The country's law and order problems are also widely publicized. In 2009, the United Nations human development index ranked PNG 148 out of 182 countries, just behind Kenya and ahead of Haiti (UNDP 2009).

PNG's health indices compare poorly in wider Asia-Pacific tabulations and are the worst in the Pacific. At 54.2 years, PNG has the Pacific's lowest life expectancy (PNG 2010, I: 10);[4] at 56.7 per 1,000, the Pacific's second worst infant mortality, while under five mortality is *c.*75 (PNG 2008: 7); and at an estimated 733 per 100,000 live births, PNG's maternal mortality ratio is exceptionally high – second only to Afghanistan's in the Asia-Pacific region (PNG 2010, I: 10, 11). Only 40 per cent of Papua New Guineans have access to safe water (SOPAC 2007: 8). Although the population has almost trebled since independence, in 2006 over 40 per cent of PNG's 2,633 aidposts (nearly all dating from the colonial era) were considered closed (PNG 2008: 8). In some provinces, the proportion is higher (PNG 2010, IIb: 45). The health of rural people, especially women and children, is worst affected. Although complete, basic vaccination has increased overall from 39 per cent in 1996 to 52 per cent in 2006, in some places the last immunizations were in the 1990s (PNG 2009: 117; Haley 2010: 222). Public health education is thwarted by many factors, including some 800 languages and generally low levels of schooling (WB 2007: 14–16). The 2000 census reported that 40 per cent of men and 50 per cent of women were illiterate, but functional literacy may be around 30–40 per cent (PNG 2003: 42; RN 2011).

The human geography and disease ecologies of PNG pose challenges of long-standing to human health. It can be useful to think of three zones: a coastal zone, where the advantages of generally superior protein supplies are compromised by malaria; a highlands zone, where the advantages of intense sweet potato cultivation and, until recently, the absence of malaria (now epidemic) were offset by scarce protein supplies; and a marginal zone, often on mountain sides, where gardening is difficult, protein supplies are scarce, and malaria is often present (Attenborough and Alpers 1995: 190–191; Denoon 1989: 11–12). Human biologists suggest that PNG populations have, over long spans of time (human settlement in PNG dates back 50,000 years or more) adapted to a diet low in calories and protein (Heywood and Jenkins, 1992: 261–262). Coastal peoples have also evolved genetic defences against malaria (Cattani 1992: 306–307), though this remains a major impediment to health. The infectious diseases that could persist in small human populations tended to be chronic – such as yaws and hepatitis B (Taylor 2008: 281), or skin diseases like tinea. Others (such as insect-borne malaria and filariasis) spend part of their lifecycle in other hosts or (such as hookworm) in the soil. Childbirth and infant survival everywhere were always risky. Wear-and-tear, injuries, accidents, septic wounds, and snake bite would always have been common causes of disability, sickness, or death. Nutritional deficits and occasional famine affected health and survival. PNG is also prone to natural calamities – earthquakes, tsunamis, volcanic eruptions, cyclones, floods, frosts, and droughts.

The influence of these old patterns and long-standing factors remain strong, but since the second half of the nineteenth century, when missions, plantations, and colonial administrations began operating in coastal locations, much has changed. Increasing interconnection within PNG and between PNG and the wider world enabled some infections already endemic in parts of the country to spread more widely while exotic infections from beyond PNG were introduced (Luker 2008: 254–257). These 'new' infections, whether from nearby or far away, initially caused many lowland populations to decline (Scragg 1977: 102–109; Ulijaszek 2006: 67–89). The existence of highlanders – then perhaps over one million people – was unknown to colonial administrations until the interwar period. But lowland and highland communities directly or indirectly affected by fierce fighting between Japanese and Allied forces during the Second World War suffered food shortages and wartime epidemics (Allen 1983: 218–235). After the war, when the process of integrating the highlands strengthened, antibiotics and immunizations, campaigns against malaria, and the expansion of basic health services contributed to substantial reductions in mortality and extensions of life expectancy (Scragg 2010: 71–75). Infant mortality fell to a national average of 100 in the mid 1960s (Bell 1973: 134). Nutritional improvements due to new crops and food imports as well as the capacity of modern agencies to mitigate the effects of some disasters probably helped lower mortality too (Luker 2008: 259–263). From the 1960s urban centres, mining and later logging enclaves, and the cash economy also grew, but development has been uneven. Much of the rural majority lags behind, large parts of the urban population are disadvantaged, while other problems, including violence, scarce money-making opportunities, and declining services have been exacerbated. Currently, the population is growing at 2.7 per cent per year (PNG 2003: 7).

A few points should be stressed about health data. In PNG, birth and death registration is very limited. Most health data derive from hospitals. Yet much sickness and death is experienced outside these facilities and the quality of hospital data is often open to doubt. Demographic and health surveys and other studies also yield information. Although it is common to hear that one condition or another is 'underreported', this warning can apply to most conceivable conditions. Some, however, are even less likely than others to be counted.

## NCDs

The modern NCDs have been virtually absent from PNG communities that depend on traditional subsistence (Sinnett and Whyte 1981: 171–187; Sinnett *et al.* 1992: 374–376). If urbanization is one of their chief determinants, unsurprisingly their risk factors were first detected in Port Moresby. Ian and Patricia Maddocks ran a clinic in the peri-urban village of Pari from 1968 to 1974: while infant mortality had declined, they found it difficult to conclude that the health of Pari's young adults, whose lifestyle shared 'many features in common with the life of the great affluent cities of the West', had improved (Maddocks and Maddocks 1977: 116). They noted several changes: less physical exercise; new energy-dense, processed foods; excessive alcohol consumption, particularly by young men; new kinds of anxiety and frustration no longer manageable through traditional ritual; and new patterns of marriage and parenthood, entailing tensions (Maddocks and Maddocks 1977: 115–116). Most conspicuous was the gain in body size by young adults: the Maddocks conjectured that 'the Pari population may be shifting from a weight pattern resembling that of rural New Guinea to one which is closer to that of the USA, and shifting at a striking rate' (Maddocks and Maddocks 1977: 113).

Obesity is now recognized, globally, as a major factor in diabetes, coronary heart disease, stroke, and certain cancers (WHO 2011a: 22–23). For decades, obesity has been seen as 'a major, if not *the* major' risk for NCDs in the Pacific (Coyne 1984: 93; Coyne 2000: 171–224). As early as the 1960s, increased body size in several Island populations had been linked with diabetes and coronary heart disease among other NCDs (Zimmett and Whitehouse 1981: 210–213). Today, obesity in the Islands is a problem 'too big to ignore' and some nations report extraordinary levels (Gill *et al.* 2002).

In PNG, the emergence of overweight has been noted in urban communities, especially Port Moresby (Maddocks and Maddocks 1977: 113; Martin *et al.* 1981: 192; Benjamin 2007: 163–171). A recent survey of 2,988 people (public sector employees, private sector employees, urban settlement dwellers, and the residents of a peri-urban village) found public servants were the fattest: 30 per cent were obese (PIN 2010: 6). Yet as that study suggests, obesity is linked with urbanized and moneyed minorities in a country where relatively few people are in waged employment – in 2000 only 15 per cent of men and 5 per cent of women were formally employed (PNG 2003: 56). That 'fatness' is seen as the attribute of the modern 'big man' – a sign of his power to consume whatever he desires (Gewertz and Errington 2010: 114) – corroborates this association.[5] Although diet has changed – Saweri traces a shift to rice, new crops and imported foods (2001: 151–163) – a strong reliance on garden produce continues, and chronic energy deficiency is likely more common nationwide than an energy surplus. Data from a national survey in 1996 indicated that 42 per cent of PNG's population failed to get 2,000 calories a day and that more women suffered a shortfall than men (Gibson 2001: 408, 410). In 2005, 18 per cent of children under five years were underweight for age (Countdown 2008), but unlike some other countries, including some Pacific Islands, where underweight children often grow into obese adults, conditions in PNG are not generally conducive to this result.

Mature onset or type II diabetes, which is increasing globally and is a bane of many Pacific Islands populations, has increased in PNG too (Zimmet and Alberti 2006: 1–3; Ogle 2001a: 81–87). In early 1962, when four urban communities with 'modernized' dietary habits were examined, diabetes was still very rare. The authors noted that in all four groups, despite increased consumption of purchased foods, overall calorie intake was still inadequate and concluded that more diabetes would have been detected if this was not so (Price and Tulloch 1966: 647). By the 1970s, admissions to hospital for diabetes had increased but were still few. Though 27 per cent of the male diabetics and 49 per cent of the females seen in major hospitals between 1974 and 1977 were obese (and most of these obese patients were from the capital), the majority were either thin or of normal weight (Martin 1978: 320). Patients presented late and fared poorly. Commonest causes of death were diabetic coma, gangrene, and infection (Martin 1978: 318). Further steep increases in diabetes were tracked in some groups over the next decade. In 1977, prevalence in Koki, a middle class suburb of Port Moresby, was exceptionally high: 15.6 per cent (Martin *et al.* 1981: 188). Within 14 years, diabetes prevalence among Koki residents had further doubled – to a level then the second highest ever documented in a population anywhere in the world (Dowse *et al.* 1994: 767–774).

Genetic differentials were initially thought to explain the extreme variation in diabetes prevalence recorded among different PNG communities. Thus many coastal Papua New Guineans, like the residents of Koki, who shared in the Austronesian heritage of Islanders in Micronesia and Polynesia, were thought more susceptible, in contrast to PNG highlanders regarded as purely 'Melanesian'

(Zimmet and Whitehouse 1981: 205, 219). However, the degree and length of 'modernization' appears to offer a better explanation. 'Modernization' came later to highlanders, but in 1985 outside Goroka, the capital of the Eastern Highlands Province, the first signs of glucose intolerance were detected within a highlands population (King 1992: 369). Subsequent studies of 'modern' highlanders in Port Moresby versus their more 'traditional' relatives in home villages identified higher glucose levels in the former (Kende 2001: 135). Among highlanders resident in Port Moresby attending health clinics, diabetes is prevalent (Benjamin 2001: 101).

A good estimate of diabetes prevalence in PNG remains elusive. For the year 2000, Ogle favoured an estimate of 181,000 people living with diabetes, equivalent to 7.4 per cent of adults over 20 years of age; but only 5,000 diabetics were known to health services (Ogle 2001b: 80). According to the current national health plan, only in Manus Province is diabetes among the top ten causes of hospital deaths (PNG 2010, IIb: 95).[6] The World Health Organization (WHO) estimates that 2 per cent of PNG's mortality is now attributable to diabetes (WHO 2011b: 146) – though WHO's mortality estimates are cited in this chapter mainly because they influence perceptions, not because they can be taken as accurate.[7] The survey of urbanized populations, mentioned above in relation to obesity, found that 8.8 per cent had hypertension (often caused by diabetes) and 14.4 per cent had diabetes. No single case of either had previously been diagnosed (PIN 2010: 6). But even allowing for undiagnosed levels and underestimates of hospital-based mortality involving diabetes, these figures are unlikely to represent the status of most Papua New Guineans who still depend on more traditional livelihoods.

Coronary heart disease (CHD), which ranks first or second as a cause of death in most Pacific Islands (Coyne 2000: 99), has also increased in PNG. The earliest case report of myocardial infarction suffered by an indigenous Papua New Guinean was only published in 1971, and around that time Powell remarked, 'Ischaemic heart disease does occur but it is very uncommon indeed' (1973: 355). Within 20 years, CHD in Papua New Guineans was observed more frequently. Of the 20 patients diagnosed with acute myocardial infarction at Port Moresby General Hospital from 1985 to 1987, Dr (now Professor Sir) Isi Kevau noted the following risk factors: urban residence, male gender, smoking, and diabetes; but hypertension did not seem significant (Kevau 1990b: 276, 278). The median age of this group was 45 and eight died – with a high in-hospital mortality of 35 per cent (Kevau 1990b: 278). While CHD has been noted among waged workers in the public and private sectors, in towns and development enclaves (Flew and Paika 1996: 1), the deaths of prominent Papua New Guineans from CHD have attracted public and political attention. In 2008, when the then Minister for Health and HIV/AIDS, Sasa Zibe, declared 'war' on 'lifestyle' diseases, he stressed that they had claimed hundreds of people in PNG since 1989, including valuable members of the nation's elites (Anon. 2008).

But how common is CHD among the bulk of PNG's population? WHO estimates that 21 per cent of PNG's mortality is caused by cardiovascular disease

(CVD) (WHO 2011b: 146) and in only four of PNG's 20 provinces is CVD missing from the top ten causes of death (PNG 2010, IIb: 53, 59, 71, 113). Yet CHD does not cause most of these deaths; nor do strokes, though doctors at Port Moresby General Hospital now deal with stroke patients every week (Lindeberg 2003: 273).[8] The main diseases of the heart, aside from congenital defects, are rheumatic heart disease and cor pulmonale. Staphlyccocal infection causes the former and repeated respiratory infections and domestic wood-smoke are factors in the latter. Most of the heart disease suffered in PNG does not conform to the stereotypical NCD syndrome on the 'modern' side of the 'double disease burden', where coronary heart disease and stroke normally weigh in so heavily.

WHO currently attributes 8 per cent of PNG's mortality to cancer (WHO 2011b: 146). But cancers typically regarded as 'modern', such as cancers of the lung (often linked to smoking), breast and colon (both linked to obesity) (WHO 2011a: 13) do not predominate in PNG, where the main cancer for men is oral and for women is cervical. The chief cause of the former is betelnut-chewing, and of the latter, the sexually transmitted human papilloma virus (HPV). Both cancers have increased with the spread of betelnut-chewing to the highlands and the wide transmission of sexually transmitted infections (STIs). Other common cancers are, like cervical cancer, also associated with prior infection: skin cancers tend to grow in the depigmented scar tissue from tropical ulcers; Burkitt's Lymphoma, a common childhood cancer in the coastal regions, is linked with infection by the Epstein Barr Virus, to which malaria has perhaps lowered immunity; while liver cancer follows hepatitis B infection, highly endemic and likely an ancient infection in PNG (and also a cause of cirrhosis) (Martin *et al.* 1992: 2949; Shann *et al.* 2003: 205; Taylor 2008: 281). PNG thus illustrates the pattern of cancers in low and lower-middle income countries where a larger proportion are attributed to infectious agents (WHO 2011a: 26). Of the archetypal 'modern' cancers, breast cancer is increasing, but is still less common than cervical and oral cancers for women, and not far ahead of liver cancer (Halder *et al.* 2001: 590; Moore *et al.* 2011: 101). Lung cancer, a leading cancer throughout most of the Pacific Islands especially among men, is rarely reported in PNG (Moore *et al.* 2010: 101, 102). The current health plan predicts cancer to increase with more people living beyond 65 (PNG 2010, I: 12).

Chronic respiratory disease (CRD) also figures in the top ten causes of hospital death in PNG provinces, fourth in Enga and Madang, fifth in Central and Oro (PNG 2010, IIb: 17, 29, 47, 77); and WHO estimates that noncommunicable respiratory disease accounts for 5 per cent of mortality nationwide (WHO 2011b: 146). CRD encompasses several conditions – chronic cough (without chronic airway limitation), chronic obstructive pulmonary disease (COPD), and asthma. Internationally, tobacco is a major risk factor – 75 per cent of COPD cases globally are attributed it (Aït-Khaled *et al.* 2001: 972). But Anderson and Woolcock could find no relationship between COPD and tobacco smoking in the PNG coastal and highland populations they studied, and indicated other possible causes, including domestic wood-smoke, repeated childhood acute respiratory infection (ARI), and domestic pollutants in thatch and other building materials

(1992: 293–295). ARI is a large problem in PNG, and most Papua New Guineans live in housing built of traditional materials and rely on wood for fuel.[9] The domestic house-mite may also be behind the surge of asthma (Anderson and Woolcock 1992: 298). Thus the character of CRD in PNG, as with heart disease and cancer, rather differs from that experienced in high income countries and much of the urbanized, developing world.

Some standard risk factors for the archetypically 'modern' NCDs are not yet spread widely enough, or for long enough, in PNG. Most people are dying from other causes first. Obesity is not as highly prevalent as elsewhere. Most people still need to exert themselves physically to survive. Smoking has grown in popularity since the 1960s (Temu 1991: 3–4; PNG 2010, I: 14; PIN 2010: 6) but has not started an epidemic of lung cancer, perhaps partly because tobacco's effects are still to unfold. Alcohol is a big public health problem (Marshall 1990: 101–117) but mainly for its role in morbidity, disability, and mortality from alcohol-associated trauma (Maddocks and Maddocks 1977: 112, 115) and for stymieing 'safe sex' necessary for preventing the spread of STIs.

Other risk factors that loom large in PNG have no profile in the global message against modern NCDs. Betelnut-chewing, for instance, is the biggest factor behind PNG's main cancer, of the oral cavity, but deserves more attention for that, and also for other direct and indirect health effects: on diet (through the suppression of hunger and the diversion of cash from other purchases), on cognitive development (in many parts of PNG school-aged children chew betel), and periodontal health more generally. Betelnut-chewing may also be a risk factor for diabetes and possibly other 'modern' NCDs (Benjamin 2001: 101; Lin *et al.* 2008: 1204–1211). While PNG's efforts to tackle tobacco or the importation of fatty lamb flaps are definitely to be supported and align with regional and international efforts to manage the risks for modern NCDs, locally significant factors can be overlooked, or seen primarily in relation to internationally major but locally less important risks.

Three underlying determinants proposed for modern NCDs – longer lives, globalization and urbanization (WHO 2005: 48) – warrant some reflection. PNG's life expectancy at birth, even on more generous estimates (not favoured by the current national health plan) that push it above 60 years, is still below the regional and global average (WHO 2010b, 1; PNG 2010, I: 10). Globalization, particularly of markets, has not yet incorporated, to a great degree, large sections of PNG's populace. In fact, some communities participate in less exchange with the wider world than formerly. PNG's urban populations, although they have grown absolutely and may now be set to grow more strongly relative to rural populations (Storey 2010: 2), are still small by comparison with cities in most other countries, while the urban proportion did not significantly increase over the 20 years to 2000.[10] Contrasts with sub-Saharan Africa are suggestive: there 37.23 per cent of the population (as against PNG's 13 per cent in 2000) is urban, and continues to grow apace (UN Habitat 2010: 242). Although infectious disease in that region still accounts, as in PNG, for most sickness and death, an urban base for NCDs is larger.

PNG's current health plan downplays the significance of modern NCDs. It states that hospital data show no real increase in these conditions (PNG 2010, I: 12). Although this position seems at odds with international and regional concerns about the mounting challenge of new NCDs, and advocacy within PNG to tackle these diseases (Temu 1991: 1–5; Anon. 2008; Vinit 2009), it is not inconsistent with assessments that have stressed PNG's very short history of halting development, the deterioration of the health system, and the stagnation or regression of key conventional health indices during recent decades (Thomason *et al.* 1991: 3–7; Connell 1997: 271–279; Attenborough 2007: 289–291; Luker 2008: 263–267). Under five mortality has remained largely unchanged (PNG 2008: 7). Infant survival rates fell in the 1990s before more recent gains (Duke 1999: 1,291; Duke 2004: 659–724). Estimates of maternal mortality have escalated, from a high 330 per 100,000 live births in 1996 to a giddy 733 in 2006 (PNG 2010, I: 10).

If the prevalence of the modern NCDs is patchy and overall low, still their importance must not be discounted. In countries like PNG they exact disproportionate costs to national development from the loss of scarce human resources embodied in educated minorities (McMurray and Smith 2001: 10–12). The disability or death of a money-earning adult from an NCD can set back a multitude of dependants, since those with a cash income tend to have many.[11] Modern NCDs also help draw attention to bigger questions of men's health and men's role in health because certain modifiable risk factors such as smoking and excessive alcohol consumption, are predominantly masculine habits while coronary heart disease affects men at a younger age more often than women. Almost 20 years ago Jack and Patricia Caldwell remarked that once countries attain a life expectancy in the 50s, and assuming that health gains to date are secure, the greatest scope for further extensions is in reducing premature adult mortality – especially male mortality (Caldwell and Caldwell 1993: 267–268) – but already in some Pacific nations, premature adult mortality from NCDs has slowed gains or even reversed life expectancy at birth by cancelling the effects of decreased infant mortality (Haberkorn 2004: 6). The youthful age structure of populations in developing countries also now offers an historic but brief opportunity to prevent emerging NCDs (Leeder *et al.* 2004: 15).

## Infectious diseases

The greater burden of PNG's 'modern' disease comprises not the 'modern' NCDs but the diversifying range of infectious diseases. These include exotic infectious diseases which had evolved in the 'crowd' conditions of other human ecologies and were introduced from the late nineteenth century, such as acute respiratory infections and tuberculosis (TB), as well as endemic infectious diseases, such as malaria, that have changed and spread through local developments since then. These three diseases alone – ARI, malaria, and TB – account for about one-third of PNG's morbidity and mortality. According to one study, in PNG malaria and pneumonia account for the most years lost to disability and death (the disability adjusted life years or DALYs that integrate measures of both mortality and morbidity (Lopez *et al.* 2006: 2–4) – followed by accidents and injuries, CRD, and maternal death (Izard and Dugue 2003: 21).

High mortality in PNG from epidemics of exotic, airborne diseases such as measles, influenza, and whooping cough, was observed early under colonialism (Riley *et al.* 1992: 282–285). Today no class of disease causes more hospital admissions or deaths than ARI. The chief killer remains pneumonia. In PNG it afflicts all ages including young adults, but is a leading cause of infant mortality. Half of newborn deaths in hospital are attributed to ARI, which is often a fatal complication of other airborne infections (WB 2007: 42). Because pneumonia has perhaps received less attention than it deserves as a killer in developing countries, important pneumonia research conducted in PNG since the 1960s should be mentioned. Researchers at the PNG Institute of Medical Research discovered the first penicillin-resistant strains, isolated the bacteria chiefly responsible in children and adults, and invented a vaccine that reduces morbidity and mortality – although this has not been adopted internationally (Riley *et al.* 1992: 283–286).[12]

Second to pneumonia as a disease causing hospital admissions and death is malaria. Though strains have been present in parts of PNG for aeons, from the colonial era malaria has spread to new coastal regions and into the highlands, and, following post-war control efforts, has resurged and diversified (Cattani 1992: 308–309; Attenborough 2007: 281–286). The World Bank reports that 60 per cent of Papua New Guineans live with endemic malaria, the remainder in areas of epidemic malaria (WB 2007: 42). In three of PNG's northern coastal provinces – Madang, West New Britain, Bougainville – malaria is the greatest single cause of reported deaths; in East Sepik, Sandaun, and East New Britain, it comes second (PNG 2008, IIb: 77, 113, 119, 83, 89, 107); while outbreaks in the highlands have increased in frequency and severity (Dapeng 2004: 135). Malaria tends to be lethal more often to adults subject to malarial epidemics and to small children (accounting for 7 per cent of child deaths (PNG 2008: 7)). It also damages maternal health (Gillett 1991: 71–80). Today the severer falciparum strain predominates and resistance to chloroquine is widespread (Hetzel 2009: 2). WHO finds no evidence of malaria decreasing in PNG over the period 2001–2008, but since 2003 the Global Fund has invested heavily in anti-malaria initiatives. The Fund's award of US$147 million to PNG for malaria work in 2009–2014 was the greatest outside Africa (WHO 2009: 138).

As a cause of death from disease, tuberculosis ranks third in PNG and accounts for 13 per cent of hospital bed-stays, more than any other disease (PNG 2010, I: 12). TB appears to have spread rapidly from the nineteenth century,[13] but despite colonial countermeasures, was never stamped out. It too has resurged. PNG currently has the highest TB prevalence in the Pacific. Each year, 16,000 new cases are reported, 1.9 per cent of which are multi-drug resistant (WHO 2011c). HIV is a contributing factor since TB is one of the main expressions of AIDS in PNG; but unfortunately TB patients are not routinely tested for HIV (in 2009, the HIV status was known in only 10 per cent of TB patients (WHO

2011c; PNG NACS 2010: 271)).The Global Fund's US$19 million programme to deliver TB treatment and prevention to 80 per cent of PNG's population by 2012 is not expected to reach target (IRIN 2010). PNG citizens, often with severe and drug resistant TB, are crossing the Torres Straits in dinghies to seek treatment within Australian borders (Chandler 2011b).

Diarrhoeal and enteric diseases and STIs also are leading causes of hospital admission and fatalities. In both categories, infections not 'traditionally' part of PNG's disease ecology predominate. Dysentery epidemics in the Second World War caused much fatality (Allen 1983: 218–215). Typhoid has become a major endemic killer since the 1980s (Passey 1995a; Shann *et al.* 2003: 373). Since 2009, epidemics of cholera, unknown in PNG since the 1960s, have swept parts of the country, prompting Australia to close its Torres Strait border in late 2010 (IRIN 2011; Elks 2010). Cholera, typhoid, and several other enteric diseases infect via contaminated water supplies and, more often, the faecal–oral route, frequently even where water is safe (Passey 1995b: 257–261).

PNG's most fatal STI is HIV, a global newcomer first identified and named in the early 1980s. It rides on a wave of other introduced STIs. Gonorrhoea was observed spreading from the late nineteenth century when men went to work on plantations, where women were few. Syphilis began spreading from the late 1950s following the wide suppression of yaws (which had provided some immunity) and the construction, in the 1960s, of PNG's main thoroughfare, the Highlands Highway (Hughes 1997: 238–239). The growth of extractive industries and, since the 1960s, urban centres, has been associated with other introductions (Lombange 1984: 145–147). While STIs (with the exception of HIV) rarely cause death, syphilis can prove fatal for infants congenitally infected (Frank and Duke 2000: 124), and some are disfiguring. Widespread female infertility is attributed to high levels of STI (Jenkins 1993: 79–81) while cervical cancer follows from HPV infection. But STIs, particularly ulcerating STIs, also facilitate the transmission of HIV (Passey 1996: 252).

HIV is now listed among the top ten causes of hospital deaths in five of the PNG's 20 provinces; fifth in the National Capital District and Eastern Highlands Province, sixth in Western Highlands Province, and ninth in Enga and Simbu (also in the Highlands) (PNG 2010, 11b: 23, 47, 53, 59, 65). HIV elevates infant mortality, but its effect on productive adults including those with professional skills is of special concern. From 2003 to 2008, 25–55 per cent of deaths recorded by the Nambawan Superannuation Scheme for public sector employees were attributed to HIV (CAP 2009: 49). Yet earlier projections for HIV in PNG, modelled on severe sub-Saharan epidemics, have not so far materialized.[14] PNG's first reported case was in 1987, and more than two decades later the estimated national prevalence is 0.9 per cent (UNAIDS 2010) – in contrast to say, South Africa, where prevalence rose from low levels to an estimated 12 per cent in the decade to 2000 (Dorrington *et al.* 2001: 21) and is now 17.8 per cent (UNAIDS 2011). Overall HIV incidence in PNG is said to have peaked, but the experience varies in different provinces, and the effects of resource exploitation over the coming years could boost HIV's spread. Owing to dedication and donor funding, 74.5 per cent of persons with advanced HIV who need anti-retroviral treatment are estimated to receive it (PNG NACS 2011: 6).

Other widespread infectious causes of sickness do not figure so prominently in hospital statistics, and fail to receive so much attention because they rarely in themselves cause death, are undiagnosed, or are accepted by sufferers as a normal part of life. Many number among the recently labelled 'Neglected Tropical Diseases' (NTDs), which tend to be chronic, often highly prevalent in afflicted populations, co-endemic, and major contributors to debility, ill health, and poverty, especially rural poverty (Hotez 2008: 5–10). In PNG they include hookworm, filariasis, and, to a much lesser extent, resurgent yaws. The latter can sometimes leave permanent disfigurement, hookworm and other intestinal parasites can gravely sicken children and impair physical and cognitive development (Barnish 1992: 345–354; King and Mascie-Taylor 2004: 181–191), and in some areas, filariasis is a major cause of disability (Bell 1973: 363–367).

The contribution of infectious diseases to disability in PNG is difficult to measure. Basic data on disability – a category variously conceptualized and encompassing heterogenous conditions, some permanent, others possibly passing – are lacking (Tnines 2010: 15–19; PNG 2005: 6). So the term is used here in its broadest sense. While leprosy and polio are considered eradicated from PNG, other preventable or treatable infectious diseases, including cerebral malaria, meningitis, measles, and chronic ear infections (Danaya 1999: 159–161; Veenstra *et al.* 2010: 209) often bequeath blindness, deafness, and other impairments. Malnutrition and infectious disease together – as in cycles of childhood infection and malnutrition (Lehmann *et al.* 1988: 109–116) – also retard development. Anaemia, due to multiple factors, including diet and diseases such as malaria and hookworm, is a serious health problem, especially prevalent among women (Gillett 1991: 60–64). Yet one in three men in PNG is anaemic too, and anaemia is among the top ten causes of hospital-based mortality (PNG 2010, I: 14).[15] Other causes of disability, aside from congenital factors, include complications during delivery (only 53 per cent of births are medically attended (PNG 2009: 112)), stark nutritional deficits (though less marked than formerly, iodine deficiency still causes goitre and cretinism (Heywood 1992: 355–362)), and septic wounds and trauma that lead to limb loss. While some recent literature highlights the global contribution of 'modern' NCDs to disability (WHO 2011d: 33), within PNG the contribution of infectious disease is huge.

Infectious diseases thus remain an enormous and multi-faceted challenge for PNG. They have diversified, fuel morbid and mortal synergies, are highly ramified in their effects (on NCDs too), and are in practice if not theory difficult to medically prevent and control. The gains against them are not secure, as many examples cited here have shown – including resurgent malaria, tuberculosis, and immunizable ARI. Nor is PNG exempt from the threats of new pandemics of infectious diseases, as inroads by HIV or recent concerns in PNG and internationally about global airborne pandemics indicate. While pronouncements about the MDGs can be glib and the goals themselves problematic, as the 2015 deadline approaches, PNG is utterly off-track. It is certainly not expected to meet the three explicitly health-related goals for reducing child mortality, improving maternal health, and combating HIV, malaria, and TB (UN 2010).

Returning to those determinants said to underlie NCDs – globalization, urbanization, and increasing life expectancy (WHO 2005: 48) – in PNG so far these seem to have done more to promote communicable disease. Thus globalization has established the networks and patterns of interaction that have introduced and reintroduced infectious diseases, which could not have evolved in PNG and which often could not be locally sustained without repeated introductions. Urbanization in PNG – if still on a relatively small scale – affords conditions for some communicable diseases to thrive and to be carried from towns to villages by circular migration. While cities figure in the recent rise of NCDs, they have a longer human history, highly pertinent to PNG, as 'spawning grounds' of infectious disease (Burnet and White 1972: 13). And although literature on NCDs and development often emphasize the vulnerabilities to them of the urban disadvantaged, Sims's study found most of the poor in his sample from settlements in Port Moresby died of chronic infections, especially TB and AIDS (2004: 194, 196). PNG's reduction in infant mortality from earlier levels may ironically have 'fed' infectious diseases that prey on adults, since more survive infancy to reach that age – a sequence noted in the health change of other societies (Riley 2001: 25)

In many parts of the world, health change diverges from Omran's theory of epidemiological transition, based as it is on Western Europe (Riley 2001: 24). Shortly before PNG's independence, Sinnett predicted that new NCDs would not replace infectious diseases, but just 'increase the total spectrum of disease with which the health services of this country will be forced to cope' (Sinnett 1973: 394). PNG's experience since has been described as a 'protracted' transition, 'with a mixture of traditional and modern influences acting together and with different parts of its society at different stages' (PNG IMR 2006). Looking forward, several researchers have speculated that both within the broader Asia-Pacific and within PNG itself, the epidemiological transition may have divergent endpoints (Ulijaszek and Ohtsuka 2007: 1–20; Attenborough 2007: 290–291; Luker 2008: 268). Attenborough has even warned against assuming that modern NCDs in PNG will ever outweigh infectious disease (2007: 290). Yet PNG seems on the cusp of a new era and resource bonanza (Callick 2011). Effects on development, epidemiology, and health services cannot be divined.

Looking back on PNG's version of the transition, distinctive features include its late integration with the modern world, its sudden but internally staggered transition into 'the global disease pool',[16] its sparse, dispersed, and to date relatively un-urbanized population, the patchy, halting, and uneven nature of development since independence, and the late colonial introduction of modern medicine (Luker 2008: 250–275). In other times or places, nutrition, sanitary engineering, environmental improvements, better education, a higher status for women, and influential changes in practices outside the strict domain of health services have contributed heftily to reductions in sickness and death from infectious diseases. In PNG, however, while nutritional improvements have played a likely part, modern medicine appears to have been pivotal in the health gains that have occurred. Although medical services at best are only one of many factors in producing better health population-wide, in PNG, partly by default, much continues to hinge on them.

## Back to basics?

Health in PNG is a state responsibility. Some mining and other companies, as 'quasi-states', provide health services to their constituencies. A small private sector caters to the elite, who often access treatment in Australia too. But the vast majority depends on state services provided through government- or church-run facilities. Overseas development assistance accounts for roughly one-quarter of total health spending (WHO 2010c: 347) and per capita funding for health has fluctuated mostly well below WHO's recommended levels for a basic package (PNG 2010, I: 15). Decentralization commenced before independence and has contributed to administrative disintegration (Thomason *et al.* 1991: 3–7). The health workforce is ageing, human resources are short, and most doctors congregate in Port Moresby (PNG 2008: 8; WHO 2010c: 348; PNG 2010, I: 15). Many facilities, including about one aidpost in three, are currently closed (PNG 2010, I: 14). Law and order problems have been a factor in some closures (Allen and Vail 2002: 4; PNG 2010, IIb: 45), and add to the difficulty of recruiting staff and accessing facilities –both by suppliers and patients. Despite population growth, the national health plan notes a downward trend in inpatient bed numbers and outpatient visits per person to health clinics, while village outreach visits that provide referrals, family planning, antenatal care, nutrition monitoring, and immunizations 'have stalled from an already unacceptably low level' (PNG 2010, I: 14). This fall-away in primary health services is reflected in health indices.

The 'double disease burden' in PNG encapsulates a perceived dilemma for PNG's health provision: whether on one hand, to deploy resources against infectious diseases, which is inextricable from primary health, or on the other, to improve treatment of 'modern' NCDs, which tends to concentrate in secondary and tertiary levels of health provision and prove increasingly expensive per patient. While wealthy countries too struggle to keep pace with demands to treat NCDs, the experience of PNG's Pacific Island neighbours, where the burden of NCDs is so much bigger, illustrates the cost and impossible difficulties (Khalegian 2001: I, 13–16; Doran 2003: v, 57–60). Some patients, as in PNG, manage to access treatment in the health systems of wealthier rim countries. Most do not.

The call for resources to go to 'modern' NCDs commands some political advantages. The international and regional agenda on NCDs is strengthening. PNG representatives must attend NCD fora. A ready-made international and regional discourse on NCDs can easily be applied to PNG, even if it may not accurately reflect local conditions. Politically influential citizens are likely to be more attuned to – and personally interested in – the threat of modern NCDs (Kevau 1990a: 271). Most health workers would prefer to work in, say, a coronary unit than a health centre in a remote village or urban settlement. And doctors and nurses want training and professional experience of an international standard (Kevau 1990a: 273).

In PNG, medical interventions taken for granted elsewhere are absent. Thus the operation of PNG's only radiotherapy machine, in Lae, has been intermittent since installation in 2004 (IRIN 2008; Nebas 2010). Pap smears for screening against cervical cancer are impracticable because PNG's ten gynaecologists are so busy with emergency and other work that colposcopies would waste their time and histological backup is lacking (FPI 2009: 17). While local capacity continues to be weak, overseas medical teams, on goodwill, charity, and donor support, fly in to perform procedures on a lucky few and then fly out (Anon. 2010: 8–9; Anon. 2011: 8–9). Yet even simpler services, for many Papua New Guineans, are unavailable or becoming harder to get.

Kevau acknowledged the dilemma in 1990: 'If a large portion of the health budget is devoted to the establishment of coronary care units, it is frightening to imagine what might happen to rural health services' (1990a: 271). In 2010, a proposal for a new tertiary hospital in Port Moresby provoked uproar. Opponents argued that it would suck resources from the government's commitment to rebuild and extend primary health (ABC 2010). And the national health plan, as its subtitle states, stresses a policy of 'back to basics' (PNG 2010, I: 1).

But 'basics' today have to be less basic. The 'spray gun' approach for dispensing antibiotics, quinine, and other medicines (Allen 1989: 61), which once worked so splendidly against infectious diseases, is no longer effective, partly because it promoted the evolution of new and drug-resistant strains. The immunization campaigns, which still promise to deliver the biggest and widest health returns on investment and can be designed to deliver other services too, must operate on a larger scale, with more sophisticated offerings, in greater logistical complexity, and often in less secure environments than before (Duke 2003: 1–7; Clements *et al.* 2006: 13). The 'maternal' in maternal and child health services was always a pitfall, but PNG's current estimates of maternal mortality indicate an abyss, while the spread of STIs, including HIV, together with continuing unmet needs for family planning (PNG 2009: 85), confirm the need for comprehensive sexual and reproductive health services. Demands on medical facilities for the treatment of trauma – which now accounts for 11 per cent of hospital admissions (PNG 2010, I: 12) – have grown as contributors to injury (cars, guns, alcohol, fighting, and domestic violence) increase. Infectious diseases and various other conditions previously sidelined, such as care for the disabled and mentally ill, are now on the global development agenda. And new diseases – both communicable and noncommunicable – have appeared.

But perhaps more illuminating than the contrast between communicable and noncommunicable disease is an older contrast between acute and chronic conditions. To paraphrase the reflections of a doctor back in 1968, in PNG this dichotomy is clear: whereas doctors can generally intervene quickly to save patients from acute afflictions and then return them to productive lives, 'What a different picture we see in nephrotic syndrome, cirrhosis of the liver, polyarthritis, chronic anaemia and cor pulmonale!' Patients of the first group are 'a shining example of the benefits of modern medicine', whose treatment is cheap and simple, hospital stays short, and requirements for maintenance therapy or supervision after discharge zero. But patients of the second group, who suffer chronic diseases, need protracted and often costly treatment, stay long in hospital, require supervision and maintenance therapy on discharge, return for repeat treatments, and often remain economically unproductive. '[T]he results of treatment', Douglas concluded, 'certainly inspire no confidence in the health service' (1968: 49). Thus the challenges posed by modern NCDs to health services are not new. They were posed before and continue to be widely posed by chronic infectious diseases, 'traditional' NCDs, and other disabling conditions, regardless of the modern NCDs.

Demands for treating chronic conditions in poor communities require a health response different from that launched against acute infectious diseases. They point to a basic need for sustained kinds of services, involving collaboration with patients, kin, and other allies, to promote prevention, manage care (more often in the community), and mobilize local resources. This basic need is recognized internationally for twenty-first century primary health, especially in low and middle-income countries (Beaglehole *et al.* 2008: 941, 943–945; Aikins *et al.* 2010: 4–5). It was unmet even in the hallowed days of late colonial and early independence primary health, a point that historian Denoon was at pains to stress (1989: 122). And many examples in PNG, including community-based projects for AIDS, point to integrative possibilities (Aggleton *et al.* 2011: 10–11; Reid 2010: 265–273).[17] The 'strong, cooperative and innovative partnerships' seen as imperative by the current health plan will also require of health workers on the periphery special qualities of commitment and human skill (PNG 2010, I: viii; Swartz and Dick 2002: 914–915). The challenges are myriad. But a restored, enhanced, and extended primary health system, with capacity to address both acute and chronic conditions, would hopefully better handle the multiplicity of PNG's disease burdens elided by the dualism of this chapter's guiding metaphor.

## Notes

1 'Papua New Guinea' or 'PNG' will be terms used throughout this chapter to refer to the area that now comprises the nation of Papua New Guinea.
2 Individual nations, however, have the scope to specify particular diseases as their targets.
3 The 2000 figures, from the national census, are given by Attenborough (2007: 257). Preliminary results from the 2011 census are not yet available. In the last few years, with the great expansion of the resource sector, the population of greater Port Moresby may have amply exceeded the figure given here (Callick 2011), while Lae too is said to be growing rapidly. Census-taking in PNG is difficult, and as Storey notes, urban populations tend to be 'best guesstimates' and often exclude informal settlements and periurban 'villages' further out (2010: 3). These communities, however, may have greater involvement in agriculture and husbandry (Storey 2010: 2), which can be a crucial economic difference from urban communities that lack access to land.

4 The figure cited by the PNG's current National Health Plan is for the year 2000. Other sources give higher figures (WHO 2010b) which might reflect some improvements in infant mortality rates over the last decade (Duke 2004: 659–724; PNG 2010, I: 11).

5 WHO estimates that in 2008, 16.2 per cent of PNG's population were obese and 48.3 per cent were overweight (WHO 2011b: 146). These seem implausible as national figures, as data from studies of body size in four locations, conducted 1999 to 2002, suggest (Benjamin 2007: 163–171).

6 The high diabetes mortality reported from Manus also correlates with the high reported levels of hypertension (Benjamin 2006: 137) and of overweight and obesity (Benjamin 2007: 163).

7 For a discussion of comparable problems, see Carter *et al.* (2010: 4).

8 Dr G. Tau, then Chief Medical Officer of Port Moresby General Hospital (PMGH), noted that in 2000 the most common cause for admissions to PMGH was infectious disease, but hypertension, coronary heart disease, and diabetes were addressed against this background (Naraqi *et al.* 2003: 8).

9 Of the 5,136,031 persons enumerated in the 2000 census, 3,722,932 lived in traditional and 305,621 in makeshift housing (PNG 2003: 79).

10 The urban proportion of the population in 1980 was estimated to be 10 per cent; 20 years later that proportion had only grown by 3 per cent (Attenborough 2007: 256).

11 Ironically, the costs of premature adult morbidity and mortality to families, communities, and national development were elaborately scoped with respect to HIV (Barnett and Whiteside 2001: 159–347), which in the 1990s and early 'noughties' overshadowed the growing problem of NCDs.

12 For personal accounts of this research, see particularly Douglas (2010), Riley (2010) and Alpers (2010). Other achievements of medical research in PNG are surveyed in Scragg (2010). While these research achievements typically bear on very prevalent diseases, the research that is perhaps best known, because it won a Nobel Prize, discovered the cause of the disease kuru, limited to the Fore people in the Eastern Highlands Province. For a full account, see Anderson (2008).

13 Though some believe it existed in PNG long before and only flourished under modern conditions (Wigley 1990: 167).

14 For instance, one influential report by the Centre for International Economics modelled possible scenarios for PNG on the experience of Kenya, South Africa, and Zimbabwe (CIE 2002: *passim*).

15 Where provinces report anaemia as one of the top ten causes of hospital mortality, malaria is invariably another of the top ten (PNG 2010, IIb: 17, 29, 35, 41, 71, 89, 95, 101, 107, 113, 119).

16 The phrase adapts the metaphor of 'disease pools' used by McNeill in his classic study (1979).

17 For comparable international examples, see Beaglehole *et al.* 2008: 944.

# References

ABC (Australian Broadcasting Commission) (2010) 'Prominent PNG Doctor Rejects Super Hospital Plan', *Pacific Beat*, updated 10 October. Online, available at: www.radioaustralia.nte.au/pacbeat/stories/201010/s3043756.htm (accessed 4 February 2011).

Abbot, D. and Pollard, V. (2004) *Poverty and Hardship in the Pacific*, Manila: Asian Development Bank.

Aggleton, P., Bharat, S., Coutinho, A., Dobunaba, F., Drew, R., and Saidel, T. (2011) 'Independent Review Group on HIV/AIDS: Report from an Assessment Visit 28 April – 13 May 2011'. Online, available at: aidsdatahub.org/dmdocuments/Independent_Review_Group_on_HIV_AIDS_2011_2nd_Mission.pdf (accessed 8 November 2011).

Aikins, A.de-G., Unwin, N., Agyemang, C., Allotey, P., Campbell, C., and Arhinful, D. (2010) 'Tackling Africa's Chronic Disease Burden: From the Local to the Global', *Globalization and Health*, 6(5): 1–7.

Aït-Khaled, N., Enarson, D., and Bousquet, J. (2001) 'Chronic Respiratory Diseases in Developing Couuntries: The Burden and Strategies for Prevention and Management', *Bulletin of the World Health Organization*, 79(10): 971–979.

Allen, B.J. (1983) 'A Bomb or a Bullet or the Boody Flux? Populations Change in the Aistage Inland, Papua New Guinea, 1941–1945', *Journal of Pacific History*, 18(3–4): 218–235.

Allen, B.J. (1989) 'Infection, Innovation and Residence: Illness and Misfortune in the Toricelli Foothils from 1800', in S. Frankel and G. Lewis (eds), *A Continuing Trial of Treatment: Medical Pluralism in Papua New Guinea*, Dordrecht: Kluwer Academic Publishers, 35–68.

Allen, B.J. and Vail, J. (2002) 'Health and Environment in the Tari Area', *Papua New Guinea Medical Journal*, 45(1–2): 1–7.

Alpers, M. (2010) 'The Pneumonia Research Program of the Papua New Guinea Institute of Medical Research: Its Beginnings and the Development of an Integrated Approach', in C. Leahy, G. Vilakiva, and D. Diave (eds), *Pneumonia: 40 Years of Research in PNG: Colloquium Magazine*, Goroka: Papua New Guinea Institute of Medical Research, 21–26.

Anderson, H.R. and Woolcock, A.J. (1992) 'Chronic Lung Disease and Asthma in Papua New Guinea', in R.D. Attenborough and M.P. Alpers (eds), *Human Biology in Papua New Guinea: The Small Cosmos*, Oxford: Clarendon Press, 289–301.

Anderson, W. (2008) *The Collectors of Lost Souls: Turning Kuru Scientists into Whitemen*, Baltimore, MD: Johns Hopkins University Press.

Anon. (2008) 'Health: Zibe Declares War on Lifestyle Diseases: Worrying Trend for Papua New Guineans', *Islands Business* (March). Online, available at: http://www/islandsbusiness.com/ (accessed 27 April 2011).

Anon. (2010) 'Paediatric Team Works in PNG: Fortnight in Papua New Guinea Highlights Needs of our Nearest Neighbour', *Surgical News*, 11(9): 8–9.

Anon. (2011) 'Passing on the Healing in Papua New Guinea: After Many Years of Helping Restore Sight to People in Papua New Guinea, Dr Michael Scobie is Reluctantly Passing on the Gauntlet', *Surgical News*, 12(1): 8–9.

Attenborough, R. (2007) 'Health Changes in Papua New Guinea: From Adaptation to Double Jeopardy?' in R. Ohtsuka and S.J. Ulijaszek (eds), *Health Change in the Asia-Pacific Region: Biocultural and Epidemiological Approaches*, Cambridge: Cambridge University Press, 254–302.

Attenborough, R.D. and Alpers, M.P. (1995) 'Change and Variability in Papua New Guinea's Patterns of Disease', in A.J. Boyce and V. Reynolds (eds), *Human Populations: Diversity and Adaptation*, Oxford: Oxford University Press, 189–216.

Barnett, T. and Whiteside, A. (2002) *AIDS in the Twenty-First Century: Disease and Globalization*, Houndmills, Basingstoke: Palgrave Macmillan.

Barnish, G. (1992) 'The Epidemiology of Intestinal Parasites in Papua New Guinea', in R.D. Attenborough and M.P. Alpers (eds), *Human Biology in Papua New Guinea: The Small Cosmos*, Oxford: Clarendon Press, 345–354.

Beaglehole, R., Epping-Jordan, J., Patel, V., Chopra, M., Ebrahim, S., Kidd, M., and Haines, A. (2008) 'Improving the Prevention and Management of Chronic Disease in Low-income and Middle-income Countries: A Priority of Primary Health Care', *Lancet*, 372(13 September): 940–949.

Bell, C.O. (1973) 'Filariasis', in C.O. Bell (ed.), *The Diseases and Health Services of Papua New Guinea*, Port Moresby: Department of Health, 363–367.

Benjamin, A.L. (2001) 'Community Screening for Diabetes in the National Capital District, Papua New Guinea: Is Betelnut Chewing a Risk Factor for Diabetes?' *Papua New Guinea Medical Journal*, 44(3–4): 101–107.

Benjamin, A.L. (2006) 'Community Screening for High Blood Pressure among Adults in Urban and Rural Papua New Guinea?' *Papua New Guinea Medical Journal*, 49(3–4): 137–146.

Benjamin, A.L. (2007) 'Body Size of Papua New Guineans: A Comparison of the Body Mass Index of Adults in Selected Urban and Rural Areas of Papua New Guinea', *Papua New Guinea Medical Journal*, 50(3–4): 163–171.

Bourke, M. and Allen, B. (2008) 'Poverty in Rural Papua New Guinea', Powerpoint presentation, Research School of Pacific and Asian Studies, Australian National University, Canberra, 3 July.

Burnet, F. and White, D.O. (1972) *Natural History of Infectious Disease*, London: Cambridge University Press.

Caldwell, J.C. (2001) 'Population Health in Transition', *Bulletin of the World Health Organization*, 79(2): 159–160.

Caldwell, J.C. and Caldwell, P. (1993) 'Roles of Women, Families and Communities in Providing Health Services in Developing Countries', in J.N. Gribble and S.H. Preston (eds), *The Epidemiological Transition: Policy and Planning Implications for Developing Countries*, Washington, DC: National Academy Press, 352–371.

Callick, R. (2011) 'PNG is on the Cusp of an Extraordinary Economic, Social and Political Expansion', *Weekend Australian*, 26–27 March.

CAP (Commission on AIDS in the Pacific) (2009) *Turning the Tide: An OPEN Strategy for a Response to AIDS in the Pacific*, Suva: Commission on AIDS in the Pacific.

Carter, K., Rao, C., Taylor, R., and Lopez, A. (2010) 'Routine Mortality and Cause of Death Reporting and Analysis in Seven Pacific Island Countries', Health Information Systems Knowledge Hub, Documentation Note Series No. 8, School of Population Health, University of Queensland.

Cattani, J. (1992) 'The Epidemiology of Malaria in Papua New Guinea', in R.D. Attenborough and M.P. Alpers (eds), *Human Biology in Papua New Guinea: The Small Cosmos*, Oxford: Clarendon Press, 302–312.

Chandler, J. (2011a) 'Papua New Guinea Teeters on a Wide Political Faultline', *Sydney Morning Herald*, 3 September.

Chandler, J. (2011b) 'Aid Failing to Prevent PNG's Health Catastrophe', *Sydney Morning Herald*, 9 September.

CIE (Centre for International Economics) (2002) 'Potential Economic Impacts of an HIV/AIDS Epidemic in Papua New Guinea'. Online, available at: www.ausaid.gov.au/publications/pdf/hivaids_png.pdf (accessed 14 May 2002).

Clements, C.J., Morgan, C., Posanai, E., Polume, H., and Sakamoto, C. (2006) 'A Qualitative Evaluation of the Immunization Program in Papua New Guinea', *Papua New Guinea Medical Journal*, 49(1–2): 5–13.

Connell, J. (1997) 'Health in Papua New Guinea: A Decline in Development', *Australian Geographical Studies*, 35(3): 271–279.

Countdown to 2015 (2008) 'Papua New Guinea'. Online, available at: www.countdown-2015mnch.org/documents/countryprofiles/papua_new_guinea_20080311.pdf (accessed 26 April 2011).

Coyne, T. (1984) *The Effect of Modernisation and Western Diet on the Health of Pacific Island Populations*, Noumea: Secretariat of the Pacific Community.

Coyne, T. (2000) *Lifestyle Diseases in Pacific Communities*, Noumea: Secretariat of the Pacific Community.

Crosby, A.W. (1997) 'Papua New Guinea, its Demographic History and Infectious Diseases', in H.J. Hiery and J.M. MacKenzie (eds), *European Impact and Pacific Influence: British and German Colonial Policy in the Pacific Islands and the Indigenous Response*, London: I.B. Tauris Publishers, 151–167.

Danaya, R.T. (1995) 'Childhood Disabilities in Papua New Guinea', *Papua New Guinea Medical Journal*, 38(3): 159–162.

Dapeng, L. (2004) 'Editorial: Malaria Epidemics in the Highlands of Papua New Guinea', *Papua New Guinea Medical Journal*, 47(3–4): 135–137.

Denoon, D. (with Dugan, K. and Marshall, L.) (1989) *Public Health in Papua New Guinea: Medical Possibility and Social Constraint, 1884–1984*, Cambridge: Cambridge University Press.

Doran, C. (2003) 'Economic Impact Assessment of Non-communicable Diseases on Hospital Resources in Tonga, Vanuatu and Kiribati', Report funded under the Pacific Action for Health Project, Secretariat of the Pacific Community and AusAID (unpublished).

Dorrington, R., Bourne, D., Bradshaw, D., Laubscher, R., and Timaeus, I.M. (2001) 'The Impact of HIV/AIDS on Adult Mortality in South Africa', Technical Report, [Capetown]: Burden of Disease Research Unit, South African Medical Research Council.

Douglas, B. (2010) 'Pneumonia in Papua New Guinea and the Licensure of Pneumococcal Polysaccharide Vaccines 1967–1990', in C. Leahy, G. Vilakiva, and D. Diave (eds), *Pneumonia: 40 Years of Research in PNG: Colloquium Magazine*, Goroka: Papua New Guinea Institute of Medical Research, 12–15.

Douglas, R.M. (1968) 'Legitimate Objectives in the Management of Chronic Disease in Papua and New Guinea', *Papua and New Guinea Medical Journal*, 11(2): 49–51.

Dowse, G.K., Spark, R.A., Mavo, B., Hodge, A.M., Erasmus, R.T., Gawlimu, M., Knight, L.T., Koki, G., and Zimmet, P.Z. (1994) 'Extraordinary Prevalence of Non-insulin-dependent Diabetes Mellitus and Bimodal Plasma Glucose Distribution in the Wanigela People of Papua New Guinea', *Medical Journal of Australia*, 160(12): 767–774.

Duke, T. (1999) 'Decline in Child Health in Rural Papua New Guinea', *Lancet*, 354(9 October): 1,291–1,294.

Duke, T. (2003) 'The Crisis of Measles and the Need to Expand the Ways of Delivering Vaccines in Papua New Guinea', *Papua New Guinea Medical Journal*, 46(1–2): 1–7.

Duke, T. (2004) 'Slow but Steady Progress in Child Health in Papua New Guinea', *Journal of Paediatrics and Child Health*, 40(12): 659–724.

Elks, S. (2010) 'Border Sealed against Cholera from PNG', *The Australian*, 25 November.

Flew, S.J. and Paika, R.L. (1996) 'Health and Major Resource Developments in Papua New Guinea: Pot of Gold or Can of Worms at the End of the Rainbow?' *Papua New Guinea Medical Journal*, 39(1): 1–5.

FPI (Family Planning International) (2009) 'Cervical Cancer in the Pacific', Discussion Paper. Online, available at: www.fpi.org.nz/info_resources/submissions (accessed 8 November 2011).

Frank, D. and Duke, T. (2000) 'Congenital Syphilis at Goroka Base Hospital: Incidence, Clinical Features and Risk Factors for Mortality', *Papua New Guinea Medical Journal*, 43(1–2): 121–126.

Gewertz, D. and Errington, F. (2010) *Cheap Meats: Flap Food Nations in the Pacific Islands*, Berkeley, CA: University of California Press.

Gibson, J. (2001) 'The Nutritional Status of PNG's Population', in R.M. Bourke, M.G. Allen, and J.G. Salisbury (eds), *Food Security for Papua New Guinea*, Canberra: Australian Centre for International Agricultural Research, 407–413.

Gill, T., Hughes, R., Tunidau-Schultz, J., Nishida, C., Gauden, G., and Cavilli-Sforza, T. (2002) *Obesity in the Pacific: Too Big to Ignore*, Noumea: Secretariat of the Pacific Community.

Gillett, J.E. (1991) *The Health of Women in Papua New Guinea*, Goroka: Papua New Guinea Institute of Medical Research.

Haberkorn, G. (2004) 'Current Pacific Population Dynamics and Recent Trends', SPC Demography/Population programme, July. Online, available at: www.spc.int/demog/en/stats/2004/ (accessed 16 September 2005).

Halder, A., Morewya, J., and Watters, D.A. (2001) 'Rising Incidence of Breast Cancer in Papua New Guinea', *ANZ Journal of Surgery*, 71(10): 590–593.

Haley, N. (2010) 'Witchcraft, Torture and HIV', in Vicki Luker and Sinclair Dinnen (eds), *Civic Insecurity: Law, Order and HIV in Papua New Guinea*, Canberra: ANU E Press, 219–235.

Hetzel, M.W. (2009) 'An Integrated Approach to Malaria Control in Papua New Guinea', *Papua New Guinea Medical Journal*, 52 (1–2): 1–7

Heywood, P. (1992) 'Iodine-deficiency Disorders in Papua New Guinea', in R.D. Attenborough and M.P. Alpers (eds), *Human Biology in Papua New Guinea: The Small Cosmos*, Oxford: Clarendon Press, 355–372.

Heywood, P.F. and Jenkins, C. (1992) 'Human Nutrition in Papua New Guinea', in R.D. Attenborough and M.P. Alpers (eds), *Human Biology in Papua New Guinea: The Small Cosmos*, Oxford: Clarendon Press, 249–267.

Hotez, P.J. (2008) *Forgotten People, Forgotten Diseases: The Neglected Tropical Diseases and their Impact on Global Health and Development*, Washington, DC: ASM Press.

Howden, G.F. (1984) 'The Cariostatic Effect of Betel Nut Chewing', *Papua New Guinea Medical Journal*, 27(3–4): 123–131.

Hughes, J. (1997) 'A History of Sexually Transmitted Infections in Papua New Guinea', in M. Lewis, S. Bamber, and M. Waugh (eds), *Sex, Disease, and Society: A Comparative History of Sexually Transmitted Diseases and HIV/AIDS in Asia and the Pacific*, Westport CT: Greenwood Press, 231–248.

IRIN (UN Office for the Coordination of Humanitarian Affairs) (2008) 'Papua New Guinea: Health Services Fail to Cope with Cancer Increase', 11 November. Online, available at: www.irinnews.org/Report.aspx?ReportID=81396 (accessed 26 April 2011).

IRIN (UN Office for the Coordination of Humanitarian Affairs) (2010) 'Papua New Guinea: MDR-TB an Emerging "|Health Emergency"', 16 November. Online, available at: www.irinnews.org/Report.aspx?ReportID=91096 (accessed 29 March 2011).

IRIN (UN Office for the Coordination of Humanitarian Affairs) (2011) 'Papua New Guinea: Cholera "Going from Bad to Worse"', 5 February. Online, available at: www.irinnews.org/Report.aspx?Reportid=88011 (accessed 30 October 2011).

Izard, J. and Dugue, M. (2003) *Moving Toward a Sector-wide Approach: Papua New Guinea: The Health Sector Development Program Experience*, Manila: Asian Development Bank.

Jenkins. C. (1993) 'Fertility and Infertility in Papua New Guinea', *American Journal of Human Biology*, 5(1): 75–83.

Kende, M. (2001) 'Superiority of Traditional Village Diet and Lifestyle in Minimising Cardiovascular Disease Risk in Papua New Guineans', *Papua New Guinea Medical Journal*, 44(3–4): 135–150.

Kevau, I.H. (1990a) 'Cardiology in Papua New Guinea in the Twenty-First Century', *Papua New Guinea Medical Journal*, 33(4): 271–274.

Kevau, I.H. (1990b) 'Clinical Documentation of Twenty Cases of Acute Myocardial Infarction in Papua New Guineans', *Papua New Guinea Medical Journal*, 33(4): 275–278.

Khaleghian, P. (2001) 'Non Communicable Diseases in Pacific Island Countries: Disease Burden, Economic Cost and Policy Options', Report prepared for the Secretariat of the Pacific Community and the World Bank (unpublished).

King, H. (1992) 'The Epidemiology of Diabetes Mellitus in Papua New Guinea and the Pacific: Adverse Consequences of Natural Selection in the Face of Sociocultural Change', in R.D. Attenborough and M.P. Alpers (eds), *Human Biology in Papua New Guinea: The Small Cosmos*, Oxford: Clarendon Press, 363–372.

King, S.E. and Mascie-Taylor, C.G.N. (2004) '*Strongyloides Fuelleborni Kellyi* and other Intestinal Helminths in Children from Papua New Guinea: Associations with Nutritional Status and Socioeconomic Factors', *Papua New Guinea Medical Journal*, 47(3–4): 181–191.

Leeder, S., Raymond, S., and Greenberg, H. (2004) *A Race against Time: The Challenge of Cardiovascular Disease in Developing Economies*, New York: Center for Global Health and Economic Development, Columbia University.

Lehmann, D., Howard, P., and Heywood, P. (1988) 'Nutrition and Morbidity: Acute Lower Respiratory Tract Infections, Diarrhoea and Malaria', *Papua New Guinea Medical Journal*, 31(2): 109–116.

Lin, W.Y., Chiu, T.Y., Lee, L.T., Lin, C.C., Huang, C.Y., and Huang, K.C. (2008) 'Betel Nut Chewing is Associated with Increased Risk of Cardiovascular Disease and All-cause Mortality in Taiwanese Men', *American Journal of Clinical Nutrition*, 87(5): 1,204–1,211.

Lindeberg, S. (2003) 'Stroke in Papua New Guinea', *Lancet Neurology*, 2(5): 273.

Lombange, C.K. (1984) 'Trends in Sexually Transmitted Disease Incidence in Papua New Guinea', *Papua New Guinea Medical Journal*, 27(3–4): 145–157.

Lopez, A.D., Mathers, C.D., Ezzati, M., Jamison, D.T., and Murray, C.J.L. (2006) 'Measuring the Global Burden of Disease and Risk Factors, 1990–2001', in A.D. Lopez, C.D. Mathers, M. Ezzati, D.T. Jamison, and C.J.L. Murray (eds), *Global Burden of Disease and Risk Factors*, New York: Oxford University Press and the World Bank, 1–13.

Luker, V. (2008) 'Papua New Guinea: Epidemiological Transition, Public Health and the Pacific', in M.J. Lewis and K.L. MacPherson (eds), *Public Health in Asia and the Pacific: Historical and Comparative Perspectives*, London: Routledge, 250–275.

McMurray, C. and Smith, R. (2001) *Diseases of Globalization: Socioeconomic Transitions and Health*, London: Earthscan.

McNiell, W.H. (1979) *Plagues and Peoples*, Harmondsworth: Penguin Books.

Maddocks, D.L. and Maddocks, I. (1977) 'The Health of Young Adults in Pari Village', *Papua New Guinea Medical Journal*, 20(3): 110–116.

Marshall, M. (1990) 'Alcohol as a Public Health Problem in Papua New Guinea', in B.G. Burton-Bradley (ed.), *A History of Medicine in Papua New Guinea: Vignettes from an Earlier Period*, Kingsgrove, NSW: Australasian Medical Publishing Company, 101–117.

Marshall, S.J. (2004) 'Developing Countries face Double Burden of Disease', *Bulletin on the World Health Organization*, 82(7): 556.

Martin, F.I.R. (1978) 'The Clinical Characteristics of Diabetes Mellitus in Papua New Guinea', *Papua New Guinea Medical Journal*, 21(4): 317–322.

Martin, F.I.R., Wyatt, G.B., Griew, A.R., Mathews, J.D., and Campbell, D.G. (1981) 'Diabetic Surveys in Papua New Guinea: Results and Implications', *Papua New Guinea Medical Journal*, 24(3): 188–194.

Martin, W.M.C., Sengupta, S.K., Murthy, D.P., and Barua, D.L. (1992) 'The Spectrum of Cancer in Papua New Guinea: An Analysis based on the Cancer Registry 1979–1988', *Cancer*, 70(12): 2,942–2,950.

Moore, M.A., Bauman, F., Foliaki, S., Goodman, M.T., Haddock, R., Maraka, R., Koroivueta, J., Roder, D., Vinit, T., Whippy, H.J.D., and Sobue, T. (2010) 'Cancer Epidemiology in the Pacific Islands: Past, Present and Future', *Asian Pacific Journal of Cancer Prevention*, 11(suppl. 2): 99–106.

Naraqi, S., Feling, B., and Leeder, S.R. (2003) 'Disease and Death in Papua New Guinea: Infectious Diseases are still the Dominating Cause of Death', *Medical Journal of Australia*, 178(1): 7–8.

Nebas, F. (2011) 'Cancer Patients Dying! Six Dead as Cancer Treatment Centre Sits Idle at Angau Hospital', *Post Courier*, 2 July.

Ogle, G.D. (2001a) 'Type 2 Diabetes Mellitus in Papua New Guinea: An Historical Perspective', *Papua New Guinea Medical Journal*, 44(3–4): 81–87.

Ogle, G.D. (2001b) 'Editorial: Diabetes in Papua New Guinea', *Papua New Guinea Medical Journal*, 44(3–4): 79–80.

Omran, A.R. (1971) 'The Epidemiological Transition: A Theory of the Epidemiology of Population Change', *Milbank Memorial Fund Quarterly*, 49(4): 509–538.

Passey, M. (1995a) 'The New Problem of Typhoid Fever in Papua New Guinea: How do We Deal with It?' *Papua New Guinea Medical Journal*, 38(4): 300–304.

Passey, M. (1995b) 'Social and Ecological Considerations in the Prevention of Enteric Infections', *Papua New Guinea Medical Journal*, 38(4): 257–261.

Passey, M. (1996) 'Issues in the Management of Sexually Transmitted Diseases in Papua New Guinea', *Papua New Guinea Medical Journal*, 39(3): 252–260.

PIFS (Pacific Islands Forum Secretariat) (2011) Forum Leaders' Statement on Non-Communicable Diseases, Annex 2, Forum Communique, 42nd Pacific Islands Forum, Auckland, New Zealand, 7–8 September. Online, available at: http://forum.forumsec.org/pages.cfm/newsroom/press-statements/2011/forum-communique-42nd-pif-auckland-new-zealand.html (accessed 19 September 2011).

PIN (2010) 'Time is Running Out: Papua New Guinea', *PIN Pacific Islands NCDs*, October: 6.

PNG (Papua New Guinea) (2003) *National Census 2000: National Report*, Port Moresby: National Statistical Office.

PNG (Papua New Guinea) (2005) *Papua New Guinea National Policy on Disability*, Port Moresby: Department for Community Development.

PNG (Papua New Guinea) (2008) 'Child Health Plan 2008–2015'. Online, available at: www.adi.org/upload/PNG_Child_Health_Plan_2008–2015.pdf (accessed 8 November 2011).

PNG (Papua New Guinea) (2009) *Demographic and Health Survey 2006: National Report*, Port Moresby: National Statistical Office.

PNG (Papua New Guinea) (2010) *National Health Plan 2011–2020: Transforming our Health System towards Vision 2050*, 2 Vols, Waigani: National Department of Health.

PNG IMR (Papua New Guinea Institute of Medical Research) (2006) 'Modernisation

Diseases'. Online, available at: www.pngimr.org.pg/disease_of_modernization.htm (accessed 19 November 2006).

PNG NACS (Papua New Guinea AIDS Council Secretariat and Partners) (2011) *UNGASS 2010 Country Progress Report Papua New Guinea*, Reporting Period January 2008 to December 2010. Online, available at: www.unaids.org/en/regionscountries/countries/papuanewguinea/ (accessed 26 April 2011).

Powell, C.O. (1973) 'Cardiovascular Disease', in C.O. Bell (ed.), *The Diseases and Health Services of Papua New Guinea*, Port Moresby: Department of Health, 355–356.

Price, A.V.G. and Tulloch, J.A. (1966) 'Diabetes Mellitus in Papua New Guinea', *Medical Journal of Australia*, 2(14): 645–648.

Reid, E. (2010) 'Rethinking Human Rights and the HIV Epidemic: A Reflection on Power and Goodness', in Vicki Luker and Sinclair Dinnen (eds), *Civic Insecurity: Law, Order and HIV in Papua New Guinea*, Canberra: ANU E Press, 265–273.

Riley, I. (2010) 'Establishing a Research Site in Tari', in C. Leahy, G. Vilakiva, and D. Diave (eds), *Pneumonia: 40 Years of Research in PNG: Colloquium Magazine*, Goroka: Papua New Guinea Institute of Medical Research, 16–18.

Riley, I.D., Lehman, D., and Alpers, M.P. (1992) 'Acute Respiratory Infections', in R.D. Attenborough and M.P. Alpers (eds), *Human Biology in Papua New Guinea: The Small Cosmos*, Oxford: Clarendon Press, 281–288.

Riley, J.C. (2001) *Rising Life Expectancy: A Global History*, Cambridge: Cambridge University Press.

RN (Radio National) (2011) 'PNG Literacy in Reverse: Drops below 50%', 15 July. Online, available at: www.radioaustralia.net.au/pacbeat/stories/20117/s3270032 (accessed 20 July 2011).

Saweri, W. (2001) 'The Rocky Road from Roots to Rice: A Review of the Changing Food and Nutrition Situation in Papua New Guinea', *Papua New Guinea Medical Journal*, 44(3–4): 151–163.

Scragg, R. (2010) 'Science and Survival in Paradise', *Health and History*, 12(2), 57–78.

Scragg, R.F.R. (1977) 'Historical Epidemiology in Papua New Guinea', *Papua New Guinea Medical Journal*, 20(3): 102–109.

Shann, F., Biddulph, J., and Vince, J. (2003) *Paediatrics for Doctors in Papua New Guinea: A Guide for Doctors Providing Health Services for Children*, [no publication place cited]: Department of Health with funding assistance from AusAID.

Sims, P. (2004) 'How the Poor Die in the Settlements of Port Moresby, 2003–2004', *Papua New Guinea Medical Journal*, 47(3–4): 192–201.

Sinnett, P. (1973) 'Heart Disease, Obesity, Diabetes and Cancer', in C.O. Bell (ed.), *The Diseases and Health Services of Papua New Guinea*, Port Moresby: Department of Public Health, 392–396.

Sinnett, P. and Whyte, M. (1981) 'Papua New Guinea', in H. Trowell and D.P. Burkitt (eds), *Western Diseases: Their Emergence and Prevention*, London: Edward Arnold, 171–187.

Sinnett, P.F., Kevau, I.H., and Tyson, D. (1992) 'Social Change and the Emergence of Degenerative Cardiovascular Disease in Papua New Guinea', in R.D. Attenborough and M.P. Alpers (eds), *Human Biology in Papua New Guinea: The Small Cosmos*, Oxford: Clarendon Press, 373–386.

SOPAC (2007) National Integrated Water Resource Management Diagnostic Report: Papua New Guinea. Draft SOPAC miscellaneous report 2433. Online, available at: http:www.pacificwater.org/pages.cfm/country-information/papua-new-guinea.html via link to diagnostic report (accessed 10 October 2011).

SPC (Secretariat of the Pacific Community) (2010) *2010 Pocket Statistical Summary*, Noumea: Secretariat of the Pacific Community.

SPC (Secretariat of the Pacific Community) (2011) 'NCD Statistics for the Pacific Islands Countries and Territories', Healthy Pacific Lifestyle Section, Public Health Division, Secretary of the Pacific Community. Online, available at: www.spc.int/hpl/ (accessed 3 April 2011).

Storey, D. (2010) 'Urban Poverty in Papua New Guinea', National Research Institute Discussion Paper 109, Boroko: National Research Institute.

Swartz, L. and Dick, J. (2002) 'Managing Chronic Diseases in Less Developed Countries: Healthy Teamworking and Patient Partnership are Just as Important as Adequate Funding', *BMJ*, 325(7370): 914–915.

Taylor, R. (2008) 'History of Public Health in Pacific Island Countries', in M.J. Lewis and K.L. MacPherson (eds), *Public Health in Asia and the Pacific: Historical and Comparative Perspectives*, London: Routledge, 276–307.

Temu, P. (1991) 'Adult Medicine and the New Killer Diseases in Papua New Guinea', *Papua New Guinea Medical Journal*, 34(1), 1–5.

Thomason, J.A., Newbrander, W.C., and Kolemainen-Aitken, R.-L. (1991) 'Introduction', in J.A. Thomason, W.C. Newbrander, and R.-L. Kolemainen-Aitken (eds), *Decentralization in a Developing Country: The Experience of Papua New Guinean and its Health Service*, Canberra: National Centre of Development Studies, Australian National University, 3–7.

Tnines, M. (2010) 'Introduction', in M. Tnines (ed.), *Making Sense of Disability in Papua New Guinea: Perceptions and Treatment of Disability in PNG*, Goroka: Melanesian Institute, 15–19.

Trowell, H. (1981) 'Hypertension, Obesity, Diabetes Mellitus and Coronary Heart Disease', in H. Trowell and D.P. Burkitt (eds), *Western Diseases: Their Emergence and Prevention*, London: Edward Arnold, 3–32.

Trowell, H. and Burkitt, D. (1981) 'Preface', in H. Trowell and D.P. Burkitt (eds), *Western Diseases: Their Emergence and Prevention*, London: Edward Arnold, xiii–xvi.

Ulijaszek, S.J. (2006) 'Purari Population Decline and Resurgence across the Twentieth Century', in S.J. Ulijaszek (ed.), *Population, Reproduction and Fertility in Melanesia*, New York: Berghahn Books, 67–89.

Ulijaszek, S.J. and Ohtsuka, R. (2007) 'Health Change in the Asia-Pacific Region: Disparate End-points?' in R. Ohtsuka and S.J. Ulijaszek (eds), *Health Change in the Asia-Pacific Region: Biocultural and Epidemiological Approaches*, Cambridge: Cambridge University Press, 1–20.

UN (2010) 'Papua New Guinea', MDG Monitor. Online, available at: www.mdgmonitor. org/country_progress.cfm?c=PNG&cd=598 (accessed 27 September 2011).

UN Habitat (2010) *The State of African Cities: Governance, Inequality and Urban Land Markets*, Nairobi: UN Habitat.

UNAIDS (2010) 'Papua New Guinea Releases New HIV Prevalence Figures', 26 August. Online, available at: http://unaids.org/en/resources.presscentre/featurestories/2010/August/20100826fspng/ (accessed 29 October 2011).

UNAIDS (2011) 'South Africa'. Online, available at: unaids.org/en.regionscountries/countries/southafrica (accessed 29 October 2011).

UNDP (United Nations Development Programme) (2009) 'Human Development Report 2009: HDI Rankings'. Online, available at: http://hdr.undp.org/statistics/ (accessed 29 July 2010).

Veenstra, N., Byford, J., and Gi, S. (2010) 'Disability in the Middle Ramu, Madang Province: Perceptions, Prevalence and the Role of Community Based Rehabilitation', in M. Tnines (ed.), *Making Sense of Disability in Papua New Guinea: Perceptions and Treatment of Disability in PNG*, Goroka: Melanesian Institute, 198–237.

Vinit, T. (2009) 'Burdens of Illness from Diseases', *Post Courier*, 31 March. Online, available at: www.postcourier.com.pg/20009033l/focus.htm (accessed 27 April 2011).

WB (World Bank) (2007) *Strategic Directions for Human Development in Papua New Guinea*, Washington, DC: World Bank.

WHO (World Health Organization) (2005) *Preventing Chronic Diseases: A Vital Investment*, Geneva: WHO.

WHO (World Health Organization) (2007) *Noncommunicable Disease and Poverty: The Need for Pro-poor Strategies in the Western Pacific Region*, Geneva: WHO Western Pacific Region.

WHO (World Health Organization) (2009) *World Malaria Report 2009*, Geneva: WHO.

WHO (World Health Organization) (2010a) *Noncommunicable Disease Risk Factors and Socioeconomic Inequalities: What Are the Links?* Geneva: WHO Western Pacific Region.

WHO (World Health Organization) (2010b) 'Papua New Guinea: Health Profile'. Online, available at: www.who.int/gho/countries/png.pdf (accessed 26 April 2011).

WHO (World Health Organization) (2010c) 'Papua New Guinea', *Western Pacific Country Health Information Profiles, 2010 Revision*, Geneva: WHO.

WHO (World Health Organization) (2011a) *Global Status Report on Noncommunicable Diseases*, Geneva: WHO.

WHO (World Health Organization) (2011b) *Noncommunicable Diseases: Country Profiles*. Geneva: WHO.

WHO (World Health Organization) (2011c) 'Papua New Guinea Tuberculosis Profile'. Online, available at: http://ww.who.int/gho/countries/png/country_profiles/en/index. html (accessed 26 April 2011).

WHO (World Health Organization) (2011d) *World Report on Disability*, Geneva: WHO.

Wigley, S.C. (1990) 'Tuberculosis and New Guinea: Historical Perspectives with Special Reference to the Years 1871–1973', in B.G. Burton-Bradley (ed.), *A History of Medicine in Papua New Guinea: Vignettes of an Earlier Period*, Kingsgrove, NSW: Australasian Medical Publishing Company, 167–204.

Zimmet, P.Z. and Alberti, M.M. (1992) 'Introduction: Globalization and the Noncommunicable Disease Epidemic', *Obesity*, 14(1): 1–3.

Zimmet, P. and Whitehouse, S. (1981) 'Pacific Islands of Nauru, Tuvalu and Western Samoa', in H.C. Trowell and P.D. Burkitt (eds), *Western Diseases: Their Emergence and Prevention*, Cambridge, MA: Harvard University Press, 204–224.

# 15 The double disease burden in Pacific Island states (except Papua New Guinea)

*Richard Taylor*

*Sub sole nihil novi est.*

## Introduction

### Diversity of Pacific Islands

The Pacific Island states of Melanesia, Micronesia and Polynesia encompass populations that vary greatly in size, from over five million in Papua New Guinea (PNG), around 800,000 in Fiji, and down to 1,000 or fewer in some small Polynesian entities. There are extensive variations in land mass and geography from substantial high islands with rich volcanic soil in Melanesia and parts of Micronesia and Polynesia, to tiny atolls consisting of little more than sand in parts of Micronesia and Polynesia, and as Melanesian outliers. While some populations are concentrated on main islands, others are scattered through rugged mountainous terrain or across far flung archipelagos. Many islands have plentiful water from rainfall, whereas those near the equator, in the 'doldrums', are severely drought prone. The range of the malaria mosquito (Anopheles species), extends southwest to the Buxton line to encompass PNG, the Solomon Islands and Vanuatu, but not beyond; all other Pacific Island states are malaria free (Taylor 2008: 276–307).

There are differences in language and culture within and between Pacific Island states. Melanesian society is traditionally based on 'big men', who have advanced to this position through strategic alliances; and there is a plethora of local languages – in PNG over 800 local languages, over 100 in the Solomon Islands and in Vanuatu, and 28 in New Caledonia. This poses challenges for national integration and for social cohesion in towns composed of diverse and sometimes antagonistic language groups (especially the 'wontok' system in PNG; literally 'one talk'). National but related versions of pidgin are widespread in PNG, the Solomons and Vanuatu, and have become the local lingua franca – along with imported European languages: English and French. Polynesian societies tend to be hierarchical with hereditary nobility, and with one local language; they are part of the Austronesian diaspora through South East Asia that probably spread from Taiwan. Although Fijians are racially considered Melanesian, their language and culture are more Polynesian. Micronesians are also Austronesian speakers, with a generally egalitarian social organisation and often matrilineal inheritance.

Colonial history also differs significantly, and hence the cosmopolitan language and cultural influence: the United Kingdom (UK), France, the United States (USA), Australia, New Zealand (NZ); and, earlier, Spain, Germany and Japan. Some states remain territories of metropolitan countries, such as Guam and American Samoa (USA), and New Caledonia and French Polynesia (France); others have very close ties (including migration) such as Cook Islands and Niue (NZ) and northern Micronesian states (USA). Other Pacific Island states are 'independent' but function within economic, geopolitical and migration spheres of influence, usually exercised by their former colonial masters. As a consequence of colonial history and continuing attachments, some Pacific Island states contain substantial immigrant communities; most notably in Fiji where the Indian population (derived from indentured labourers and immigrants from British India) peaked at 51 per cent of the population in 1966, but from coup-related emigration and reduced fertility was down to 37 per cent in 2007. There are also substantial communities derived from immigrants, or inter-mixed with them, in New Caledonia (Europeans, Vietnamese and Polynesians from other French territories), Guam (Europeans and Asians) and French Polynesia (*les demis*). While Christianity is widespread from European colonisation, there are still areas of animist belief in Melanesia, and Indo-Fijians are determinedly Hindu or Moslem.

There is a diversity of natural resources and industries (agriculture, tourism, minerals, fishery and forestry), but also, in many Island states, significant reliance on external economic aid, externally funded bureaucracy (most notably in French territories) and remittances from expatriate workers (Watters and Bertram 2008: 254–282). Differences in the type and extent of economic activity are reflected in considerable differences in gross domestic product (GDP) per capita. Further, there are variations in the extent of current immigration of Europeans and Asians, and current emigration of the skilled workforce and the size of particular ethnic groups (such as Indo-Fijians).

There are formal subregional, regional and international groups to which Pacific Island states belong, many of which undertake health-related activities. These include: the Melanesian Spearhead Group (MSG) consisting of PNG, Vanuatu and the Solomons, initially with representation from New Caledonian Kanaks, and later Fiji; the Pacific Island Forum, consisting of politically independent and 'self-governing' Pacific Island states, and Australia and New Zealand; the Secretariat for the Pacific Community (SPC), formerly the South Pacific Commission, consisting of all Pacific Island states and current or previous colonial powers (although the UK has dropped out); and regional involvement in international agencies such as WHO (World Health Organization), UNICEF (United Nations International Children's Emergency Fund), UNFPA (United Nations Fund for Population Activities) and prominent international and global non-government and donor agencies. Informal ties based on migration, economic, language and transport connections remain strong, especially among Anglophone or Francophone Island states and US-associated Micronesia, and between Pacific Island states and Australia, NZ and the USA (especially Hawaii and the West Coast). There are quite large proportions of some Polynesian and Micronesian populations resident in NZ, USA and Australia who send significant remittances back to kin in their country of origin. Many Pacific-wide joint activities in the health and other sectors have floundered or fragmented because of understandable jealousies over the site of infrastructure, and the greater difficulty of transport between Island states, compared with that between Island states and Pacific Rim countries; for example, initiatives related to bulk purchase of pharmaceuticals and the site of tertiary education institutions.

For those with little knowledge of the diversity of Pacific Island states, including some international agencies situated in distant countries, there is often for analytical purposes a desire to aggregate these relatively small populations into one group. In this case, aggregate data will reflect the situation in PNG because of its comparatively large population. Another approach is to produce statistics separately for PNG, and for the 'rest' of Pacific Island states as a single group. However, 'the rest' is exceedingly diverse, with both the Solomons and Vanuatu being malarious, Melanesian populations still dominating, and includes a variety of independent countries and states attached to metropolitan powers (with various degrees of remoteness), and at various levels of social and economic development. Another approach is to select Fiji as a 'reference' population because it is the largest after PNG, politically independent, Melanesian yet Polynesian, produces relatively good statistics on population, economic, health and other sectors, and houses the headquarters of several international and regional agencies. On the other hand, Fiji has a substantial population of Indo-Fijians who are quite different from Fiji Melanesians, and the Fiji population is mostly clustered on two main islands which have been the subject of much economic and social development activity over past decades. Although the traditional division into Melanesian, Polynesian and Micronesian makes some cultural and geographic sense, such a classification does not allow for the considerable diversity within these groups because of colonial history, present political status, geography, malaria distribution, population size, ethnic composition, and economic and social development.

It is not surprising, given this great heterogeneity, that there are differences in the timing and extent of the demographic and epidemiological transitions, and their variants, between Island states, and within the more populous countries. Yet, aggregation of Pacific Island states is inadvisable, and geo-ethnic stratification of larger Island states is desirable, although not always possible.

### Demographic and epidemiological transitions

The demographic transition was described as a sustained reduction in mortality which was followed by a sustained reduction of fertility, but not before leading to a population increase which then stabilised at a higher level, even after fertility declined to replacement rate (or below). This description was based on the Western European and North American experience (Notestein 1953: 13–31; Coal 1973: 53-72; Kirk 1996: 361–387), although the demographic transition (and variants) has been repeated in many populations subsequently. Omran described the epidemiological transition (1971: 509–538) to explain the reasons for the reduction in mortality – the driving force of the demographic transition – by examination of changes in cause of death. He posited, inter alia, three 'Ages' of the epidemiological transition: 'Pestilence and Famine' (life expectancy 20–40 years); 'Receding Pandemics' (life expectancy 30–50 years); and 'Degenerative and Man-Made Disease' (life expectancy over 50 years). He noted that reduction of mortality from infection in children and young women was particularly influential in the extension of life expectancy beyond 50 years.

It is beyond the scope of this chapter to provide a full critique of Omran's article. However, it is relevant to note that he wrote his essay when much less was known of the causes of cardiovascular disease (CVD), cancer and the like than is known at present and before the spectacular declines in some of these conditions in Western countries associated with changes in population risk factors related particularly to diet and tobacco smoking (Thom *et al.* 1992). The use of the term 'Degenerative Disease' by Omran and many subsequent observers, referring to a constellation of particular chronic and non-communicable diseases (especially in adults) is unhelpful. So-called 'degenerative disease' refers to conditions in which the structure and function of affected tissues and organs deteriorate over time and has been used to refer to a wide range of conditions (generally not microbial in origin and often of unknown cause) affecting the alimentary, nervous, genitourinary, musculoskeletal and cardiovascular systems as well as cancer and diabetes. The term does not indicate causation and is hardly ever used in modern medical textbooks. 'Degenerative' is not to be found in the index of *Harrisons' Principles of Internal Medicine* (15th edition) (Braunwald *et al.* 2001: I1–I158) and in *Cecil Textbook of Medicine* (22nd edition) (Goldman and Ausiello 2004: i–cv) is mentioned in the index once as 'Degenerative Joint Disease', but the reader is referred to 'Osteoarthritis'. There is an implication that these 'degenerative' conditions are inevitable associations of the ageing process, which in most instances is not the case, even though rates may increase with age. The loaded term 'man made' for chronic non-communicable disease (NCD) used by Omran appears to imply that previous and current diseases caused by under-nutrition or infection are not a consequence, in large part, of human agency, which is now a highly contestable proposition.

An additional, fourth 'Age' of the epidemiological transition was described by Olshansky and Ault (1986: 355–391) as 'delayed degenerative death' to accommodate the significant extension of life expectancy from the decline in premature cardiovascular mortality (and other causes) in high income countries which was evident from 1970. The non-communicable chronic diseases, which are noted in the last two 'Ages' of the epidemiological transition now mostly have known specific causes.

With the epidemiological transition there is also a transition within major disease categories. The traditional cardiovascular diseases of chronic rheumatic valvular disease (delayed consequence of streptococcal infection) and haemorrhagic stroke, change to coronary heart disease (CHD) and ischaemic stroke (both associated with arterial atheroma) and in many instances premature CVD mortality increases. Cancer is linked by similarities in pathology and biological behaviour. However, cancers of different anatomical and cell types usually have entirely different epidemiology and causes. The epidemiological transition in cancer consists of a change from traditional cancers of the upper alimentary tract (oesophagus and stomach) and liver (due to hepatitis B and C) to those of the lower alimentary tract (colon and rectum), lung and breast. These changes are due to changes in population exposure to known causative risk factors which will not be explored in detail here. Whether total cancer mortality increases or decreases during various stages of the epidemiological transition depends on the relative proportions of particular cancers with different fatalities. Further, there is an epidemiological transition in injury deaths with fewer deaths from causes prevalent among hunter gatherers or peasant farmers such as falls (from trees), injury from animals and drowning, to motor vehicle, mining and industrial injuries, and sometimes increases in suicide and homicide. If these causes balance then the total injury burden may not change. Thus the epidemiological transition is not only a change in causes of death from infection and under-nutrition (especially in children) to NCD and injury (especially in adults) but also changes within the major cause-of-death categories.

### Premature and delayed mortality from non-communicable disease

Not usually mentioned is the fundamental difference between (1) epidemics (over decades) of premature adult mortality from CVD, certain cancers (lung, breast and colorectal) and injuries (especially motor vehicle accidents) which limit increases or reduce life expectancy; and (2) the consequences of ageing of the population (structure) from reductions in previous mortality and fertility and characterised by rising life expectancy and 'delayed degenerative death' (Olshansky and Ault 1986: 355–391). The confusion arises because cause of death data are so often presented as a proportion of all deaths for all ages (and both sexes) combined whereas age-specific mortality by cause, or years of life lost (YLL) by cause, would indicate the significant causes of premature mortality. Increased numbers (and proportion) of deaths from CHD, stroke, cancers and the like due to population ageing, and associated with high and increasing life expectancy, has implications for provision of medical care for the aged, but premature mortality from these conditions that limits improvement or reduces life expectancy is a serious public health issue. The epidemiological transition is often naively stated as a change from under-nutrition and infection (especially in children) as major causes of mortality (and morbidity) to a situation where NCD and injuries (especially in adults) are the major causes without this crucial distinction being made. Complicating the issue is that they can occur together. But it is important to distinguish how much of the increase in NCD deaths is due to demographic factors (population increase and ageing) and how much it is a consequence of epidemiological factors (increases in age-specific, premature death rates) because the responses needed differ.

### Double burden of disease

The term the 'double burden of disease' appears to have been used in association with the first Global Burden of Disease study based on 1990 data (Murray and Lopez, 1997a: 1436–1442; 1997b: 1347–1352; 1997c: 1269–1276). This study showed that some world regions or countries (such as India and China) manifested excess mortality from both the pre-transitional causes of mortality (perinatal and maternal causes, under-nutrition and communicable disease or Group I conditions), and also from non-communicable disease (Group II) and injuries (Group III). The discourse on the 'double burden of disease' increased following the 2004 World Health Assembly pronouncements on diet, physical activity and health issues affecting developing countries (Marshall 2004: 556).

The double burden of disease can manifest in populations in several ways. Certainly there are well described differences between urban and rural areas with respect to the progress of the demographic and epidemiological transitions which can lead to spatial heterogeneity in major causes of premature death (van der Sande *et al.* 2001: 1641–1644). However, there is also heterogeneity in these transitions within the same geographic area and by socioeconomic class. The urban poor eking out a living on the street are in earlier stages of the transitions than the wealthier inhabitants of the high rise apartments looking down upon them; and likewise, rural landless peasants are in earlier stages of the transitions than landowners surveying their estates from the verandas of their haciendas. Further, the double burden of disease can occur within the same family, with infants and children suffering under-nutrition and communicable disease, whilst their parents are obese with diabetes and CVD disease, as is observable in some Indigenous minorities in developed countries. Within the framework of the epidemiological transition, the 'double burden of disease' is merely different stages of the epidemiological transition occurring in groups which differ in their ecological situations because of geographic, socioeconomic, age, sex, ethnic or other characteristics.

The first populations to be affected by the epidemiological transition, with declines in mortality from infection (especially from the mid-1800s) and real increases in NCD (especially from the 1920s) were countries of Western Europe, North America and Australasia. In Australia in 1935, at a life expectancy of 65 years (at birth, both sexes), the proportional mortality from infection was 25 per cent and from CVD 28 per cent – with the addition of cancer, NCD mortality becomes 40 per cent – and there was another 6 per cent from injuries. This is an example of the 'double burden of disease'. There were plateaux in life expectancy increases in males (1945–1970) and females (1960–1970) in Australia due to epidemics of coronary heart disease, followed by continuous increases in life expectancy as premature CVD (including stroke) mortality substantially declined, although the proportion of deaths from NCD increased because of population ageing (Taylor *et al.* 1998a: 27–36; 1998b: 37–44). The second group of countries to be affected by the epidemiological transition included Russia and other republics of the former USSR, and Eastern European countries (the 'Second World'), in which increases in NCD occurred mostly after 1945. NCD mortality peaked for most of Eastern Europe in the 1990s, but Russia and some former USSR republics have experienced increasing CVD disease death rates (contributing to declines in life expectancy), which by the twenty-first century are higher than ever previously observed (Mirzaei *et al.* 2009: 740–746). Again there is evidence of the 'double burden of disease' in what was known as the 'Second World' not only after 1945, as infectious disease fell and NCDs rose, but after 1990 when the collapse in health services and rising intravenous drug use led to increases in tuberculosis and HIV/AIDS, in concert with further increases in the CVD disease epidemic (especially in Russia). The third group of populations affected by the epidemiological transition are the diverse countries of what used to be termed the 'Third World', which are at various levels of socioeconomic development and demonstrate significant secular heterogeneity in the demographic and epidemiological transitions between each other and within their populations. This is certainly the situation for the various Pacific Island states.

These complex changes in particular causes of death are a result of changes in causal exposures. Although increases in exposures to risk factors for non-communicable chronic disease can be associated with urbanisation and 'global-isation', epidemics of NCDs commenced well before the present episode of 'globalisation', and decreases in NCD have occurred in many populations with no reduction in urbanisation, and continued 'globalisation'. The celebrated epi-demic of CHD in Finland was worse in rural dairy farmers than in the urban population (Jousilahti *et al.* 1998: 481–487), and CHD is higher in rural than urban Australia (Burnley 1998: 1209–1222). NCDs have particular causes, espe-cially the important risk factors of elevated serum cholesterol, glucose and blood pressure (related to diet and exercise) and tobacco smoking. These can be con-trolled in populations producing significant reductions in premature mortality (Taylor *et al.* 2006: 760–768; Tobias *et al.* 2008: 117–125), without changing most aspects of social organisation, and are not the 'inevitable price of affluence' as once thought. Since there has been significant regression of these conditions as causes of premature mortality in countries first affected by them, they are also not manifestations of 'Westernisation', 'civilisation', 'globalisation' or 'urbani-sation'. Likewise, the disastrous health effects of human aggregation in cities without potable water and sanitation, with insufficient and contaminated food supplies and inadequate housing – from infectious disease and under-nutrition – can be rectified by attention to these specific details, not de-urbanisation. In fact, urbanisation can facilitate reticulation of potable water, sewage disposal, distri-bution of electricity, implementation of building regulations and supply of health and education services. Similarly, chronic NCD in adults can be controlled by changes in population risk factors which can be easier to implement in cosmopolitan urban than rural areas.

Socioeconomic differentiation of populations in urban areas of developing countries means that conditions for inhabitants of urban slums associated with under-nutrition and infection can exist alongside conditions among other groups that lead to chronic NCD in adults. This duality in way of life leads to different phases of the epidemiological transition existing simultaneously within the same geographic area.

## The double burden of disease in Pacific Island populations

### *Progress of the epidemiological transition in the Pacific Islands*

The epidemiological transition in many Pacific Island populations has been noted for some time. By the 1970s NCDs such as CVD and diabetes were an evident cause of significant morbidity and mortality in adults in many Island populations. This was a result of a real increase in these conditions as well as the decline in infectious diseases and under-nutrition as important health issues. Numerous studies have shown NCDs to be greater problems in modernized and urban areas and less important in other places, especially in Melanesian, malarious countries.

Studies in many Island states in the 1980s demonstrated that urban subjects were more obese, had higher prevalence rates of diabetes and hypertension, higher salt intake and generally higher serum cholesterol than their rural counterparts despite a lower overall calorie intake, indicating the impact of physical exercise as well as dietary differences on cardiovascular risk factors (Taylor *et al.* 1985a: 499–501; Taylor *et al.* 1992: 283–293). Further, there were differences in infection and NCD mortality and morbidity in Pacific Island states around 1980 which correlated with modernisation, development and presence or absence of malaria (Taylor and Thoma 1985: 149–155; Taylor *et al.* 1989: 634–646; Taylor *et al.* 1991: 207–221; Taylor 1993: 266–270).

In Fiji, trends in hospital admissions revealed increases in patients admitted to hospital with CVD from the 1970s with risk factors for these conditions (Pathik and Ram 1974: 922–924; Reed and Feinleib 1983: 182–205; Tuomeilehto *et al.* 1984: 133–143). The rise of CVD prompted a national survey of risk factors in 1980 (Ram *et al.* 1983: 88–94; Tuomeilehto *et al.* 1984: 133–143) which showed significant prevalences of hypertension, diabetes, tobacco smoking and obesity. Cigarette sales in Fiji rose 273 per cent from 1956 to 1984, while the population increase was 88 per cent (Tuomeilehto *et al.* 1984: 133–143). A rising proportion of CVD mortality has been associated with a plateau in life expectancy since 1980 (Carter *et al.* 2011a: 412–420).

In the phosphate rich island of Nauru, infection was a major cause of death in the 1940s and 1950s, but decreased significantly thereafter. Maternal mortality was also significant during this period but subsequently declined. CVD and diabetes increased from a small proportion of deaths to 20 to 30 per cent following

Independence in 1970. Cancer constituted around 10 per cent of deaths by the 1980s, and external causes (mostly road accidents in males) increased from less than 10 per cent before 1970 to peak at 24 per cent in the mid-1980s (Taylor and Thoma 1983: 1–89; Taylor and Thoma 1985: 149–155; Schooneveldt *et al.* 1988: 89–95; Carter *et al.* 2011b: 10–23). Whereas under-nutrition had been noted during and before the First World War, a nutrition transition to reliance on imported foods (especially rice) had been reported in the Nauruan population from the 1950s, and a weight reduction clinic opened in 1965 (Taylor and Thoma 1983: 11).

In some instances the rise of non-communicable conditions has been associated with a decline in life expectancy, as in Nauru (Taylor and Thoma 1985: 89–95; Schooneveldt *et al.* 1988: 89–95; Carter *et al.* 2011b), and in other instances a plateau in life expectancy, as in Fiji (Carter *et al.* 2011a. Previously life expectancy had been rising because of the control of infection and under-nutrition, especially in children.

By 1980, and continuing through to the new millennium, it has been evident that Pacific Island populations are quite heterogeneous with respect to health and mortality. The demographic and epidemiological transitions are at quite different stages in various populations, with the less developed states still affected by endemic infectious disease and under-nutrition, with relatively high mortality (especially in children), and other states with relatively high life expectancy and a predominance of NCD and accidents (in adults), but with some other Island countries in the middle, with a double burden of disease; and life expectancy limited by premature mortality from both infectious and non-communicable conditions. Furthermore, there may be significant differences between rural and urban areas, or between major ethnic groups, with respect to stages of the demographic and epidemiological transitions in the one Island state. Cross-sectional patterns mirror the longitudinal progression of the demographic and health transitions within populations.

Figures 15.1 and 15.2 illustrate the epidemiological transition in Pacific Island states *circa* 1980 and *circa* 2000. Life expectancy (at birth) has been derived from published sources for 1980 (Taylor *et al.* 1989: 634–646; Taylor *et al.* 1991: 207–221) and 2000 (Taylor and Lopez 2007: 45–58; Taylor *et al.* 2005: 207–214). For causes of death, the infection category is used as an indicator of the traditional pattern, usually associated with under-nutrition, and the CVD category is used an indicator of the modernised pattern, and associated with other NCDs (including cancer), especially in adults. For 1980 and 2000 cause of death data have been abstracted from multiple country sources (Taylor *et al.* 1989: 634–646; Taylor *et al.* 1991: 207–221; Taylor 2008: 276–307). Circles in the figures encompass Pacific Island states in which there are particular relationships between life expectancy and major cause of death. Circles encompass states in which life expectancy is significantly limited by infection and by CVD, with the intersection of these circles indicating Pacific Island states with significant limitation of life expectancy by both (the double burden of disease). Circles also indicate Pacific Island states with some or little limitation of life expectancy

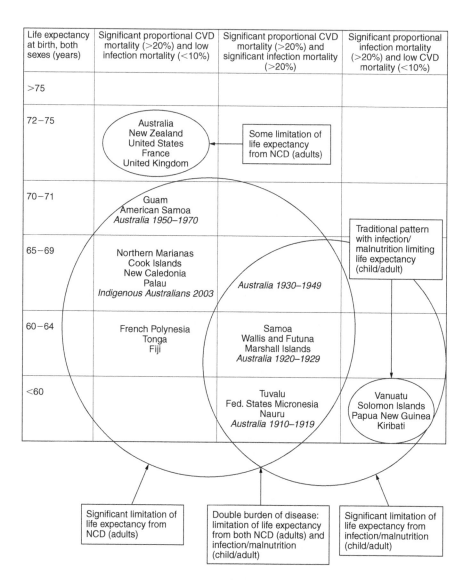

| Life expectancy at birth, both sexes (years) | Significant proportional CVD mortality (>20%) and low infection mortality (<10%) | Significant proportional CVD mortality (>20%) and significant infection mortality (>20%) | Significant proportional infection mortality (>20%) and low CVD mortality (<10%) |
|---|---|---|---|
| >75 | | | |
| 72–75 | Australia<br>New Zealand<br>United States<br>France<br>United Kingdom | Some limitation of life expectancy from NCD (adults) | |
| 70–71 | Guam<br>American Samoa<br>*Australia 1950–1970* | | Traditional pattern with infection/ malnutrition limiting life expectancy (child/adult) |
| 65–69 | Northern Marianas<br>Cook Islands<br>New Caledonia<br>Palau<br>*Indigenous Australians 2003* | *Australia 1930–1949* | |
| 60–64 | French Polynesia<br>Tonga<br>Fiji | Samoa<br>Wallis and Futuna<br>Marshall Islands<br>*Australia 1920–1929* | |
| <60 | | Tuvalu<br>Fed. States Micronesia<br>Nauru<br>*Australia 1910–1919* | Vanuatu<br>Solomon Islands<br>Papua New Guinea<br>Kiribati |

Significant limitation of life expectancy from NCD (adults)

Double burden of disease: limitation of life expectancy from both NCD (adults) and infection/malnutrition (child/adult)

Significant limitation of life expectancy from infection/malnutrition (child/adult)

*Figure 15.1* Double burden of disease in Pacific island states based on life expectancy and proportional mortality from infections and CVD as indicators, *c.*1980 (except where otherwise indicated) (sources: Taylor *et al.* 1989: 634–646; Taylor *et al.* 1991: 207–221; Taylor *et al.* 2005: 207–214; Taylor and Lopez 2007: 45–58; Taylor 2008: 276–307; Taylor *et al.* 1998a: 27–36; Taylor *et al.* 1998b: 37–44; Vos *et al.* 2007: 27–49).

Note
Niue and Tokelau are not included because their populations are fewer than 1,500.

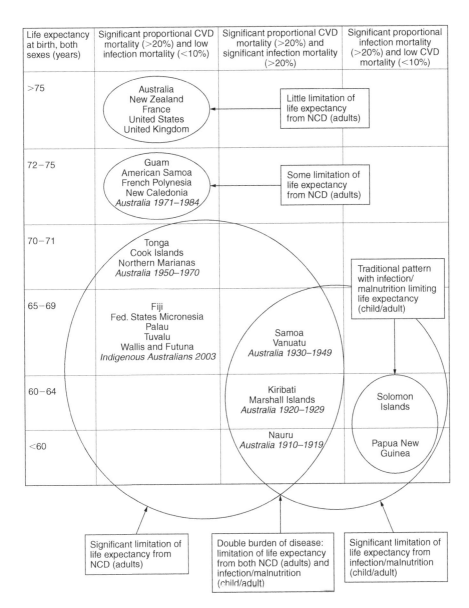

| Life expectancy at birth, both sexes (years) | Significant proportional CVD mortality (>20%) and low infection mortality (<10%) | Significant proportional CVD mortality (>20%) and significant infection mortality (>20%) | Significant proportional infection mortality (>20%) and low CVD mortality (<10%) |
|---|---|---|---|
| >75 | Australia New Zealand France United States United Kingdom | Little limitation of life expectancy from NCD (adults) | |
| 72–75 | Guam American Samoa French Polynesia New Caledonia *Australia 1971–1984* | Some limitation of life expectancy from NCD (adults) | |
| 70–71 | Tonga Cook Islands Northern Marianas *Australia 1950–1970* | | Traditional pattern with infection/ malnutrition limiting life expectancy (child/adult) |
| 65–69 | Fiji Fed. States Micronesia Palau Tuvalu Wallis and Futuna *Indigenous Australians 2003* | Samoa Vanuatu *Australia 1930–1949* | |
| 60–64 | | Kiribati Marshall Islands *Australia 1920–1929* | Solomon Islands |
| <60 | | Nauru *Australia 1910–1919* | Papua New Guinea |

Significant limitation of life expectancy from NCD (adults)

Double burden of disease: limitation of life expectancy from both NCD (adults) and infection/malnutrition (child/adult)

Significant limitation of life expectancy from infection/malnutrition (child/adult)

*Figure 15.2* Double burden of disease in Pacific island states based on life expectancy and proportional mortality from infections and CVD as indicators, *circa* 2000 (except where otherwise indicated) (sources: Taylor *et al.* 1989: 634–646; Taylor *et al.* 1991: 207–221; Taylor *et al.* 2005: 207–214; Taylor and Lopez 2007: 45–58; Taylor 2008: 276–307; Taylor *et al.* 1998a: 27–36; Taylor *et al.* 1998b: 37–44; Vos *et al.* 2007: 27–49).

Note
Niue and Tokelau are not included because their populations are fewer than 1,500.

from CVD (but not infection), and those with the traditional pattern with significant limitation of life expectancy from infection, but not CVD. For comparative purposes, the metropolitan countries associated with Pacific Island states are included in both figures for 1980 and 2000; and comparative positioning is also provided for Australia during the twentieth century and for Indigenous Australians for 2003 (Taylor *et al.* 1998a: 27–36; 1998b 37–44; Vos *et al.* 2007: 1–178).

These figures illustrate the cross-sectional and longitudinal trajectory of Pacific Island states and metropolitan countries with respect to the epidemiological transition. Between 1980 and 2000 many Pacific Island states moved across the epidemiological transition with increasing life expectancy and decreasing proportional mortality from infection. PNG and Nauru remained in the same categories in 2000 as they were in 1980 (although life expectancy increased somewhat in PNG). The most developed Island states experienced increased life expectancy but significant mortality from CVD. Metropolitan countries all exceeded life expectancy of 75 years by 2000 but with significant proportional mortality from CVD. Australia experienced a 'double burden of disease' from the early years of the twentieth century to 1949, before moving to predominant CVD proportional mortality and increasing life expectancy once these diseases were controlled as a cause of significant premature mortality. Indigenous Australians in 2003 show significant limitation of life expectancy from CVD similar to some Pacific Island states such as Fiji.

### Responses to under-nutrition and communicable disease

Responses to communicable disease and under-nutrition in Pacific countries has been partly through the traditional public health methods of improved nutrition, water supply and sanitation, food hygiene and preservation, vector control, quarantine and isolation, housing and electrification, and the effects of education and health promotion, and partly through disease-specific prevention (especially immunisation, micronutrient supplementation) and treatment (especially antimicrobials) which were not generally available on a mass scale until after the Second World War. Both infection and under-nutrition are particularly important problems in children, and Omran (1971: 509–538) noted that the decline in mortality which first pushed life expectancy (at birth) over 50 years was from reductions in death rates in childhood (and also in young women).

Following independence it was apparent in many Island countries that expensive hospital- and doctor-based medical services could not be sustained at former levels, and, coinciding with the WHO and UNICEF Primary Health Care (PHC) initiative of Alma Ata in 1978, which was accepted by most Pacific Island states, many outer-island or peripheral hospitals were consolidated or closed and replaced by PHC centres staffed by nurses or health extension officers. Supervision of primary health care and evacuation for secondary and tertiary care have continued to present significant problems because of dispersed populations and the archipelagic nature or rugged terrain of some Pacific Island states. PHC waned during the 1990s and early years of this century, and was replaced by an emphasis on private-provider services, fee-for-service payment, non-universal health insurance, and reduction of government health sector funding and service provision, which was collectively known as 'Health Sector Reform', often part of more general 'structural adjustment' economic policies pushed by the World Bank (WB), International Monetary Fund (IMF) and the World Trade Organization (WTO). Disillusionment with coverage and effectiveness of private provision, especially for the most needy, and doubt as to whether the Millennium Development Goals (MDGs) could be achieved with the health services available in many countries following 'Health Sector Reform' (enhanced by the 2007 financial crisis that demonstrated major private sector failings and which required massive public sector intervention) led to the miraculous resurrection of PHC in 2008 as the dominant paradigm for developing country (if not all) health systems, albeit in a form different from the 1978 original.

*Responses to under-nutrition*

Under-nutrition is generally prevented and remedied by adequate food intake. While hunter gatherers usually have a varied diet, although they are none the less limited by the food sources which are available, peasant farmers and those with inadequate means in urban areas or in labour lines on plantations or mining developments, are often reliant on an irregular or insufficient supply of carbohydrate stapes (such as rice, wheat flour and root crops). These may also be deficient in particular nutrients (such as protein, minerals and vitamins). Knowledge of nutrition accumulated over the early years of the twentieth century and has been used to prevent and treat calorie and specific deficiencies by dietary recommendations, rationing where needed and supplementation (with vitamins or minerals), including fortification of manufactured food. Under-nutrition is nearly always a consequence of lack of availability or affordability of food, and thus is primarily a development and economic issue (Sen 1981: xii, 257). With development, food can be supplied to nutritionally marginal areas in the Pacific such as atolls and highlands and when intermittent disasters strike, especially cyclones that destroy crops and salt water inundation that can render agricultural land barren for years. While cash crops may replace food crops for local consumption to some extent, they also provide money for purchase of a more diverse range of foods which can often be stored for quite long periods; food such as rice, wheat flour and canned meat and fish.

Many Island countries have imported significant amounts of food for some time paid for through local industry, including tourism, cash crop production (especially sugar, copra and palm oil), mining, fisheries and forestry, the ubiquitous direct and indirect aid flows which in many Island states are quite large in per capita terms as well as remittances from relatives abroad. Furthermore, there has been relentless nutrition education and promotion through Maternal and Child Health (MCH) services, and also through primary and secondary schools, stressing an adequate intake of nutrients. Stress on breast feeding and growth monitoring of children under five years have become a standard part of MCH services encapsulated by the UNICEF GOBI programme (growth monitoring, oral rehydration, breast feeding and immunisation).

Vitamin supplementation has been undertaken in several countries: vitamin A supplements in Micronesia where vitamin A deficiency has been documented in Kiribati, the Federated States of Micronesia and the Marshall Islands (Gamble *et al.* 2004: 336–340; Yamamura *et al.* 2004: 16–19; Schaumberg *et al.* 1996: 761–774), iodinisation of salt, especially for populations in inland mountainous areas such as in PNG (Temple *et al.* 2005: 45–48) and the Sigatoka valley of Fiji (King *et al.* 1983: 112–115); fortification of flour with iron in Fiji (Hughes 2006: 1–28); and even emergency import of 'Vegemite' (an Australian yeast extract spread rich in thiamine) to quell beriberi in Nauru in the 1930s (from drought affecting the flow of thiamine-rich coconut sap) (Grant 1933: 113–118). The main effect of macro- and micro-nutrient deficiency is that it engenders susceptibility to serious infection, especially in children. Under-nutrition is no longer a major problem in many Pacific Island states, but there are still some problems, particularly in some urban areas, highland regions in Melanesia and outer atolls in Micronesia.

## Responses to communicable diseases

Prior to the Second World War responses to communicable disease involved quarantine (which delayed rather than prevented disease introduction) and segregation of diseased individuals (e.g. leprosy and tuberculosis), protection of the water supply from faecal contamination (which required infrastructure), personal hygiene, food hygiene and prevention of adulteration, control of mosquito breeding and personal protection with nets, quinine for expatriates if infected with malaria, vaccination against smallpox, attempts at hookworm control (probably ineffective) and topical antiseptics for skin infection. Coupled with reduction of macro- and micro-nutrient deficiency (which improved resistance to serious infection) and reduction of over-crowding (which reduced transmission of infection) through improved housing, these measures had a remarkable effect on population mortality such that by the mid-1930s, prior to availability of antibiotics and mass immunisation, life expectancy (at birth) had reached 65 years in some developed countries including Australia, New Zealand, some Scandinavian countries and the Netherlands; although its advance was limited by CVD and other non-communicable conditions and by residual infection and under-nutrition.

In Pacific Island countries the population decline, from introduced infectious disease mortality and reduced fertility, consequent upon European contact and colonisation, had ceased by the end of the first quarter of the twentieth century despite the dire predictions of mass extinction of Pacific Island peoples. Formerly epidemic diseases had become endemic, armed conflict ended, food supplementation in marginal areas and in times of emergency was provided, and rudimentary public health measures were introduced (Taylor 2008: 276–307).

The last great epidemic was influenza in 1918. Although the population of Fiji finally started to increase during the First World War after continued decline since at least 1891, the influenza epidemic dealt another blow; by 1927 the population had only recovered to that of a decade earlier (Hermant and Cilento 1929: 34–35)

In 1928 the mortality situation in malarious Melanesia (PNG, the Solomon Islands and Vanuatu) was that the major causes of death were: malaria, especially in children, followed by pneumonia, then tuberculosis, dysentery and under-nutrition (including beriberi that was especially rife among indentured labourers). Yaws was common. Filariasis was multi-focal, and hookworm 'almost universal' but of little clinical significance. In non-malarious Melanesia (New Caledonia and Fiji) there was pneumonia, dysentery, enteric fevers, filariasis, yaws, childhood infections, tuberculosis and leprosy. Quarantine was strenuously undertaken in the non-malarious countries to prevent introduction of anopheles mosquitoes and cases of malaria as well as other infectious diseases (Hermant and Cilento 1929: 34–35).

During the Second World War various measures were introduced in order to protect troops: improved hygiene including a clean water supply and sanitation; vector control including chemical insecticides such as DDT (from 1943); new anti-malarial and antibiotic chemotherapy; and improvements in surgery and blood transfusion. The post-war period marked the beginning of serious population-wide economic and social development for the Pacific, and the application to populations of the public health methods, and new drugs and insecticides, that had been developed during the War. Yaws eradication by mass penicillin administration is one of the more spectacular ventures of the early post-war era. But without the immunity provided by yaws the next generation would be susceptible to venereal syphilis (Willcox 1980: 204–209). In 1955 the WHO adopted malaria eradication as a global strategy (Trigg and Kondrachine 1998: 11–16). Eradication proved possible in areas where the disease was seasonal and focal and in developed countries such as Australia, but while there was considerable success in reducing mortality and morbidity, global eradication proved to be beyond reach. By 1993 eradication formally gave way to control as WHO policy (Trigg and Kondrachine 1998: 11–16), with the objective of reducing and controlling morbidity and mortality from the disease by personal protection though bed nets (impregnated with insecticide) and treatment of symptomatic cases with anti-malarials. Malaria declined in the Solomon Islands during the 1990s from a combination of DDT spaying, insecticide impregnated bed nets and health education (Over *et al*. 2004: 214–223).

However, malaria has not been eradicated from PNG, the Solomon Islands or Vanuatu, although elimination is being attempted currently in the latter two countries through the Pacific Malaria Initiative Support Centre (PacMISC 2010).

Antibiotics became available and cures for previously untreatable diseases could be offered: pneumonia, tuberculosis and leprosy, intestinal infections, meningitis as well as malaria. Furthermore, vaccines became available, especially for childhood diseases: diphtheria, pertussis, polio, tetanus and later measles and hepatitis B. For diarrhoeal diseases, there was oral rehydration salts since most are viral and unresponsive to antibiotics and mortality is due to dehydration.

Besides being affected by global paradigms and programmes affecting health systems such as PHC, Pacific Island states were swept up in the continued stream of disease-specific control initiatives which flowed out of WHO Geneva to be implemented by regional and country WHO offices, collaborating international or regional agencies, international and national non-government organisations and national health departments, often funded through bilateral and multi-lateral donors. The Expanded Programme on Immunisation (EPI) commenced in 1974 by WHO and ten years later a standard immunisation schedule was established. The Global Alliance for Vaccines and Immunisation (GAVI) was established in 2000 from multiple international and private foundation donors to support vaccine production and distribution.

Oral rehydration therapy for diarrhoea, which could be prescribed by PHC workers and administered to children by family members, was introduced in Pacific Island countries from the late 1970s. The 1980s were also the International Decade of Drinking Water Supply and Sanitation. In the 1980s, programmes were introduced for control of mortality from acute respiratory infection (pneumonia) in children by the judicious prescription of antibiotics by PHC workers; they were based on simple physical signs. TB control was rejuvenated through the Stop TB initiative (1998) based on DOTS (Directly Observed Therapy, Short course) which had been adopted by WHO earlier in the decade. Likewise, malaria control was strengthened by the Roll Back Malaria campaign commenced in 1998. It relied on mosquito protection through insecticide-impregnated bed nets (long lasting by the mid-2000s), and case management, with diagnosis often including use of rapid diagnostic tests (by the mid-2000s) and treatment often by artemisin combination therapy (by the mid-2000s). During the mid-1990s WHO and UNICEF developed the Integrated Management of Childhood Illnesses (IMCI) approach that focused on pneumonia, diarrhoea, measles, malaria and malnutrition; these frequently occur together or in rapid succession. Prevention and control of HIV and AIDS were begun in the 1980s in developed countries, and then promoted through WHO when the nature and huge extent of the infection became clear; UNAIDS was formed in 1996 to provide a strengthened and more multi-sectoral response and because of some disquiet with the effectiveness of what some termed WHO's 'medical' approach.

Pacific Island states were recipients of these programmes through WHO regional (Manila), sub-regional (Port Moresby, Suva and Apia) and national offices, but also through associated agencies, especially UNICEF and the Secretariat for the Pacific Community (SPC). In many instances small Island countries were bewildered and overloaded by the steady stream of disease-specific and vertical control initiatives flowing out of international and regional agencies; and their success varied by time and place.

The Global Fund for Control of AIDS, Tuberculosis and Malaria was established in 2002 with funding from a number of bilateral aid donors, philanthropic foundations and international agencies to support in-country programmes for the control of these three communicable diseases. Funding was based on technical assessment of detailed proposals and these had to include significant participation from non-government sectors while continued funding was contingent on the outcome of detailed monitoring and audit. These requirements were beyond most Pacific Island states and regional international Pacific agencies often handled proposal development and reporting which consumed a significant amount of the budget. The flow of resources for control of these three particular diseases often led to a bias in infectious disease control efforts since many important conditions were not covered, especially diarrhoea, pneumonia and most vaccine-preventable disease particularly relevant to children; there was also a bias towards infectious rather than non-communicable chronic disease and injury, which were the most important causes of premature mortality in many Island states. Even in the few Pacific Island states with significant problems with AIDS, TB and malaria (especially PNG), it was often difficult to spend the money available, to recruit specialised staff and to implement such vertical, disease-specific, control programmes at the village level through health services which had suffered from chronic lack of support for Primary Health Care in the era of 'Health Care Reform'.

The MDGs said to relate specifically to health, namely, 'Goal 4: Reduce child mortality; Goal 5: Improve maternal health; and Goal 6: Combat AIDS, malaria and other diseases' relate primarily to pre-transitional conditions. NCD could be fitted into Goal 6, although it is not specifically mentioned. All of the eight MDGs relate directly or indirectly to health, but mostly to under-nutrition and infection. Thus the relentless push by many international agencies for achievement of these goals by 2015, while appropriate for some countries, is not particularly helpful for populations with significant premature mortality from NCDs but relatively low child and maternal mortality and morbidity, as is the case in some Pacific Island states.

### Response to non-communicable conditions

Non-communicable chronic disease has received rather belated recognition as a significant cause of premature mortality in developing countries. The WHO produced a Global Strategy for Prevention and Control of Non-communicable Disease in 2000, a Framework Convention on Tobacco Control in 2003, a Global Strategy on Diet, Physical Activity and Health in 2004, a document on *Preventing Chronic Disease: A Vital investment* in 2005 (WHO 2005: 1–182), and an implementation plan for prevention and control of non-communicable diseases in 2008 (WHO 2008: 1–21). However, there are WHO reports dating back to the 1950s on coronary heart disease, stroke, diabetes, hypertension, obesity and their relation to diet and other determinants, although these focus on developed countries.

The first response to the appearance of non-communicable conditions as notable causes of illness and mortality in the more modernised Pacific Islands states from the 1970s was to investigate it, especially though sample surveys of risk factors and precursors. Researchers from developed countries, where these diseases had already become significant health problems, were interested in investigating causative factors and significant urban–rural and ethnic differences in Pacific populations, since no solutions were in sight from their own countries. A rather naive paradigm which linked modernisation of 'lifestyle' with NCD as an 'inevitable price of affluence' was paramount among researchers working on Pacific Islands countries; much nihilism concerning health improvement resulted and the call was for a return to a 'traditional lifestyle' and/or inter-marriage with other races to dilute the effects of presumed genetic susceptibilities in Pacific Islanders, particularly to diabetes. There were complaints from some Pacific Islanders that the large numbers of surveys undertaken led to published articles for the researchers, but did not result in effective prevention programmes for the subjects of these studies. Certainly the somewhat unexpected declines in risk factors and premature mortality from CVD seen in Australia, New Zealand and the United States from 1970 (although not documented until later) were not replicated in most Pacific Island countries.

NCD control programmes started in the Pacific Islands, mostly during the 1980s, at the national level and, through SPC and WHO, at regional inter-country level. These efforts involved epidemiological evaluation and monitoring, health and nutrition education and promotion, and PHC and outpatient management of cases of CVD and diabetes. Prevention programmes have continued, but have been diluted somewhat following the flood of resources for communicable disease control through the Global Fund (AIDS, TB and malaria), and for containment of possible respiratory virus pandemics (such as influenza A and avian influenza) which occurred in the wake of the epidemic of SARS (severe acute respiratory syndrome). Thus in Island countries where non-communicable conditions and injury are major causes of premature mortality, public health priorities can be influenced by the flow of resources for infectious disease as a consequence of global policy that may not be locally relevant.

The response to epidemics of NCD (especially CVD and diabetes) is problematic because effective primary prevention (and much secondary prevention) involves active, independent contributions from non-governmental organisations, universities and professional associations, sophisticated health promotion strategies, and structural changes in marketing and advertising of potentially health-damaging products. Governments and their health departments are seriously handicapped in control of NCD by understandable reluctance to act to change individual behaviours which lack obvious direct effects on others (unlike infectious diseases), and are wont to ascribe consumption behaviour related to diet, alcohol and tobacco, and participation in activities involving physical exertion, solely to individual 'choice'; the traditional, market economic view. On this analysis unhealthy behaviours are manifestations of the individual failings of gluttony (diet), laziness (lack of exercise), intemperance (alcohol) and self-indulgence (tobacco). Governments are reluctant to intervene in markets through price manipulation of healthy and unhealthy products because of neo-liberal, economic orthodoxy and the policies of international and global agencies that implement these: the World Bank, IMF and the World Trade Organization. In addition, governments are subject to lobbying by their own manufacturers, traders and distributors of consumption products such as tobacco, alcohol, dairy products and red meats, and by large national and transnational corporations that manufacture, market and trade in these products. Thus strong, independent contributions from non-governmental organisations, universities and professional associations are required, but these are often lacking in small developing countries like Pacific Island states. Further, the success of health promotion depends not only on the dissemination of relevant messages, but also on the extent of formal school education of the population and in particular their health literacy.

Injury is a cause of significant premature mortality in many countries, and, with modernisation, motor vehicle accidents (often associated with alcohol) and industrial, mining and farm-based injuries replace more traditional injuries such as falls (from trees) and drowning. There are standard approaches to control of injuries from these causes, but implementation may be difficult in resource-poor settings (road improvement, for example). Suicide in young adults has been noted, particularly in Indo-Fijians, in Samoans and in Micronesians.

Evaluation of the extent and trajectory of the NCD epidemic is difficult in many Pacific Island states because of unreliable statistics on trends in population risk factors and NCD mortality, although this situation is starting to improve in some states with WHO STEPS surveys for risk factors (Government of Republic of Nauru and World Health Organization 2004: 1–59; Government of American Samoa and World Health Organization 2007: 1–67; Government of Federated States of Micronesia and World Health Organization 2008: 1–124; Government of Kiribati and World Health Organization 2009: 1–108) and critical analysis of cause of death data (Carter *et al.* 2011a, 2011b).

Some of the more developed states appear to have enjoyed improving life expectancy over the period, 1980–2000 (Guam, American Samoa, French Polynesia, New Caledonia and, to a lesser extent, Tonga, the Cook Islands and the Northern Marianas). This has occurred despite significant proportional mortality from NCD, implying a reduction in the premature mortality from these causes, while others manifest more modest improvements, with a heavier burden of NCD and injury mortality as probably the main reason for limitation in improvement in life expectancy (see Figures 15.1 and 15.2). Most recent data indicate that several countries have life expectancies in the 60s because of premature mortality from NCD (similar to Indigenous Australians) or with a 'double burden of disease', similar to Australia prior to 1950 (see Figure 15.2).

## Conclusions

A combination of infectious and non-communicable conditions, limiting growth of life expectancy and known as the 'double burden of disease', is not new, even if the designation is relatively recent. This situation is evident in many Pacific Island states, although some have moved to a predominant NCD burden, while others remain with infectious disease mortality as the major pattern. Predominant approaches to health improvement in Pacific Island states, and those pursued by regional and international agencies over the last 50 years, have stressed infectious disease control and adequate diet. However, programmes for NCD control, especially through health promotion aiming to change risk factors, have been undertaken in the Pacific since the 1980s. These endeavours appear to have met with some success, as judged by improvements in life expectancy (presumably due to declines in premature adult mortality) in some of the more modernised states that have strong links to metropolitan countries. These linkages may facilitate import of successful NCD and injury control strategies. But there are other states where considerable premature mortality from NCD and injuries poses a significant restraint on improvements in life expectancy, in some instances in combination with continued excessive mortality from infectious disease and perinatal conditions despite continued national and international programmes.

## References

Braunwald, E., Fauci, A., Kasper, D., Hauser, S., Longo, D. and Jameson, J. (2001) *Harrisons' Principles of Internal Medicine* (15th edn), New York: McGraw Hill.

Burnley, I.H. (1998) 'Inequalities in the Transition of Ischaemic Heart Disease Mortality in New South Wales, Australia, 1969–1994', *Social Science and Medicine*, 47(9): 1209–1222.

Carter, K., Cornelius, M., Taylor, R., Ali, S., Rao, C., Lopez, A., Lewai, V., Goundar, M. and Mowry, C. (2011a) 'Mortality trends in Fiji', *Australian and New Zealand Journal of Public Health*, 35(5): 412–420.

Carter, K., Soakai, S., Taylor, R., Gadabu, I., Rao, C., Thoma, K. and Lopez, A. (2011b) 'Mortality Trends and the Epidemiological Transition in Nauru', *Asia Pacific Journal of Public Health*, 23(1): 10–23.

Coal, A. (1973) 'The Demographic Transition', International Union for the Scientific Study of Population International Population Conference, Liège, Belgium.

Gamble, M.V., Palafox, N.A., Dancheck, B., Ricks, M.O., Briand, K. and Semba, R.D. (2004) 'Carotenoid Status among Preschool Children with Vitamin A Deficiency in the Republic of the Marshall Islands', *Asia Pacific Journal of Clinical Nutrition*, 13(4): 336–340.

Goldman, L. and Ausiello, D. (2004) *Cecil Textbook of Medicine* (22nd edn), Philadelphia: Saunders.

Government of Republic of Nauru and World Health Organization, Western Pacific Region (2004) *Nauru NCD Risk Factors STEPS Report*, Suva: WHO.

Government of American Samoa and World Health Organization, Western Pacific Region (2007) *American Samoa NCD Risk factors STEPS Report*, Suva: WHO.

Government of Federated States of Micronesia and World Health Organization, Western Pacific Region (2008) *Federated States of Micronesia (Pohnpei) NCD Risk Factors STEPS Report*, Suva: WHO.

Government of Kiribati and World Health Organization, Western Pacific Region (2009) *Kiribati NCD Risk Factors STEPS Report*, Suva: WHO.

Grant, A. (1933) 'A Medical Survey of the Island of Nauru', *Medical Journal of Australia*, 1(4): 113–118.

Hermant, P. and Cilento, R. (1929) *Report of the Mission Entrusted with a Survey on Health Conditions in the Pacific Islands*, Geneva: League of Nations Health Organization.

Hughes, R.G. (2006) 'The Feasibility of Micronutrient (Iron) Food Fortification in Pacific Island Countries'. Report prepared for the WHO Western Pacific Regional Office, Division of International and Indigenous Health, School of Population Health, University of Queensland, Brisbane, April.

Jousilahti, P., Vartiainen, E., Tuomilehto, J., Pekkanen, J. and Puska, P. (1998) 'Role of Known Risk Factors in Explaining the Difference in the Risk of Coronary Heart Disease between Eastern and Southwestern Finland', *Annals of Medicine*, 30(5): 481–487.

King, H., Taylor, R., Zimmet, P., Collins, V., Ram, P., Maberly, G., Eastman, C. and Hetzel, B. (1983) 'Endemic Goitre in the Sigatoka Valley, Fiji', *Proceedings of the Nutrition Society of New Zealand*, 8: 112–115.

Kirk, D. (1996) 'Demographic Transition Theory', *Population Studies*, 50: 361–387.

Marshall, S. (2004) 'Developing Countries face Double Burden of Disease', *Bulletin of the World Health Organization*, 82(7): 556.

Mirzaei, M., Truswell, A.S., Taylor, R. and Leeder, S. (2009) 'Coronary Heart Disease (CHD) Epidemics: Not All the Same', *Heart*, 95: 740–746.

Murray, C.J. and Lopez, A.D. (1997a) 'Global Mortality, Disability, and the Contribution of Risk Factors: Global Burden of Disease Study', *Lancet*, 349(9063): 1436–1442.

Murray, C.J. and Lopez, A.D. (1997b) 'Regional Patterns of Disability-free Life Expectancy and Disability-adjusted Life Expectancy: Global Burden of Disease Study', *Lancet*, 349(9062): 1347–1352.

Murray, C.J. and Lopez, A.D. (1997c) 'Mortality by Cause for Eight Regions of the World: Global Burden of Disease Study', *Lancet*, 349(9061): 1269–1276.

Notestein, F. (1953) 'Economic Problems of Population Change', in *Proceedings of the Eigth International Conference of Agricultural Economists*, London: Oxford University Press, 13–31.

Olshansky, S. and Ault, A. (1986) 'The Fourth Stage of the Epidemiological Transition: The Age of Delayed Degenerative Diseases', *Milbank Memorial Fund Quarterly*, 64(3): 355–391.

Omran, A.R. (1971) 'The Epidemiological Transition: A Theory of the Epidemiology of Population Change', *Milbank Memorial Fund Quarterly*, 49(4): 509–538.

Over, M., Bakote'e, B., Velayudhan, R., Wilikai, P. and Graves, P.M. (2004) 'Impregnated Nets or DDT Residual Spraying? Field Effectiveness of Malaria Prevention Techniques in Solomon Islands, 1993–1999', *American Journal of Tropical Medicine and Hygiene*, 71(2 Suppl.): 214–223.

PacMISC (2010) Online, available at: www.pacmisc.net/pacmisc/ (accessed 3 February 2010).

Pathik, B. and Ram, P. (1974) 'Acute Myocardial Infarction in Fiji: A Review of 300 Cases', *Medical Journal of Australia*, 2(26): 922–924.

Ram, P., Collins, V., Zimmet, P., Taylor, R., King, H., Sloman, G. and Hunt, D. (1983) 'Cardiovascular Disease Risk Factors in Fiji: The Results of the 1980 Survey', *Fiji Medical Journal*, 11(7/8): 88–94.

Reed, D. and Feinleib, M. (1983) 'Changing Patterns of Cardiovascular Disease in the Pacific Basin: Report of an International Workshop', *Journal of Community Health*, 8(3): 182–205.

Schaumberg, D.A., O'Connor, J. and Semba, R.D. (1996) 'Risk Factors for Xerophthalmia in the Republic of Kiribati', *European Journal of Clinical Nutrition*, 50(11): 761–764.

Schooneveldt, M., Songer, T., Zimmet, P. and Thoma, K. (1988) 'Changing Mortality Patterns in Nauruans: An Example of Epidemiological Transition', *Journal of Epidemiology and Community Health*, 42(1): 89–95.

Sen, A. (1981) *Poverty and Famines: An Essay on Entitlement and Deprivation*, Oxford: Oxford University Press.

Taylor, R. (1993) 'Non-communicable Disease in the Tropics', *Medical Journal of Australia*, 159(4): 266–270.

Taylor, R. (2008) 'History of Public Health in Pacific Island Countries', in M.J. Lewis and K.L. MacPherson, eds, *Public Health in Asia and the Pacific: Historical and Comparative Perspectives*, London: Routledge, 276–307.

Taylor, R. and Lopez, A. (2007) 'Differential Mortality among Pacific Island Countries and Territories', *Asia-Pacific Population Journal*, 22(3): 45–58.

Taylor, R. and Thoma, K. (1983) *Nauruan Mortality 1976-81 and a Review of Previous Mortality Data*, Nouméa: South Pacific Commission.

Taylor, R. and Thoma, K. (1985) 'Mortality Patterns in the Modernized Pacific Island Nation of Nauru', *American Journal of Public Health*, 75(2): 149–155.

Taylor, R., Badcock, J., Pargeter, K., Lund, M., Fred, T., Ringrose, H., King, H., Zimmet, P., Bach, F., Wang, R.-L. and Sladden, T. (1992) 'Dietary Intake, Exercise, Obesity and Non-communicable Disease in Rural and Urban Populations of Three Pacific Island Countries', *Journal of American College of Nutrition*, 11(3): 283–293.

Taylor, R., Brampton, D. and Lopez, A. (2005) 'Contemporary Patterns of Pacific Island Mortality', *International Journal of Epidemiology*, 34(1): 207–214.

Taylor, R., Dobson, A. and Mirzaei, M. (2006) 'Contribution of Changes in Risk Factors to the Decline of Coronary Heart Disease Mortality in Australia over Three Decades', *European Journal of Cardiovascular Prevention and Rehabilitation*, 13(5): 760–768.

Taylor, R., Henderson, B., Levy, S., Kolonel, L. and Lewis, N. (1985b) *Cancer in Pacific Island Countries*, Noumea: South Pacific Commission.

Taylor, R., Lewis, M. and Powles, J. (1998a) 'The Australian Mortality Decline: All-cause Mortality 1788–1990', *Australian and New Zealand Journal of Public Health*, 22(1): 27–36.

Taylor, R., Lewis, M. and Powles, J. (1998b) 'The Australian Mortality Decline: Cause-specific Mortality 1907–1990', *Australian and New Zealand Journal of Public Health*, 22(1): 37–44.

Taylor, R., Lewis, N. and Levy, S. (1989) 'Societies in Transition: Mortality Patterns in Pacific Island Populations', *International Journal of Epidemiology*, 18(3): 634–646.

Taylor, R., Lewis, N. and Sladden, T. (1991) 'Mortality in Pacific Island Countries around 1980: Geopolitical, Socioeconomic, Demographic, and Health Service Factors', *Australian Journal of Public Health*, 15(3): 207–221.

Taylor, R., Zimmet, P., Levy, S. and Collins, V. (1985a) 'Group Comparisons of Blood Pressure and Indices of Obesity and Salt Intake in Pacific Populations', *Medical Journal of Australia*, 142(9): 499–501.

Temple, V., Mapira, P., Adeniyi, K. and Sims, P. (2005) 'Iodine Deficiency in Papua New Guinea (Sub-clinical Iodine Deficiency and Salt Iodization in the Highlands of Papua New Guinea)', *Journal of Public Health*, 27(1): 45–48.

Thom, T.J., Epstein, F.H., Feldman, J.J., Leaverton, P.E. and Wolz, M. (1992) *Total Mortality and Morbidity from Heart Disease, Cancer and Stroke from 1950 to 1987 in 27 Countries*, Washington, DC: National Heart, Lung and Blood Institute, National Institutes of Health.

Tobias, M., Taylor, R., Yeh, L., Huang, K., Mann, S. and Sharpe, N. (2008) 'Did It Fall or Was It Pushed? The Contribution of Trends in Established Risk Factors to the Decline in Premature Coronary Heart Disease Mortality in New Zealand', *Australian and New Zealand Journal of Public Health*, 32(2): 117–125.

Trigg, P.I. and Kondrachine, A.V. (1998) 'Commentary: Malaria Control in the 1990s', *Bulletin of the World Health Organization*, 76(1): 11–16.

Tuomeilehto, J., Ram, P., Eseroma, R., Taylor, R. and Zimmet, P. (1984) 'Cardiovascular Diseases and Diabetes Mellitus in Fiji: Analysis of Mortality, Morbidity and Risk Factors', *Bulletin of the World Health Organization*, 62(1): 133–143.

van der Sande, M.A., Ceesay, S.M., Milligan, P.J., Nyan, O.A., Banya, W.A., Prentice, A., McAdam, K.P. and Walraven, G.E. (2001) 'Obesity and Undernutrition and Cardiovascular Risk Factors in Rural and Urban Gambian Communities', *American Journal of Public Health*, 91(10): 1641–1644.

Vos, T., Barker, B., Stanley, L. and Lopez, A.D. (2007) *The Burden of Disease and Injury in Aboriginal and Torres Strait Islander Peoples 2003*, Brisbane: School of Population Health, University of Queensland.

Watters, R. and Bertram, I. (2008) 'The MIRAB Economy in South Pacific Microstates', in R. Watters ed., *Journeys Towards Progress: Essays of a Geographer on Development and Change in Oceania*, Wellington: Victoria University Press, 254–282.

Willcox, R.R. (1980) 'Venereal Diseases in the Islands of the South Pacific', *British Journal of Venereal Diseases*, 56(4): 204–209.

World Health Organization (2005) *Preventing Chronic Disease: A Vital Investment*, Geneva: WHO.

World Health Organization (2008) *Prevention and Control of Non-communicable Diseases: Implementation of the Global Strategy*, Geneva: WHO.

Yamamura, C.M., Sullivan, K.M., van der Haar, F., Auerbach, S.B. and Iohp, K.K. (2004) 'Risk Factors for Vitamin A Deficiency among Preschool Aged Children in Pohnpei, Federated States of Micronesia', *Journal of Tropical Pediatrics*, 50(1):16–19.

# 16 Asia and Pacific health transitions

## Retrospect and prospect

*Milton J. Lewis and Kerrie L. MacPherson*

In our introductory chapter we argued that more historical information – more attention to the particular historical experience of individual nations – was needed to understand better the modern health transition (including the double disease burden) in countries of the Asia-Pacific region. We believe our contributors have gone a long way towards achieving that goal.

We argued further that identification of the determinants of the modern transition to higher health status was needed. In this respect, and prompted by James C. Riley's concern with the historical role of social growth in raising health status in some developing countries, we noted that both economic and social development may be drivers of health transitions. We also noted that Richard Wilkinson and Michael Marmot have proposed that above a certain level of per capita income, social (rather than economic) factors come to the fore as determinants of health status – particularly, differences in social status.

In truth, we need both a generalisable, conceptual account – a theory – of the health transition as well as historically oriented, contextually rich, 'empirical' accounts of particular transitions in individual countries, if we are to advance our understanding of the transition (and its determinants), and thereby construct better informed policy.

Global forces, especially economic and cultural forces, increasingly influence nation states. But the nation state remains a significant player because it can employ policy to counter, to some extent, the impact of global forces. Moreover, it is still the main venue for health policy development and execution (as well as development and implementation of other domains of policy influencing health). One might even argue, as Lincoln Chen and colleagues do, that change at the global level (or indeed at the regional level) should be seen as the net result of different historical processes – economic, cultural and political – taking place in 'local worlds of human experience' (nation states and local communities) which are characterised by 'diversity and pluralism' (Chen *et al.* 1994: xiv). Clearly, global influences on health are mediated through nation states.

What might a theory of the health transition and its determinants look like? We draw on the work of Julio Frenk and colleagues (1994) to outline below such a theory.

First, to capture the full range of determinants of health status, we must order them in a hierarchical way. The most fundamental determinants are the population genome, the physical environment and a country's socioeconomic organisation (economy, culture, science and technology and political institutions). Policy interventions can be made at any level of the hierarchy and no level is more important than another.

As we observed in the introductory chapter (see Note 5), a 'deep' history of population health would allow for a significant role for genetic adaptations not only in the earlier eras of human history like the Palaeolithic, hunter gatherer and the Neolithic, agricultural periods but, if Gregory Cochran and Henry Harpending (2010) are correct, even in the last 400 years.

At the next level down are the structural (societal) determinants: a nation's level of wealth, its social stratification system, occupational structure and any wealth redistributive mechanisms like welfare payments. This set of determinants will limit the variation in the set below it – the proximate (institutional and household) determinants. These are living conditions, working conditions, lifestyles and the health care system itself. Individual health status will then be the outcome of an interaction between exposure to disease agents (biological, chemical or physical) and individual susceptibility resulting from a complex network of risks which in turn result from the above hierarchically organised sets of socioeconomic, cultural and biological determinants.

Significant among proximate determinants are living conditions which themselves are dependent on differential 'entitlements' to goods and services; both entitlements arising from the market and those from the state. Of market-related entitlements, sufficient and nutritious food is particularly important to health status. We have seen how much weight scholars like Thomas McKeown, seeking to explain the modern mortality decline from communicable diseases (CDs) in developed countries, placed on the advent of mass access to better diets (in particular more meat) in the nineteenth century; and how much weight contemporary epidemiologists have placed on over-nutrition in developed, and now in developing, countries as a cause of significant, chronic noncommunicable diseases (NCDs).

Among state-related entitlements very important are education services. The authors of the chapter on Australia in this book, Milton Lewis and Stephen Leeder, discuss the emphasis placed by demographer, John Caldwell, on the elementary education of women in reducing infant and child mortality from CDs in some developing countries like Ceylon/Sri Lanka even when per capita income remained comparatively very low.

Lewis and Leeder go on to argue that elementary education of women played a noteworthy role in helping bring down infant mortality from CDs in late nineteenth and early twentieth century Australia; a wealthy country. Other scholars have also proposed that maternal schooling has played a significant role in the reduction of child mortality in other national populations, both past and present (LeVine *et al.* 1994: 303, 331–335).

Various contributors to this volume, discussing policy responses to the advance of NCDs, have pointed to the need for basic changes in health care systems: much greater emphasis on prevention and health promotion; and better resourced, community-based, primary care facilities for management of patients (often aged and suffering from multiple NCD conditions) to forestall more expensive hospitalisation. Efficient and effective allocation of resources between primary care and hospital services is also seen as critical.

In our hierarchy of determinants discussed above, the causality operates not just in one direction. There are feedback loops, and one such involves the health care system. Thus, the system may impact directly upon fundamental and structural determinants, for example, via environmental health services; upon proximate determinants via health promotion; upon the susceptibility of individuals by individually oriented, preventive measures like vaccination; and directly upon health status through treatments.

The dominance of NCDs in mortality and morbidity involves a notable change in the meaning of disease; from acute and curable to chronic and incurable but manageable. Professional, policymakers' and popular ideas about disease will need to change accordingly if individual and collective responses are to be effective.

Individual and collective action to reduce mortality and illness has historically taken the following forms:

- avoidance;
- prevention and health promotion;
- treatment; and
- management.

Avoidance was at the heart of the mid-nineteenth century, English public health movement's strategy of washing away 'filth' (and so the disease-causing 'miasmas') from the environment to prevent the spread of CDs. It is also at the centre of modern health promotion efforts to induce people to adopt healthier lifestyles (including healthy diets) to prevent the onset of major NCDs.

Vaccination, first for a limited number of people against smallpox in the eighteenth century and then on a mass scale from the twentieth century for a number of CDs, is a classic form of prevention. Clearly, avoidance and prevention often overlap.

Treatment aims to reduce the deleterious effects of a disease in an individual, and in modern times, commonly, it results in cure.

Management, however, foreswears cure for moderation of harmful effects and prolongation of life with varying degrees of disability. Thus, contemporary drugs for patients with heart disease may not cure but they will act against deleterious effects and lower the risk of death or serious disablement. The goal of management is to control not cure (Frenk *et al.* 1994: 28–36; Riley 2001: 26–27).

Improvement in health status may be slowed or even interrupted and the direction of epidemiological change challenged, as with the emergence of new CDs like HIV/AIDS (in 2009, worldwide, there were 33 million people infected and 1.8 million deaths) or the resurgence of old ones like malaria or tuberculosis.

TB is out of control in 22 countries with India having the highest incidence in the world (*Worldwide HIV & AIDS Statistics*; Zumla 2011: 10; John *et al.* 2011: 255). Stages of the transition may overlap as with the continuing predominance of CDs among the rural poor when NCDs become predominant among the urban middle and upper classes in developing countries. These processes of change may happen at different speeds among different social classes and regions within different countries (as has been noted in the chapters on developing countries in Asia and the Pacific in this volume) (Frenk *et al.* 1994: 30–44).

We believe with Lincoln Chen and colleagues (1994: xi) that a robust theory of the health transition and its determinants along with detailed historical accounts of how transitions manifest in particular countries will help provide the basis for more effective policy; and we might expect national policy to improve in at least three areas: allocation of resources such as the distribution of funds between hospital and primary care services; appreciation of problems hitherto unrecognised like the need to reorient the health system from acute to chronic care; and understanding of the significance of non-health factors like urban planning for health improvement (Bell and Chen 1994: 491).

Policy at the national level has been extensively discussed by our contributors. Policy at the international level has been less fully addressed.

Recently, there has been an awakening of concern, in international bodies dealing with health and economic development, about the formidable problem presented by NCDs in developing countries. As we have seen, improved health status has long been attributed to economic growth. Much more recently, it has been argued the effect also operates in the reverse direction. It is widely recognised that serious illness or death can markedly reduce the circumstances of poor families: consumption including food purchases will be reduced as will spending on health support; and children, especially girls, will be taken out of school. On the other hand, better health improves the productivity of labour. Moreover, higher life expectancy at birth (LEB) encourages investment in human capital and saving for retirement (Ahlburg and Flint 2001: 9).

In 2000 the World Health Assembly (WHA), noting that 77 per cent of NCD deaths occurred in developing countries and calling for WHO collaboration with the United Nations (UN), other major international agencies, nongovernmental organisations (NGOs), professional and research bodies, and the private sector, endorsed a Global Strategy for the Prevention and Control of Noncommunicable Diseases. The strategy relied on surveillance of NCDs and their determinants, health promotion and prevention, and health care innovations, to rein in the advance of NCDs.

Increasing its engagement with NCD prevention, WHA adopted the WHO Framework Convention on Tobacco Control in 2003 and a Global Strategy on Diet, Physical Activity and Health in 2004. By late 2008, 160 parties had accepted the tobacco control convention, making it one of the UN's most successful treaties. In 2007, WHA asked WHO to develop a plan to implement the global strategy on NCDs and the next year WHA endorsed an Action Plan for the Global Strategy to be pursued, with particular reference to developing nations, over the following six years.

The action plan has six objectives:

- to increase recognition in global and national policy that NCDs and social and economic growth are critically linked and all government departments, not just health, must be involved;
- to promote development of policy on prevention and control including reduction of gender, ethnic and socioeconomic inequalities;
- to promote interventions to reduce risk from the primary, modifiable risk factors – tobacco use, unhealthy diets, physical inactivity and harmful alcohol use;
- to encourage research on prevention and control;
- because the primary determinants of NCDs are located outside the health sector, to encourage intersectoral collaboration at the national and international levels;
- to improve surveillance and standardized collection of data on risk factors, disease incidence and mortality, and regularly to evaluate progress at the national, regional and global levels.

(WHO 2008: v, 2–18, 24–28)

Formulation of such global strategies and policies is to be applauded but implementation in developing countries the health systems of which have very limited resources and face many competing demands is another matter. The WHO stepwise approach has been developed as a planning framework and has been endorsed by a number of poorer Asia-Pacific countries including Indonesia, Vietnam, the Philippines and Tonga.

The first planning step is to establish the national risk factor profile and burden of disease. Although Indonesia's proportional NCD mortality had doubled from 25 to 49 per cent in 1980–2001, the scale of the problem was not officially appreciated until this step was taken. The next step is to develop a policy of prevention and control applicable at all levels from the national down to reduce the growing mortality and morbidity. The third step is to identify the population and individual interventions that will have the largest impact for the investment made and are feasible given local conditions. The Health Ministry will implement some but non-health, government departments or the legislature might pursue others such as measures concerning the built environment or taxes on 'fatty' foods.

Vietnam with 80 million people and Tonga with only 100,000 have both pursued a stepwise approach. In Tonga in 2003 and in Vietnam the following year, the approach was adopted in meetings and consultations involving many organisations with an interest in the problem of NCDs. Soon after, an action plan was adopted by the Tongan government and in Vietnam the Ministry of Health began testing in pilot provinces a model arising from the stepwise approach (Epping-Jordan *et al.* 2005: 1667–1670).

However, the speed with which governments and international agencies were responding to the dauntingly large and growing problem of NCDs (and their impact on economic and social development) was not great enough for some health professional and research bodies and NGOs.

In 2003 the Bill and Melinda Gates Foundation provided support for the Grand Challenges in Global Health (GCGH) research initiative; and in 2007, taking up the theme of globally important health challenges and to promote policy development and research into NCDs in developing countries, the Grand Challenges Global Partnership (GCGP) was set up jointly by the Oxford Health Alliance (itself focussed on NCDs), the UK Medical Research Council, the Canadian Institutes of Health, the Indian Council of Medical Research and the US National Institutes of Health. Unlike the GCGH initiative which involved funding of US$450 million, the GCGP would not provide research funds but focus on forwarding information to funding bodies and foundations to encourage support for research on NCDs (Daar *et al.* 2007: 494–496).

This initiative was taken further in mid-2009 when at a meeting of the heads of international biomedical research organisations the Global Alliance for Chronic Diseases was formed by the following significant research councils that together provide about 80 per cent of global, public research funding: Australia's National Health and Medical Research Council, the Canadian Institutes of Health, the Chinese Academy of Medical Sciences, the UK Medical Research Council and the US National Institutes of Health; the Indian Council of Medical Research was also expected to join, and WHO obtained observer status. While the new body would continue to be concerned with Grand Challenges priorities, it would, in addition, assess priorities set under the WHO 2008–2013 Action Plan (Daar *et al.* 2009: 1642).

Policy at the international level was further advanced when at the same time the WHO announced the establishment of a new network of organisations and experts, the Global Noncommunicable Diseases Network (NCDnet), to bring together cancer, CVD, diabetes and respiratory disease interest groups and tobacco control, healthy diets and physical activity advocates. The World Bank, the World Economic Forum and NGOs like the International Diabetes Federation pledged their support. Dr Alan Alwan, WHO Assistant Director General for NCDs and Mental Health, called for NCD prevention to be made integral to national and global development agendas in developing countries.

In September 2010, at the UN's Millenium Development Goals Summit, control of NCDs was discussed as a priority in development work and related investment decisions. It was noted that NCDs were increasing so quickly, reducing productivity so notably and running down family resources so markedly, they were now a significant threat to developing countries' economic and social development. And everywhere it was the poor who suffered the most. In the World Economic Forum's 2010 ranking of global risks, NCDs were ranked third; only surpassed by the effect of food price volatility (first) and oil price spikes (second).

WHO and relevant UN departments worked in cooperation to prepare for the meeting on 19–20 September 2011 of the UN General Assembly on the prevention and control of NCDs. The UN has only once before held such a summit on a global health matter – the HIV/AIDS summit in 2001. Thirty Presidents and Prime Ministers and 100 Ministers spoke at the historic meeting on NCDs.

The political declaration that has emerged from the NCDs summit does not include specific targets as did the declaration following the HIV/AIDS summit; and at the moment it seems unlikely that it will produce the great commitment to action by governments and the very large funding (the Global Fund of $22 billion to combat AIDS, TB and malaria) that the 2001 summit generated. Only Australia and Russia pledged funds. The significant donor countries – the United States, the United Kingdom, Japan and the European Union – have yet to do so, and the global financial crisis will likely have a dampening effect.

Moreover, physical NCDs, principally CVD, cancers, chronic respiratory diseases and diabetes, are the focus and mental disorders receive only very brief mention despite the fact that these conditions represent a very substantial proportion of the full global economic cost of NCDs; about one-third of US$47 trillion.

Nevertheless, WHO is to prepare recommendations for voluntary global targets by 2012 and there will be a review of progress in implementing the political declaration in 2014; and the declaration does mean the seriousness of the threat to health (and economic and social development) presented by NCDs has been recognised at the highest level as has the need to formulate appropriate policy not only in the health area itself but in other relevant areas like trade, agriculture, food manufacturing, urban planning and the natural environment.

That the UN General Assembly (in addition to WHO) has become involved is a major political achievement. The post-2001 HIV/AIDS strategy has shown that with sustained political commitment, appropriate policy and adequate funding, measures on a global scale can be successfully implemented (WHO 2010: 1–2; WHO 2009; Alwan 2010; Patel 2011; Russell 2011; Al-Nasser 2011: 4; Moodie 2011: 508–509).

While much progress seems to have been made in the last few years in increasing the visibility of the problem of NCDs on international health and economic and social development agendas, very much more needs to be done in poorer countries to implement effective, national policy in health and health-related areas; and in particular to restructure national health systems. One indicator of the need for much greater effort is that in 2007 only an estimated 2.3 per cent (US$503 million) of total development aid for health was intended for NCDs when, by 2030, a projected 69 per cent of global deaths will be caused by NCDs and 80 per cent of such deaths will take place in low and middle income countries (Samb *et al.* 2010: 1785–1788, 1792–1793).

## References

Ahlburg, D.A. and Flint, D.J. (2001) 'Public Health Conditions and Policies in the Asia Pacific Region', *Asia-Pacific Economic Literature*, 15(2): 1–17.

Al-Nasser, N.A. (2011) 'Remarks by H.E. Mr Nassir Abdulaziz Al-Nasser, President of the 66th Session of the General Assembly at the Closing Plenary of the High-level

Meeting on the Prevention and Control of Non-communicable Diseases, 20 September 2011, New York'. Online, available at: www.who.int/nmh/events/un_ncd_summit2011/en/index.html (accessed 2 October 2011).

Alwan, A. (2010) 'Why Developing Countries must Commit to Action against Noncommunicable Diseases', International Conference on the Emerging Burden of Noncommunicable Diseases and Its Impact on Developing Countries, Copenhagen, 15–16 April 2010. Online, available at: www.who.int/entity/nmh/events/2010/adg_ppt_denmark_en.pdf (accessed 20 May 2011).

Bell, D.E. and Chen, L.C. (1994) 'Responding to Health Transitions', in L.C. Chen, A. Kleinman and N.C. Ware, eds, *Health and Social Change in International Perspective*, Boston, MA: Harvard University Press, 491–501.

Chen, L.C., Kleinman, A. and Ware, N.C. (1994) 'Overview', in L.C. Chen, A. Kleinman and N.C. Ware, eds, *Health and Social Change in International Perspective*, Boston, MA: Harvard University Press, vi–xv.

Cochran, G. and Harpending, H. (2010) *10,000 Year Explosion: How Civilization Accelerated Human Evolution*, New York: Basic Books.

Daar, A.S., Nabel, E.G., Pramming, S.K., Anderson, W., Beaudet, A., Liu, D., Katoch, V.M., Borysiewicz, L.K., Glass, R.I. and Bell, J. (2009) 'The Global Alliance for Chronic Diseases', *Science*, 324(26 June): 1642.

Daar, A.S., Singer, P.A., Persad, D.L., Pramming, S.K., Matthews, D.R., Beaglehole, R., Bernstein, A., Borysiewicz, L.K., Colagiuri, S., Ganguly, N., Glass, R.I., Finegood, D.T., Koplan, J., Nabel, E.G., Sarna, G., Sarrafzadegan, N., Smith, R., Yach, D. and Bell, J. (2007) 'Grand Challenges in Chronic Non-Communicable Diseases', *Nature*, 450(22 November): 494–496.

Epping-Jordan, J.E., Galen, G., Tukuitonga, C. and Beaglehole, R. (2005) 'Preventing Chronic Diseases: Taking Stepwise Action', *Lancet*, 366(5 November): 1667–1671.

Frenk, J., Bobadilla, J.-L., Stern, C., Frejka, T. and Lozano, R. (1994) 'Elements for a Theory of the Health Transition', in L.C. Chen, A. Kleinman and N.C. Ware, eds, *Health and Social Change in International Perspective*, Boston, MA: Harvard University Press, 25–49.

John, J., Dandona, L., Sharma, V.P. and Kakkar, M. (2001) 'Continuing Challenge of Infectious Diseases in India', *Lancet*, 377(15 January): 252–256.

LeVine, R.A., LeVine, S.E., Richman, A., Merdado Tapia Uribe, F. and Sunderland Correa, C. (1994) 'Schooling and Survival: The Impact of Maternal Education on Health and Reproduction in the Third World', in L.C. Chen, A. Kleiman and N.C. Ware, eds, *Health and Social Change in International Perspective*, Boston, MA: Harvard University Press, 303–338.

Moodie, A.R. (2011) 'The Slow-Motion Disaster that is Breaking the Bank', *MJA*, 195(9): 508–509.

Patel, A. (2011) 'Lots of Talk, Little Action from Crucial UN Summit on Deadly Diseases'. Online, available at: www.smh.com.au/opinion/lots-of-talk-little-action-from-cruc (accessed 24 September 2011).

Riley, J.C. (2001) *Rising Life Expectancy: A Global History*, Cambridge: Cambridge University Press.

Riley, J.C. (2008) *Low Income, Social Growth, and Good Health: A History of Twelve Countries*, Berkeley, CA: University of California Press.

Russell, L. (2011) 'Non-communicable Diseases Pose UN Challenge'. Online, available at: www.canberratimes.com.au/news/opinion/editorial/general/ (accessed 24 September 2011).

Samb, B., Desai, N., Nishtar, S., Mendis, S., Bekedam, H., Wright, A., Hsu, J., Martiniuk, A., Celletti, F., Patel, K., Adshead, F., McKee, M., Evans, T., Alwan, A. and Etienne, C. (2010) 'Prevention and Management of Chronic Diseases: A Litmus Test for Health-Systems Strengthening in Low-Income and Middle-Income Countries', *Lancet*, 376(20 November): 1785–1797.

WHO (2008) *2008–2013 Action Plan for the Global Strategy for the Prevention and Control of Noncommunicable Diseases*, Geneva: World Health Organization.

WHO (2009) 'New Network to Combat Noncommunicable Diseases'. Online, available at: www.who.int/mediacentre/news/releases/2009/noncommunicable _diseases_2009 (accessed 8 February 2011).

WHO (2010) *Background Paper: Raising the Priority Accorded to Non-Communicable Diseases in Development Work and in Related Investment Decisions*, Geneva: World Health Organization.

*Worldwide HIV & AIDS Statistics.* Online, available at: www.avert.org/worldstats.htm (accessed 1 February 2011).

Zumla, A. (2011) 'The White Plague Returns to London: With a Vengeance', *Lancet*, 377(1 January): 10–11.

# Index

Page numbers in *italics* denote tables, those in **bold** denote figures.

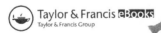